HEMOSTATIC MECHANISMS
AND METASTASIS

DEVELOPMENTS IN ONCOLOGY

F.J. Cleton and J.W.I.M. Simons, eds.: Genetic Origins of Tumour Cells. 90-247-2272-1.

J. Aisner and P. Chang, eds.: Cancer Treatment Research. 90-247-2358-2.

B.W. Ongerboer de Visser, D.A. Bosch and W.M.H. van Woerkom-Eykenboom, eds.: Neuro-oncology: Clinical and Experimental Aspects. 90-247-2421-X.

K. Hellmann, P. Hilgard and S. Eccles, eds.: Metastasis: Clinical and Experimental Aspects. 90-247-2424-4.

H.F. Seigler, ed.: Clinical Management of Melanoma. 90-247-2584-4.

P. Correa and W. Haenszel, eds.: Epidemiology of Cancer of the Digestive Tract. 90-247-2601-8.

L.A. Liotta and I.R. Hart, eds.: Tumour Invasion and Metastasis. 90-247-2611-5.

J. Banoczy, ed.: Oral Leukoplakia. 90-247-2655-7.

C. Tijssen, M. Halprin and L. Endtz, eds.: Familial Brain Tumours. 90-247-2691-3.

F.M. Muggia, C.W. Young and S.K. Carter, eds.: Anthracycline Antibiotics in Cancer. 90-247-2711-1.

B.W. Hancock, ed.: Assessment of Tumour Response. 90-247-2712-X.

D.E. Peterson, ed.: Oral Complications of Cancer Chemotherapy. 0-89838-563-6.

R. Mastrangelo, D.G. Poplack and R. Riccardi, eds.: Central Nervous System Leukemia. Prevention and Treatment. 0-89838-570-9.

A. Polliack, ed.: Human Leukemias. Cytochemical and Ultrastructural Techniques in Diagnosis and Research. 0-89838-585-7.

W. Davis, C. Maltoni and S. Tanneberger, eds.: The Control of Tumor Growth and its Biological Bases. 0-89838-603-9.

A.P.M. Heintz, C. Th. Griffiths and J.B. Trimbos, eds.: Surgery in Gynecological Oncology. 0-89838-604-7.

M.P. Hacker, E.B. Double and I. Krakoff, eds.: Platinum Coordination Complexes in Cancer Chemotherapy. 0-89838-619-5.

M.J. van Zwieten. The Rat as Animal Model in Breast Cancer Research: A Histopathological Study of Radiation- and Hormone-Induced Rat Mammary Tumors. 0-89838-624-1.

B. Löwenberg and A. Hogenbeck, eds.: Minimal Residual Disease in Acute Leukemia. 0-89838-630-6.

B.W. Hancock and A.M. Ward, eds.: Immunological Aspects of Cancer. 0-89838-664-0.

HEMOSTATIC MECHANISMS AND METASTASIS

edited by

Kenneth V. Honn
Bonnie F. Sloane

Martinus Nijhoff Publishing
a member of the Kluwer Academic Publishers Group
Boston/The Hague/Dordrecht/Lancaster

Distributors for North America:
Kluwer Academic Publishers
190 Old Derby Street
Hingham, MA 02043

Distributors for all other countries:
Kluwer Academic Publishers Group
Distribution Centre
P.O. Box 322
3300 AH Dordrecht
The Netherlands

Library of Congress Cataloging in Publication Data

Main entry under title:
Hemostatic mechanisms and metastasis.

(Developments in oncology)
Includes index.
1. Metastasis. 2. Blood—Coagulation. 3. Hemostasis. I. Honn, Kenneth V. II. Sloane,
Bonnie F. III. Series. [DNLM: 1. Hemostasis. 2. Neoplasm Metastasis.
W1 DE998N/QZ 202 H489]
RC269.H46   1984   616.99′2071   84-10198
ISBN 0-89838-667-5

CONTENTS

CHAPTER 14. PROSTACYCLIN/THROMBOXANES AND TUMOR CELL METASTASIS

K.V. HONN, J.M. ONODA, D.G. MENTER, J.D. TAYLOR AND B.F. SLOANE

CHAPTER 15. EVIDENCE FOR ALTERED ARACHIDONIC ACID METABOLISM IN TUMOR METASTASIS

P. MEHTA

CHAPTER 16. CALCIUM CHANNEL BLOCKERS: INHIBITORS OF TUMOR CELL-PLATELET-ENDOTHELIAL CELL INTERACTIONS

J.M. ONODA, B.F. SLOANE, J.D. TAYLOR AND K.V. HONN

CHAPTER 20.   THE CELLULAR INTERACTIONS OF METASTATIC TUMOR CELLS WITH
SPECIAL REFERENCE TO ENDOTHELIAL CELLS AND THEIR BASAL
LAMINA-LIKE MATRIX

G.L. NICOLSON, T. IRIMURA, M. NAKAJIMA, T.V. UPDYKE AND
G. POSTE

CHAPTER 21.   INTERACTION OF TUMOR CELLS WITH THE BASEMENT MEMBRANE OF
ENDOTHELIUM

L.A. LIOTTA AND R.H. GOLDFARB

PREFACE

Numerous investigators, both in clinical and basic sciences, have postulated that platelets, platelet thrombi and/or the coagulation cascade play a role in metastasis of tumor cells. Pioneering work in this field was performed by Trousseau, Bilroth, Schmidt, Wood, Sindelar and Gasic. However, the role of hemostatic mechanisms in metastasis has been an area of controversy and any identification of causal relationships has been illusive until very recently.

The purpose of this book is to present the most up-to-date evidence for the involvement of hemostatic mechanisms in tumor metastasis. Basic science and clinical studies are presented as well as the current clinical status of anti-platelet or anti-coagulative therapy for the treatment of tumor metastasis.

We hope that this book provides both the evidence linking hemostatic mechanisms and metastasis and a rationale for the use of platelet-active or coagulation cascade-active agents as adjuvants to chemotherapy or radiation therapy in the clinic. Many relevant topics have been omitted due to space considerations and thus the topics included reflect the prejudices of the editors. We thank the contributors for the excellence of their chapters and hope the readers will find this volume of interest.

K.V. Honn
B.F. Sloane

CONTRIBUTORS

JULIAN L AMBRUS
Department of Internal Medicine
Roswell Park Memorial Institute
666 Elm Street
Buffalo, NY 14263

MICHAEL R. BUCHANAN
Department of Pathology
McMaster University Health
  Science Centre
Hamilton, Ontario
Canada L8N 3Z5

CHERYL CANO
Department of Medicine/Oncology
  Division
Milton C. Hershey Medical Center
The Pennsylvania State University
Hershey, PA 17033

PHILIP G. CAVANAUGH
Department of Biological
  Sciences
210 Science Hall
Wayne State University
Detroit, MI 48202

JOHN D. CRISSMAN
Department of Pathology
540 E. Canfield
Wayne State University and
  Harper-Grace Hospitals
Detroit, MI 48201

MARIA B. DONATI
Laboratory for Hemostasis and
  Thrombosis Research
Istituto di Ricerche
  Farmacologiche, "Mario Negri"
Via Eritrea 62
Milan, Italy

ANN M. DVORAK
Department of Pathology
Harvard Medical School and Beth
  Israel Hospital
Charles A. Dana Biomedical
  Research Institute, Beth
  Israel Hospital
Boston, MA 02215

HAROLD F. DVORAK
Department of Pathology
Harvard Medical School and Beth
  Israel Hospital
Charles A. Dana Biomedical
  Research Institute, Beth
  Israel Hospital
Boston, MA 02215

RICHARD L. EDWARDS
Department of Medicine
Veterans Administration Medical
  Center and University of
  Connecticut Health Center
Newington, CT 06111

JOYCE E. GARDINER
Department of Immunology
Scripps Clinic and Research
  Foundation
10666 North Torrey Pines Road
La Jolla, CA 92037

GABRIEL J. GASIC
Laboratory of Experimental
  Oncology
Pennsylvania Hospital
Eighth and Spruce Streets
Philadelphia, PA 19107

TATIANA B. GASIC
Laboratory of Experimental
  Oncology
Pennsylvania Hospital
Eighth and Spruce Streets
Philadelphia, PA 19107

HELMUTH GASTPAR
Department of Otorhinolaryngology
Pettenkoferstrasse 8a
University of Munich
8000 Munich 2
West Germany

RONALD H. GOLDFARB
Cancer Metastasis Research Group
Department of Immunology and
   Infectious Disease
Central Research Division
Pfizer Inc.
Groton, CT   06340

STUART G. GORDON
Department of Medicine
University of Colorado Health
   Sciences Center
4200 East Ninth Avenue
Denver, CO   80262

ROBERT R. GORMAN
Division of Experimental
   Science I
The Upjohn Company
Kalamazoo, MI   49001

JOHN H. GRIFFIN
Department of Immunology
Scripps Clinic and Research
   Foundation
10666 North Torrey Pines Road
La Jolla, CA   92037

PETER HILGARD
Department of Experimental
   Cancer Research
Asta Werke AG Degussa Pharma
   Gruppe
D-4800 Bielefeld 14
West Germany

JACK HIRSCH
Department of Medicine
McMaster University Health
   Science Centre
Hamilton, Ontario
Canada   L8N 3Z5

KENNETH V. HONN
Department of Radiation Oncology
210 Science Hall
Wayne State University
Detroit, MI   48202

TATSURO IRIMURA
Department of Tumor Biology
University of Texas System Cancer
   Center
M.D. Anderson Hospital and Tumor
   Institute
Houston, TX   77030

SIMON KARPATKIN
Department of Medicine
New York University Medical
   Center
550 First Avenue
New York, NY   10016

ALFRED S. KETCHAM
Department of Surgery
Division of Oncology
University of Miami School of
   Medicine
Miami, FL   33101

BARNETT KRAMER
Department of Medicine
Division of Medical Oncology
University of Florida
Gainesville, FL   32610

KIM LEITZEL
Department of Medicine/Oncology
   Division
Milton S. Hershey Medical Center
The Pennsylvania State University
Hershey, PA   17033

MARGARET LEWIN
Department of Medicine
The New York Hospital-Cornell
   Medical Center
525 East 68th Street
New York, NY   10021

LANCE A LIOTTA
Laboratory of Pathology
Section of Tumor Invasion
  and Metastasis
National Cancer Institute, NIH
Bethesda, MD 20205

ALLAN LIPTON
Department of Medicine/Oncology
  Division
Milton S. Hershey Medical Center
The Pennsylvania State
  University
Hershey, PA 17033

PAULETTE MEHTA
Department of Pediatrics
University of Florida College of
  Medicine
Gainesville, FL 32610

DAVID G. MENTER
Department of Biological
  Sciences
210 Science Hall
Wayne State University
Detroit, MI 48202

MOTOWO NAKAJIMA
Department of Tumor Biology
University of Texas System Cancer
  Center
M.D. Anderson Hospital and
  Tumor Institute
Houston, TX 77030

GARTH L. NICOLSON
Department of Tumor Biology
University of Texas System
  Cancer Center
M.D. Anderson Hospital and Tumor
  Institute
Houston, TX 77030

FREDERICK OFOSU
Immunochemistry Section
Canadian Red Cross Blood
  Transfusion Centre
Toronto, Ontario
Canada

JAMES M. ONODA
Department of Radiation Oncology
210 Science Hall
Wayne State University
Detroit, MI 48202

EDWARD PEARLSTEIN
Department of Pathology
New York University Medical
  Center
550 First Avenue
New York, NY 10016

GEORGE POSTE
Director of Research and
  Development
Smith Kline & French
  Laboratories
Philadelphia, PA 19104

FREDERICK R. RICKLES
Department of Medicine
Veterans Administration Medical
  Center and University of
  Connecticut Health Center
Newington, CT 06111

NICOLA SEMERARO
Istituto di Patologia Generale
University of Bari
Bari, Italy

D.R. SENGER
Department of Pathology
Harvard Medical School and Beth
  Israel Hospital
Charles A. Dana Biomedical
  Research Institute, Beth
  Israel Hospital
Boston, MA 02215

BONNIE F. SLOANE
Department of Pharmacology
540 East Canfield
Wayne State University
Detroit, MI 48201

GWENDOLYN J. STEWART
Department of Physiology
Thrombosis Research Center
Temple University Medical School
Philadelphia, PA 19140

JOHN D. TAYLOR
Department of Biological Sciences
210 Science Hall
Wayne State University
Detroit, MI 48202

WALLEY J. TEMPLE
Department of Surgery
Division of Oncology
University of Miami School of
  Medicine
Miami, FL 33101

TIMOTHY V. UPDYKE
Department of Tumor Biology
University of Texas System
  Cancer Center
M.D. Anderson Hospital and Tumor
  Institute
Houston, TX 77030

WILHELM van EIMEREN
Institut fur Medizinische
  Infomations- und System-
  forschung
Gesellschaft fur Strahlen-
  und Umweltforschung
Munich, West Germany

BRUCE A. WARREN
Department of Anatomical
  Pathology
The Prince Henry Hospital
Little Bay, New South Wales 2036
Australia

LEONARD WEISS
Department of Experimental
  Pathology
Roswell Park Memorial Institute
666 Elm Street
Buffalo, NY 14263

BABETTE B. WEKSLER
Department of Medicine
The New York Hospital-Cornell
  Medical Center
525 East 68th Street
New York, NY 10021

LEO R. ZACHARSKI
Veterans Administration Medical
  Center and Dartmouth Medical
  School
White River Junction, VT 05001

HEMOSTATIC MECHANISMS AND METASTASIS

CHAPTER 1. IS THERE CLINICAL RELEVANCE FOR THERAPIES WHICH DISRUPT THE METASTATIC CASCADE?

JOHN D. CRISSMAN

I. INTRODUCTION

It is perplexing that while emphasis has been placed on the study of factors involved in carcinogenesis and treatment of established cancers, less effort is spent on the study of invasion and metastasis (1). Obviously, it is this element of the disease which is responsible for the majority of the morbidity and mortality of malignant cancer. "Is there clinical relevance for therapies which disrupt the metastatic cascade?" This is an intriguing question and addresses an area of clinical oncology which has not been a popular area for research. A wealth of biological and clinical information is available regarding carcinogenesis and, more recently, chemoprevention of neoplastic transformation. Research in cancer treatment has generated a vast body of knowledge dealing with the ablation of cancers once they are established. There are limited efforts in clinical investigation to develop therapies that have the potential for altering the metastatic cascade; most of these studies concentrate on aspects of the coagulation or fibrinolysis scheme. Coagulation, platelet aggregation and other factors involved in hemostasis have been clearly incriminated as contributing to steps in the metastatic cascade, but the details of their involvement are not completely understood (2). At this time, considerable effort by a select, but relatively small, number of scientists has resulted in substantial progress toward unraveling the multitude of events leading to establishment of tumor metastases. Many of these investigations are represented by chapters in this volume. It is anticipated that a better understanding of the sequence of events resulting in metastases will further development and ultimately clinical application of biologic modifiers to alter and hopefully interrupt this dreaded aspect of cancer.

Many of my oncology colleagues smile when I inquire about their views regarding the sequence leading to the establishment of metastases and chuckle when asked for their views about the "clinical relevance of disrupting the metastatic cascade." The surgeons' responses imply that I have failed to comprehend that once cancer has disseminated, cure is usually not possible and some form of palliative care is in order. Radiotherapists can provide radiation to broad expanses of the body, but if metastases are outside their ports, there is little else they can do. Medical oncologists propose that one of the many combinations available in their armamentarium of toxic chemicals may impede or eradicate these metastatic deposits and presumably would also interrupt the "metastatic cascade." While it may be humorous to reflect on the prototypical responses of each of the clinical oncology specialists, in many instances (such as tumor boards) these attitudes prevail. However, there have been significant changes in the practice of clinical oncology. Surgeons no longer believe that more surgery and wider margins of tissue removal will enhance the chance of cancer cure. Radiotherapists have altered their ports and tailored their therapy to the needs of each patient. Medical oncologists use more effective drugs and it is encouraging to note that significant progress is being made in the chemotherapy of metastatic cancer. However, in many patients the use of aggressive therapy is almost as devastating to the patient as the tumor. Childhood leukemia and testicular germ cell cancer are two notable diseases which are now potentially curable even when widely disseminated. But for the most part, chemotherapy has been utilized in patients with metastatic cancer as a palliative exercise, primarily to alleviate symptoms and prolong survival. It is puzzling that oncologists have not focused on the sequence involved in the metastatic cascade and attempted to identify less toxic therapies with the potential to interrupt the metastatic sequence in the hope of prolonging survival and decreasing metastatic progression. Many of my basic science colleagues conducting investigations on various aspects of cancer are also ambivalent on why the interruption of the metastatic cascade is important. They readily agree that blocking the sequence leading to the formation of metastases is important early in the disease when the potential to prevent formation of metastases still exists. But once metastases have been established, it is their impression that the only hope is to eradicate the disseminated disease and they fail to appreciate the significant palliative value of a therapy which would potentially impede progression of metastases from established metastatic foci and presumably increase the time interval required to reach the lethal tumor burden.

At this time, the general approach in clinical oncology is to eradicate the initial (primary) cancer using surgical excision and/or radiotherapy and less commonly adjuvant chemotherapy. Once the initial neoplasm has been successfully eradicated, survival is usually dependent on whether the metastatic cascade had already been established. In patients with clinical evidence of metastases to the regional lymph nodes, surgery or radiation is directed to these nodes. Traditionally, this latter approach has been considered part of the primary therapy of cancer with the goal of achieving local and regional control of the neoplasm. During the past few years, a major body of evidence has evolved which argues that the presence of regional lymph node metastases only indicates that there is significant potential for concurrent systemic metastases having been already established (3). This is certainly the current majority opinion for adenocarcinoma of the breast (4). This new understanding of the biology of malignant neoplasia is a major departure from traditional views in which it was felt that tumors metastasize in a stepwise fashion, first to the regional lymph nodes and subsequently to distant sites. This new knowledge has significantly altered the clinical management of cancer patients (less radical local therapy with decreased patient morbidity) and serves as an example of how better understanding of the biology of cancer impacts on clinical practice.

The mainstream of basic research and clinical applications dealing with cancer has been directed towards understanding its pathogenesis and the eradication of established cancers and metastatic deposits. Relatively little attention, at least as judged by proportional representation in the cancer literature, has been directed toward understanding the complex sequence of tumor invasion and metastasis (1). The possibility of identifying therapies which alter or impede this sequence has significant clinical implication. Utilization of "biologic modifiers," hopefully with lower host toxicity, could decrease a tumor's metastatic potential and decrease the probability of establishing metastases of tumor cells dislodged into the circulation during diagnostic manipulations, surgical resections and radiation therapy. Therapies which decrease the metastatic potential of circulating cancer cells may also have a major palliative role in decreasing the natural progression of disseminated disease from the metastases of tumor cells released by existing metastatic deposits. While such potential modifiers would not be curative in these latter situations, they would have the potential of prolonging survival, a major objective of physicians treating patients with advanced cancers. However, biologic modifiers of the metastatic cascade would have immediate use as an adjuvant therapy in patients undergoing surgical resections for cancer, a known source for increased circulating tumor cells. These potential "noncytotoxic" therapies will be covered in greater detail and whenever possible clinical data will be reviewed. However, much of the supporting evidence for events of the metastatic cascade is derived from observations in animal models. Once therapeutic agents which have the potential of interfering with the metastatic sequence are identified, their testing in clinical trials will unquestionably follow closely.

II. ESTABLISHMENT OF THE PRIMARY CANCER AND VASCULAR INVASION

Once the complex sequence of carcinogenesis has evolved and a primary focus of cancer has formed, several events must occur before metastases can develop (Figure 1). Autonomous proliferating cells require host support for the tumor to maintain growth (5). Probably, the most important of these events is the stimulation of host blood vessel proliferation to provide nutrient support for the metabolically active tumor cells. A diffusible substance has been identified which stimulates blood vessel production and is referred to as tumor angiogenesis factor (TAF; 6). Once ample host blood supply is assured, the malignant neoplasm has the capacity of essentially unchecked proliferation as long as the delicate balance between tumor proliferation and host vascular supply remains intact. In addition, a protein secreted by tumors has recently been described which increases blood vessel permeability (7). It is hypothesized that this permeability factor further optimizes nutrient support of the tumor. The nature by which the neoplastic cells proliferate and the pattern in which they invade adjacent host tissue (including the TAF stimulated host vasculature) becomes critical in the sequence leading to metastasis. Tumor spread can occur when a malignant neoplasm penetrates into a body cavity but for the most part metastasis cannot occur until either the lymphatic or blood vascular compartment is invaded. A number of clinical and pathological features of cancer have been demonstrated to correlate with the propensity to develop metastases. The three most important parameters which are utilized on a clinical basis are: (1) the size of the neoplasm at the time of diagnosis and whether regional lymph node metastases are present (tumor stage), (2) the histological grade or degree of differentiation of the malignancy and (3) the tissue of origin of the neoplasm (3).

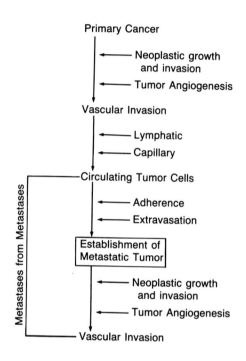

FIGURE 1. Schema for the metastatic cascade. Once extravasation and establishment of metastasis occurs, the same sequence as observed in the primary tumor is initiated. This leads to continuation of the metastatic cascade with "metastases from metastases."

A. Tumor Stage

The size of the primary tumor is extremely important in predicting whether metastasis has occurred. In general, larger tumors have the highest association with metastases to regional lymph nodes and to distant sites (3,8). However, this correlation is imperfect and it is well documented that "minimal breast cancers" (infiltrating adenocarcinomas less than 0.5 cm in diameter) have up to 17% frequency of metastases in the regional lymph node (9). Conversely, it is well established that selected cancers may grow to a large size before metastasis occurs (3). This striking observation reinforces the hypothesis that growth rate and vascular (lymph and blood) invasion are semi-independent variables. Unfortunately, the tumor characteristics which reliably predict the capability for vascular invasion are not well identified (10).

While identification of vascular invasion is considered by most observers as a poor prognostic feature (11), the most reliable predictor for the presence of systemic or distant metastases is the identification of successful regional lymph node implants (1). For this reason, the clinical or pathological assessment of the regional lymph node status is an integral part of defining tumor stage. For many years physicians felt that cancer proceeded in a logical and stepwise fashion and that cancers (especially carcinomas) first metastasized to regional lymph nodes. Subsequently, the tumor would pass through the lymphoid structures, resulting in disseminated systemic disease. Currently, the general consensus is that for most cancers the presence of regional lymph node metastases is best interpreted as an indicator for systemic metastatic potential, i.e., that if the primary cancer has the capacity to metastasize to the regional lymph nodes it probably has the potential to metastasize elsewhere (3,4,8).

The participation of the regional lymph nodes in host defense against tumor dissemination is a controversial subject. There is experimental evidence that regional lymph nodes are active in this defense for selected tumor models (3). In addition, there is considerable clinical data concluding that paracortical hyperplasia (thymic derived lymphocyte zone which participates in cell mediated immunity) predicts increased survival for a variety of neoplasms (12). Conversely, regional lymph node atrophy or reticuloendothelial and/or follicular hyperplasia predicts a poorer survival. Some surgeons have argued that regional lymph nodes are protective against the spread of cancer, but there is little clinical and no experimental evidence to support this concept (4). At this time, the rationale for regional lymph node removal during cancer surgery is twofold: (a) pathological evaluation to determine whether metastases are present in order to more accurately determine tumor stage and prognosis and (b) to remove lymph nodes obviously involved by metastatic tumor in order to enhance the maintenance of regional tumor control.

B. Histology and Differentiation

The histological grade or degree of differentiation of the malignant neoplasm is an important parameter in assessing a neoplasm's capacity for developing metastatic disease. The features that are assessed in the histological evaluation include parameters currently being studied with more sophisticated techniques. One of the most important histological parameters to assess tumor aggressiveness is nuclear size, shape and staining pattern. These features reflect abnormal chromosomal content (aneuploidy), a feature of malignant neoplasia (13). Frequency of mitoses reflects the rapidity of cell turnover or length of the cell cycle in the malignant cell population. Higher cellular turnover correlates well with tumor growth rate and to a lesser extent with the propensity to form metastases (14). Recently, many investigators are utilizing flow cytometry or tritiated thymidine uptake to measure S-phase tumor fraction, a much more sensitive method of estimating tumor cell replication cycles. Flow cytometry is also an effective tool for evaluating chromosome distributions in neoplastic cell populations (13).

The growth pattern or pattern of invasion is another valuable histological parameter that is seldom utilized in assessing tumor grade and correlates with nuclear pleomorphism, mitotic index and other indicators of increasing metastatic potential (15). Neoplasms which infiltrate in irregular cords or single cells may have the greatest cell mobility and the least intercellular cohesiveness, both of these are parameters associated with metastatic potential. TAF illicits host blood supply within the neoplasms, yet lymphatic structures are found only in the host tissue adjacent to the neoplasms and presumably are the site of tumor cell invasion which results in regional lymph node metastasis. Neoplasms infiltrating in small aggregates and single cells are associated with a much higher frequency of vascular invasion and with poorer survival (15,16). Neoplasms with a "cohesive" morphology and a "pushing" border or pattern of invasion at the tumor-host interface seldom have identifiable vascular invasion and have a significantly lower observed frequency of lymph node and systemic metastases.

There is an expanding body of evidence that a number of enzymes are released by the tumor cells which destroy host tissues allowing invasion to proceed (see Chapter 21). Many malignant neoplasms have increased activities of lysosomal acid proteinases and cytoplasmic neutral proteinases including collagenases (17-21). Neutral and acid proteinases can activate latent host collagenase, thereby increasing neoplastic invasion. Tumor cells which contain enzymes capable of basement membrane digestion gain access to the vascular space with a much greater frequency (20,22). The possibility that these same proteolytic enzymes may be important in extravasation prior to the formation of metastatic tumors is also likely (23).

C. Tissue of Origin

The organ or tissue of origin of a malignant tumor is also an important parameter in predicting how the neoplasm will behave (3). Lung carcinomas such as small cell or oat cell carcinomas almost always will have metastasized regardless of the size of the primary tumor. Conversely, basal cell carcinomas of the skin seldom metastasize no matter how large they may become. This observation would appear to indicate that not only features such as tumor size, cell turnover as indicated by S-phase fraction, pattern of invasion and vascular permeation, but also inherent factors determined by the tissue of origin are important in predicting how a malignant neoplasm will behave, both locally and in its potential for dissemination.

III. CIRCULATING CANCER CELLS

The presence of tumor cells in the lymph and blood circulation of cancer patients has been confirmed many times. Several decades ago, numerous investigators began to diligently search for cancer cells in the circulation of cancer patients and of tumor-bearing animals. In the early investigations, the neoplastic cells were primarily identified by morphological criteria after concentrating the blood sample. As one would predict, these observations were difficult to interpret and the subject of circulating cancer cells remained controversial for a number of years (24). More recently, with the advent of more specific techniques for identifying circulating cancer cells, development of better tumor markers and more sophisticated animal models, it has clearly been established that many, if not all, malignancies release cancer cells into the circulation (25,26).

Although early observations identifying cancer cells in circulation remain controversial, from recent work it appears that more cells are released into the circulation for selected tumors than had been realized. The presence of circulating cancer cells does not imply or assure either the presence or development of metastases; this is commonly referred to as metastatic inefficiency (27 and Chapter 2). The relationship of circulating cancer cells, successful extravasation and development of metastases is remarkably complex. The subsequent section is not intended as a comprehensive review of this vast body of work, but as an outline of the most important observations as they relate to circulating tumor cells and the development of metastatic disease. Several observations appear valid in regard to circulating cancer cells and these include:

1) Circulating cancer cells are not an uncommon occurrence in patients undergoing therapy for their cancers. It has been observed for many years that venous invasion in primary carcinomas predicted hematogenous spread of the neoplasm (28). Tumor cells were identified in the majority of patients and the frequency of vascular permeation correlated with the histological grade of the tumor. However, it was also noted that approximately one-half of the patients demonstrated to have circulating cancer cells survived the five to nine year period of follow-up (29). The majority of investigations documenting circulating cancer cells were performed at the time of surgery by sampling venous blood draining the tumor to be resected (30). Many of these studies demonstrated that increased numbers of cancer cells were released into the draining venous system during manipulation and resection of the primary neoplasm, an observation initially rejected by many surgeons as unimportant.

2) There are numerous studies which document that increased numbers of cells injected into the circulation of animals result in an increased number of identifiable tumor colonies (31). The majority of these studies demonstrate that in order to establish tumor colonies (usually pulmonary tumors are counted) a certain minimum number of tumor cells must be injected (normally into the tail vein) and that the subsequent number of colonies is quasi proportional to the number of cells injected (32).

3) Circulating tumor cell aggregates are more efficient in developing metastases and are more commonly associated with invasion of larger blood vessels in the primary tumor (28). Homotypic (tumor cell-tumor cell) aggregates can result from increased plasma membrane adhesiveness (33). Aggregates as small as 6-7 cells have a much higher efficiency in establishing metastases than single cell suspensions (33-35). Heterotypic aggregates (tumor cell and either other circulating cells or fibrin/platelets) also appear to increase the efficiency of establishing metastases (33,36). The role of endothelial cell-tumor cell interactions has not been clearly defined but appears to be important in selected models (37,38). One of the problems in establishing each step in the metastatic cascade is that alternate pathways may exist for different tumors. In addition, the least effective of the steps in the sequence may be the limiting factor in establishing the metastatic cascade (27).

4) Manipulation (including incisional biopsy) or massage of tumors in animals is associated with an increase (shower) of circulating cancer cells (39,40). The factors which control the release of cancer cells into the vasculature are multiple. It appears that many neoplasms constantly release cells into vessels once vascular invasion has been achieved (41). There is also some data demonstrating that larger tumors release greater numbers of cells into the circulation (34). Once vascular invasion has occurred, it is not surprising that manipulation or palpation of the primary tumor results in an increased number or shower of circulating cancer cells. Conceivably this occurs due to release of cells or, more importantly, aggregates of cells which have invaded lymphatic and venous structures.

5) Circulating cancer cells appear to be increased (released) during surgical procedures. While this observation has often been rejected in the past by our surgery colleagues, the observations are indisputable and have been reproduced by numerous investigators (42,43). Much of the work on the quantitation of circulating cancer cells and their relationship to surgical manipulation was performed by Cole and his associates (42). This work clearly demonstrated that the trauma associated with surgery results in an increase in circulating tumor cells measured in large veins draining the tumor bed. This work, while not disputed, did not appear to greatly influence the clinical practice of medicine and surgery, and some surgeons still refuse to accept the role of surgery in increasing the circulating tumor cell burden. The observation that all circulating cancer cells do not result in the successful establishment of metastases is often argued in defense of the latter view. Not until the work of Turnbull et al. (43) was there any objective evidence which clearly demonstrated that surgical techniques to isolate the vascular drainage of a cancer prior to the surgical resection resulted in superior survival. This technique for resecting carcinomas of the colon was compared to the traditional approach by two groups of surgeons in the same institution. The patients operated on using Turnbull's technique of isolating and ligating the lymph-blood vessel bundles prior to the resection of the colonic carcinoma had a 5 year survival of 51%. A comparable group of patients operated on in a conventional fashion had a 5 year survival of 35%, indicating that the isolation technique had increased survival in this nonrandomized trial. The presumption was

that the "no touch" technique with ligation of the draining vascular bed decreased the number of tumor cells released into the vascular system during the trauma of surgery.

The ability of malignant neoplasms to invade the vascular system and to release circulating cells or aggregates of cells appears to vary greatly from tumor to tumor (16,27). Observations on tumor models isolated by pedicle flaps have quantitated that up to 10% of the cells in growing and regressing MTW mammary carcinomas were discharged into the circulation in a 24 hr period (41). This translates to 3-4,000,000 cancer cells per gram of primary tumor per day, an astounding number of cells. The obviously less well controlled human studies do not appear to indicate a circulating tumor burden of this order of magnitude, yet the significance of the potential number of tumor cells capable of entering the vascular compartment must be appreciated by oncologists.

Release of cancer cells into the circulation is unquestionably enhanced by palpation (40), manipulation (44), biopsy (39) and surgical resection (42). Radiation therapy to an implanted tumor also increased the frequency of observed lung metastases in one animal study, but it was subsequently demonstrated that the manipulations associated with positioning the animal and not the radiation were responsible for this observed increase in metastases (44). The release of tumor cells during resection for colon and rectal carcinomas has been well studied in the human. The observed increase in cancer cells in the venous system draining the tumor bed has been repeatedly demonstrated and the contribution of surgical manipulation during the operation to increasing the number of tumor cells released into the vasculature, probably as homotypic aggregates, has been clearly documented. These observations have resulted in a commonly adopted surgical technique, whenever anatomically possible, that isolates and ligates the tumor vasculature prior to the primary resection. This represents a mechanical form of interfering with the metastatic cascade, a procedure that does not always avail itself to routine clinical use because of the tumor site and the anatomy of the surgical resection.

IV. METASTATIC POTENTIAL OF METASTASES

The concept of metastases originating from metastases is not considered an important problem in the clinical literature, as judged by the paucity of articles on the subject. Once metastatic foci have been clearly established, the prognosis is poor and only with rare exception is the patient considered curable. Only in the last decade have there been significant advances in the treatment of patients with demonstrated metastases. Adult testicular germ cell tumors and pediatric leukemias treated with intensive chemotherapy are the best examples of the improved efficiency of chemotherapy. However, in the majority of patients, once metastases have developed there is little effective therapy available. Two explanations for the sequence of dissemination of malignant disease, increasing tumor burden and ultimately host death are proposed. In the first, all of the secondary deposits of tumor are thought to originate from the primary cancer and either have variable growth rates or are maintained for extended periods in a dormant state. The other, and more plausible, possibility is that established metastases, in a manner analogous to primary neoplasms, develop the capacity for vascular invasion and contribute to the pool of circulating cancer cells resulting in the establishment of additional metastatic foci (45,46). It would seem logical that the biology of malignant tumors would be similar regardless of whether a primary tumor or a metastatic foci. Therefore, a similar sequence leading to vascular invasion and dissemination of cancer cells would occur (45,46).

An in-depth study of the pattern of metastases identified in autopsy examinations has been carried out by investigators at Roswell Park Memorial Institute in Buffalo, New York. Over 4,000 autopsies were performed on patients who died of disseminated cancer in order to study the pattern of spread for various types of cancer. It was determined that key sites of metastasis often occurred and these sites were usually located in the venous drainage system of the primary cancer (47). The observations were based on the fact that metastases were invariably present in the "key" organs when identified at other associated sites. An example of these observations is that in lung carcinoma, hepatic metastases are invariably present if the lung cancer has metastasized to the adrenal gland. These observations wre interpreted as evidence that malignant neoplasms disseminate in a step wise fashion, i.e., metastases are formed from metastases resulting in a predictable pattern of distribution.

While the clinical observations documenting the capacity of metastases to develop additional metastases are anecdotal, there are numerous studies utilizing animal models which clearly document metastases from metastases. The majority of studies dealing with the metastatic potential of established metastases utilize a "surgical resection" model. In general, the model consists of implantation of a tumor into the limb (usually posterior) of the animal. At a time when a high percentage of the animals will have developed systemic metastases, the leg ("primary cancer") is amputated. It has been documented that this procedure successfully ablates the "primary tumor" leaving only metastatic cancer in the animal (45). After a recovery period, it is assumed that any circulating cells or developing metastatic foci originate from the metastases. Carefully documented animal models demonstrating the capacity of metastases to metastasize include the following:

1) Circulating cancer cells have been identified in left heart blood of animals with pulmonary metastases (45). Using the previously described "surgical" model, animals with only metastatic disease were shown to release cancer cells into the circulation. The metastatic potential of these cells was documented by subsequent injection into tumor-free animals.

2) Parabiotic animals are comprised of a host with metastases but with the primary tumor excised. This host is subsequently attached to a non-tumor bearing guest. Metastatic tumors develop in the guest animal (46). Utilizing a similar technique, host animals containing only metastatic tumor were joined to tumor-free guest animals. Not

only were selected humoral and cellular aspects of "tumor immunity" passed to the guest, but numerous metastases developed in these syngeneic animals.

3) Animals with demonstrated lung metastases and eradicated (amputated) primary neoplasms will develop metastases in heterotopic isologous lung tissue implanted into soft tissue after ablation of the primary tumor. This implies that metastasis to the ectopically placed lung tissue occurred from the existing metastases (46,48). In our laboratory, we have developed an animal model of metastases from metastases. With the intravenous injection of tumor cells or the "surgical model of foot pad tumor cell injection," lung metastases are predictably produced. After four or more days, a time interval sufficient to insure the absence of residual circulating tumor cells, heterotopic isologous fetal lung tissue is implanted into soft tissue of the hind legs. Metastases readily develop in the fetal lung implants during the ensuing weeks (Figure 2). Evaluation of this model requires histological examination to quantitate the number and size of the metastatic deposits. Using a B16 tumor line results in metastases to the fetal lung implant in 100% of the animals. In addition, the number of metastases can be significantly reduced by the oral administration of nafazatrom. The proposed mechanism of action of this drug will be discussed in a subsequent chapter.

While the clinical observations dealing with the capability of metastases to disseminate is limited, there is little evidence arguing against this possibility. The animal model data, especially in our recently developed system, demonstrates unequivocally the high frequency of metastases from metastases. It appears that once metastases occur, there is an increase in the tumor's ability to form additional metastatic deposits. This ability of metastases to metastasize has been clearly demonstrated in animal models (5,48,49). There is a considerable body of evidence evolving which characterizes the variation in tumor cell population (tumor heterogeneity) of tumor metastases and which may explain the occasional failure of an isolated metastasis to disseminate further. In general, most experimental studies demonstrate increased metastatic potential of metastases, but an occasional clone of cells has the opposite behavior. This is one possible explanation for the relatively rare occurrence of successful resection of isolated metastases.

V. SUMMARY. VASCULAR INVASION AND CIRCULATING CANCER CELLS
    ORIGINATING FROM PRIMARY AND SECONDARY NEOPLASMS

There is little question that cancer cells commonly enter the vascular system. The presence of circulating cancer cells does not guarantee formation of distant metastases (metastatic inefficiency). The sequence of carcinogenesis, neoplastic expansion and invasion of host tissues, vascular permeation and development of circulating cancer cells is a complex set or sets of events. The extravasation and successful implantation of tumor cells are equally complex events and represent the topics of various chapters in this volume.

12

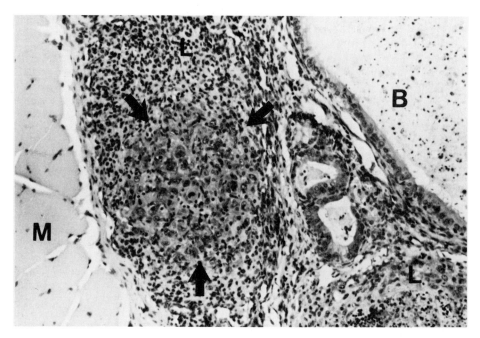

FIGURE 2. Photomicrograph of fetal lung (L) implanted in skeletal muscle (M) of syngeneic hosts. An enlarged bronchial structure is at one edge of the photomicrograph (B). A metastasis of B16 amelanotic melanoma from the host lung metastases is outlined by the arrows (Hematoxylin and Eosin stain, 300X magnification).

Up to 50% of patients presenting to a physician with cancer will already have developed systemic metastases (3). Therefore, major improvements in the treatment of patients with established metastases must obviously be directed towards the eradication of not only the primary tumor but to the microscopic or macroscopic metastases present. While the current methods of therapy directed towards the control of the primary cancer (surgery, radiation therapy and in selected instances chemotherapy) should continue to be employed, there is a body of data suggesting that many procedures utilized in cancer diagnosis and eventual therapy increase the systemic dissemination of this dreaded disease. The development of any biologic modifier which has the potential of decreasing circulating cancer cells or impeding their implantation may serve to increase the effectiveness of current therapy. In addition, these biologic modifiers may have an important role in slowing the progression of widespread metastases in disseminated cancer. The development of any biologic modifier which has the potential of decreasing metastases from metastases may serve to increase the effectivness of current therapy.

REFERENCES

1. Salomon JC. Invasion Metastasis 1:1-2, 1981.
2. Cederholm-Williams SA. Invasion Metastasis 1:85-98, 1981.
3. Sugarbaker EV. Am. J. Pathol. 97:623-632, 1979.
4. Fisher B, Redmond C and Fisher ER. Cancer (Philadelphia) 46:1009-1025, 1980.
5. Hart IR and Fidler IJ. Rev. Biol. 55:121-142, 1980.
6. Folkman J, Merler E, Abernathy C and Williams G. J. Exp. Med. 133:275-288, 1981.
7. Senger DR, Galli SJ, Dvorak AM, Perruzzi CA, Harvey VS and Dvorak HF. Science 219:983-985, 1983.
8. Lane N, Goksel H, Salerno RA and Haagensen CD. Ann. Surg. 153:483-498, 1961.
9. Smart CR, Myers MH and Gloeckler LA. Cancer (Philadelphia) 41:787-789, 1978.
10. Weigand RA, Isenberg WM, Russo J, Brennan MJ and Rich MA. Cancer (Philadelphia) 50:962-969, 1982.
11. Friedell GH, Betts A and Sommer SC. Cancer (Philadelphia) 18:164-166, 1965.
12. Tsakraklides V, Olson P, Kersey JH and Good RA. Cancer (Philadelphia) 34:1259-1267, 1974.
13. Barlogie B, Drewinko B, Schumann J, Gohde W, Dosik G, Latreille J, Johnson DA and Freireich EJ. Am. J. Med. 69:195-203, 1980.
14. Meyer JS, Bauer WC and Rao BR. Lab. Invest. 39:225-235, 1980.
15. Crissman JD, Liu WY, Gluckman J and Cummings G. Cancer (Philadelphia) (in press).
16. Nakadate T, Suzuki M and Sato H. Gann 70:435-446, 1979.
17. Sloane BF, Dunn JR and Honn KV. Science 212:1151-1153, 1981.
18. Hasimoto K, Yaminishi Y, Maeyen E, Dabbous MK and Kanzaki T. Cancer Res. 33:2790-2801, 1973.
19. Poole AR, Tiltman KJ, Recklies AD and Stoker TAM. Nature (London) 273:545-547, 1978.
20. Liotta LA, Kleinerman J, Catanzaro P and Rynbrandt D. J. Natl. Cancer Inst. 58:1427-1431, 1977.
21. Sylven B. In: Biochemical and Enzymatic Factors Involved in Cellular Detachment in Chemotherapy of Cancer Dissemination and Metastasis (Eds. Garattini J and Franchi G), Raven Press, New York, pp. 129-137, 1973.
22. Liotta LA, Tryggvason K, Garbisa S, Hart I, Foltz CM and Shafie S. Nature (London) 204:67-68, 1980.
23. Sloane BF, Honn KV, Sadler JG, Turner WA, Kimpson JJ and Taylor JD. Cancer Res. 42:980-986, 1982.
24. Salsbury AJ. Cancer Treat. Rev. 2:55-72, 1975.
25. Liotta LA, Kleinerman J and Saidel GM. Cancer Res. 34:997-1004, 1974.
26. Engell HC. Acta Chir. Scand. Suppl. 201:1-70, 1955.
27. Weiss L, Mayhew E, Rapp DG and Holmes JC. Br. J. Cancer 45:44-53, 1982.
28. Brown CE and Warren S. Surg. Gynecol. Obstet. 66:611-621, 1938.
29. Engell HC. Ann. Surg. 149:457-461, 1959.
30. Griffiths JD and Salsbury AJ. Circulating Cancer Cells, Charles C. Thomas Publisher, Springfield, IL, 1965.
31. Fisher ER and Fisher B. Cancer (Philadelphia) 12:926-932, 1959.
32. Zeidman I, McCutcheon M and Coman DR. Cancer Res. 10:357-361, 1950.
33. Fidler IJ. Cancer Res. 34:491-498, 1974.
34. Liotta L, Kleinerman J and Saidel GM. Cancer Res. 36:889-894, 1976.
35. Watanabe S. Cancer (Philadelphia) 7:215-223, 1954.
36. Gasic GJ, Gasic TB, Galanti N, Johnson T and Murphy S. Int. J. Cancer 11:704-718, 1973.
37. Nicolson GL and Winkelhake JL. Nature (London) 255:230-232, 1975.
38. Warren BA. J. Med. 4:150-177, 1973.

39. Riggins RS and Ketcham AS. J. Surg. Res. 5:200–206, 1965.
40. Jonasson OL, Long S, Robers E, McGrew E and McDonald JH. J. Urol. 85:1–12, 1961.
41. Butler TP and Gullino PM. Cancer Res. 35:512–516, 1975.
42. Roberts E, Jonasson O, Long S, McGrew EA, McGrath R and Cole WH. Cancer (Philadelphia) 15:232–240, 1962.
43. Turnbull RB, Kyle K, Watson FR and Spratt J. Ann. Surg. 166:420–425, 1967.
44. Baker D, Elkon D, Lim M, Constable W and Wanebo H. Cancer (Philadelphia) 48:2394–2398, 1981.
45. Ketcham AS, Ryan JJ and Wexler H. Ann. Surg. 169:297–299, 1975.
46. Hoover HG and Ketcham AS. Am. J. Surg. 130:405–411, 1975.
47. Bross IDJ, Viadana E and Pickren J. J. Chronic Dis. 28:149–159, 1975.
48. Kinsey DL. Cancer (Philadelphia) 11:674–676, 1960.
49. Poste G, Doll J, Brown AE, Tzeng J and Zeidman I. Cancer Res. 42:2770–2778, 1982.

CHAPTER 2. OVERVIEW OF THE METASTATIC CASCADE

LEONARD WEISS

Metastasis is one of the major problems if not <u>the</u> major problem in the diagnosis, staging and treatment of cancer. Although over the last few years, there have been major advances in our understanding of cancer, conceptual advances have often led to the recognition of many problems, where previously only comparatively few were recognized. This is particularly true for metastasis, where we are currently at the stage of recognizing at least some of the basic problems, and hopefully can begin to arrive at some of their solutions.

In dealing with metastasis, where there are major gaps in knowledge and no firm consensus of informed opinion, any brief overview cannot by definition be complete. This chapter is no exception, and consists of a short critical review of some of the major steps in the metastatic process, with emphasis on those not covered elsewhere in this volume.

I.   IS METASTASIS A RANDOM OR NON-RANDOM PROCESS?

A major problem lies in determining whether the appearance of metastases is the end result of random survival of cancer cells proceeding through a number of sequential traumatic steps of the metastatic process (Figure 1) or whether it represents the non-random

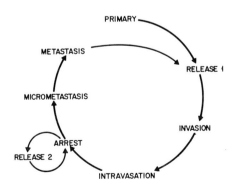

FIGURE 1. Steps in the Metastatic Process.

survival of "preexisting variant" cancer cells (1). The latter could constitute a relatively stable subpopulation within a primary tumor from which metastases are exclusively or predominantly derived (1).

Critical discussion of whether metastasis is a random or non-random process in terms of cancer cells has been limited by an apparent confusion between three issues, namely:

(A) Cancer cell heterogeneity,

(B) the significance of clones of cells with varying metastasis-related behavior derived from primary cancers and

(C) the significance of randomness or non-randomness.

A. Heterogeneity

Ever since sections of cancers have been examined with high-power light microscopy, pleomorphism has been recognized by pathologists as a diagnostic feature of cancer cells. As far as I am aware, every feature of cancer cells or indeed any other cells examined reveals population heterogeneity. This has been described with respect to cell surface components, antigenic markers, locomotion, adhesion, detachment, drug sensitivity, karyotype, etc. All of these parameters show variation on a cell-to-cell basis. Some of them may in the future be quantitated more accurately than heretofore by the use of cell-sorters in combination with monoclonal antibodies and other labeling techniques. Unfortunately, there is no direct marker for metastatic capability, and as will be seen assays of this capability have inherent limitations. Many of these properties are described in terms of means and standard errors or medians and ranges; they are not appropriately described as "subpopulations" unless the parameters in question are demonstrably heritable under defined conditions.

Various temporary changes in cell properties which may be related to metastasis (e.g., cell detachment, adhesion, deformability, surface charge, drug sensitivity) vary with metabolism, cell cycle, etc. In a solid tumor these properties could be subject to spatial and temporal variation related to vascularity, enzyme levels, necrosis and other forms of epigenetic controls (2). Obviously, any variation in the functional attributes of cancer cells under these conditions can be described as an expression of phenotype. As any cellular property can be so described, by its universality this term has become almost meaningless in the present context.

If special groups of cancer cells from the primary cancer form metastases, then initially the metastatic properties of the cancer cells in the primary and secondary lesions could be depicted as in Figure 2. In the case of random survival of the metastasizing cells, i.e., in the absence of genetically-linked metastatic heterogeneity, as shown in Figure 2a, the primary and metastatic lesions are expected to be related to each other in a manner accounted for in statistical terms reflecting random selection. The related case (Figure 2b) in which metastases arise from transient metastatic compartments (2) would result in metastases and primary tumors having similar metastatic properties and similar degrees of heterogeneity. Metastases may also arise predominantly or exclusively from the entry of <u>stable</u> "preexisting metastatic phenotypes" into the metastatic process (Figure 2c). In this case the cancer cell population would be derived from cells with high metastatic potential and metastatic lesions should on average metastasize more than comparable random samples taken from the primary tumor. The possibility that metastases are generated by heterogeneous cancer cell populations having an <u>unstable</u> metastatic phenotype is really a special case of a transient metastatic compartment (Figure 2b).

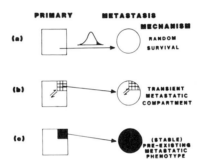

FIGURE 2. Hypothetical Relationships of the Metastatic Properties of Cancer Cells in Primary Cancers and their Metastases.

There can be no doubt that the cancer cells within a tumor are heterogeneous with respect to many parameters and it would be surprising if metastatic heterogeneity did not exist. However, comparisons of the cancer cell populations of metastases and the primary lesions generating them may not provide definitive evidence that metastases are derived predominantly or exclusively from cells with a "preexisting metastatic phenotype".

B. <u>Clones</u>

By a series of repetitive <u>in vitro/in vivo</u> passages, Fidler and his colleagues (3-5) have obtained sublines of cells from several mouse tumors. Each subline gives rise to reproducible, but different, average numbers of pulmonary colonies when injected intravenously into tumor-free recipient animals. When these sublines are maintained in culture, then development of pulmonary colonies from them following intravenous injection remains remarkably constant over prolonged periods of time. Pulmonary colonization data from my own laboratory for various sublines of the mouse B16 melanoma are given in Table 1, and are in accord with the results obtained by Fidler and his colleagues in addition to a number of other laboratories. Although in many papers, the pulmonary colonies developing after intravenous injection are referred to as "metastases," the data shown in Table 1 indicate that colonization may provide a gross overestimate of metastasis suggesting that intravasation (invasion) may constitute a major functional barrier to the realization of colonization potential. There are two major problems with respect to these lines: first, whether they really represent "preexisting metastatic phenotypes" in the tumors from which they were derived and second, the relationship of these lines to metastasis.

Table 1. Incidence of Pulmonary Tumors 21 Days after Intravenous (IV) or Intramuscular (IM) Injection of 100,000 Cancer Cells.

B16 Subline	IV		IM	
	Tumor Incidence	Median (range) Tumors/Animal	Tumor Incidence	Median (range) Tumors/Animal
Parent	12/12	240 (77–352)	25/25	6 (1–51)
F10	45/45	103 (5–400)	23/64	0 (0–19)
F10FA	12/12	27 (7–95)	48/96	1 (0–242)
F10$^{1.r-6}$	34/41	3 (0–152)	34/68	1 (0–10)
Wild	28/30	4 (0–69)	12/30	0 (0–4)

Data obtained from Weiss et al. (6).

For technical reasons, many of the lines of cancer cells used for work on metastatic heterogeneity are maintained for varying periods of time in vitro. In their work on the clonal diversity of mouse KHT sarcoma cells, Chambers et al. (7) observed the stability of 4 in vitro-isolated KHT clones with respect to lung colony formation after intravenous injection. The high colonization potential of 2 of the clones remained stable after 3 to 4 months of in vitro growth, whereas in the case of 2 clones with low colonization potential, a 10-fold increase in potential was observed over the first 30 days of culture. Thereafter these clones appeared to stabilize. This does not mean that heterogeneity of colonization potential should be dismissed as an in vitro artifact, because when in vivo cloning techniques were used a similar range of clonal diversity was detected, although the in vitro clones in general exhibited a higher colonization potential. A more extreme example of the distorting effects of combined in vitro and in vivo selection techniques is that by using such combined techniques metastasizing variants can be obtained from non-metastasizing N-methyl-N-nitrosourea-induced rat mammary adenocarcinomas (8), which evidently do not contain cells with metastatic capability. Therefore in this case the variants must be regarded as a functional artifact.

The major implication of the "preexisting metastatic phenotype" hypothesis has been that the metastatic heterogeneity observed in cloning experiments indicates the presence of stable subpopulations of cancer cells in the tumor from which they are derived. This view is consistent with Foulds' (9) view of tumor progression in which, following mutation-like events within the tumors, subpopulations of cancer cells arise which are more malignant (i.e., metastatic). Proof of Foulds' implication would indicate that metastases are normally derived from such clones. This depends on whether the cloning experiments are simply isolation procedures or whether they are in some way responsible for generating subpopulations de novo. The quantitative assessment of the generation of metastatic variants depends on the use of Luria-Delbruck fluctuation analysis of series of parallel, clonal populations. Although considerable lip-service has been paid to the use of fluctuation analysis in approaching this problem, I am only aware of two attempts to make such analyses, namely those of Cifone and Fidler (10) and Harris et al. (11). In both of these analyses metastatic potential was equated with pulmonary colonization potential following intravenous injections of cancer cells into mice.

Cifone and Fidler (10) estimated mutation rates in clonally derived mouse cancer cell lines with high and low colonization potential. These estimates were in respect to their resistance to ouabain or 6-thiopurine, but not with respect to the evolution of metastatic mutants. In each case the high potential cells had higher mutation rates (3:1 to 7:1) than the low potential cells. These results relate to the genetic stability of high and low "metastatic" clones, not to the rates of genesis of these clones. Cicone and Fidler (10) consider that while a genetic mechanism may be responsible for the process of tumor progression, their results do not exclude epigenetic effects. Harris et al. (11), in their work with the mouse KHT osteosarcoma, calculated that metastatic variants arose spontaneously in clonal lines at an apparent rate of approximately 10^{-5} per cell per generation. In calculating this rate, no correction was made for the efficiency with which intravenously injected variant cells form pulmonary colonies. Although whole populations of injected cells colonize with an overall efficiency of approximately 10^{-4}, the number of variants present is presumably small, and the estimate of a variant generation of 10^{-5} per cell per generation with respect to colonization potential appears reasonable. The possible drawbacks in calculating the efficiency of the metastatic process in terms of the total cancer cell input has been emphasized (12), but the question of developing heterogeneity in clonally derived cell lines is often overlooked. Poste et al. (13) have shown that certain B16 (F1 and F10) clones show marked heterogeneity, and that subclones with widely differing metastatic abilities rapidly emerge in these clones. However, if the subclones are co-cultured, they interact in an unspecified manner to "stabilize" the population. This might form the basis of polyclonal equilibria in tumors, and could lead to the prediction that metastases will resemble the primary cancers generating them with respect to their content of metastatic variants.

The observations made by Fidler and others on the different metastatic and metastasis-related behavior of clones or lines are not in question. However, the interpretation is rendered exceptionally difficult both by the continuous evolution of variants in vitro after the initial isolation of their progenitors from tumors and by the complicated dynamics of these cell populations. Thus, the importance of these metastatic variants in naturally occurring metastasis has yet to be established.

C. Randomness or Non-Randomness

There is a general agreement that in terms of the total numbers of available cancer cells metastasis is an inefficient process (12,14,15). Many cancer cells enter the metastatic process, yet comparatively few metastases develop. The present controversy on random or non-random events in metastasis involves the explanation for this disproportion.

If any population of cancer cells entering the metastatic cascade goes sequentially through five randomly selective (traumatic) steps as shown in Figure 1, each of which kills 90% of the cells, then only 0.001% of the initial cellular input from the primary cancer will form metastases. Therefore, survival in each step could be modified by non-random epigenetic factors, including temporary pathophysiological changes in either the cancer cells or their host. For example, clusters of cancer cells are much more efficient in forming metastases than single cells due to the greater likelihood of arrest in the microvasculature. In contrast, a metastatic efficiency of 0.001% could also be explained exclusively in terms of non-random survival. This would be true if only 0.001% of the cancer cells entering the metastatic process were of the requisite "preexisting metastatic phenotype" arising as a consequence of a mutation-like event. However, even proponents of non-random, genetically-linked metastatic mechanisms do not now rule out the possibility that epigenetic factors also affect the process (10). In addition, it must be borne in mind that even in the case of the high metastatic clones of the UV-2237 fibrosarcoma described by Cifone and Fidler (10), intravenous injection of 100,000 cells produced only 50 nodules (compared with 1 nodule per 100,000 cells with the low metastatic clone). Thus, the high metastatic clone only produced pulmonary nodules with an efficiency of 0.05%, compared with 0.001% in the case of the low metastatic clones. Even in the case of the most efficient high metastatic subclones, the efficiency was only 0.28% (280 nodules per 100,000 injected cells). These high metastatic clones are thought to represent only a very small proportion of the whole cancer cell population of a tumor. In addition, if the efficiencies could be determined in the natural process of metastasis where barriers to intravasation must also be taken into account, they would probably be even lower. It seems much more reasonable to explain the failure of more than 99% of the cancer cells to form pulmonary nodules in terms of stochastic processes resulting in cell death or dormancy, than in terms of a never-ending series of sub- or sub-sub-clones.

Studies on human tumors reveal that an important factor in metastasis propagation and pattern is the metastasis of metastases (16,17, see also Chapter 1). It is therefore of considerable practical importance to determine whether metastases are more metastatic than the primary cancers generating them. If the cells forming the metastases were derived exclusively or predominantly from a "preexisting metastatic phenotype" which according to the "progression" theory represents a more malignant state with progressive genetic instability, then it might be expected that metastases would be more metastatic than their primary cancers. This would be due to their higher proportion of metastatic variants. Describing their work with a variety of tumors, Fidler and Hart (18) observe that "The metastatic capacity of cells from the spontaneous metastases was always found to be higher than that of cells from the parent tumor." This generalization appears to be partly based on the work of Raz et al. (19) who observed that tail-vein injections of cultured cells which were originally derived from spontaneous pulmonary metastases of the UV2237 fibrosarcoma produced more colonies in the lungs of recipient hosts than cells derived from the parent tumor (19). In addition, Talmadge and Fidler (20) implanted four different tumors into mice and "several resulting spontaneous metastases were isolated and established as individual cell lines." In one case (K1735 melanoma), subcutaneous tumors derived from a parent tumor produced significantly fewer pulmonary metastases than four metastasis-derived lines. In another case (M5076 reticulum cell sarcoma), both the parent and 5 metastasis-derived lines produced hepatic metastases in "practically all of the mice." However, metastasis-derived lines gave rise to significantly more metastases per animal. Three other lines were tested for their ability to form pulmonary colonies after intravenous injection. In the case of the UV2237 and 3LL tumors, metastasis-derived lines gave rise to more pulmonary colonies than the parent tumor-derived lines. However, there was no difference in colony formation between the parent UV2237 C-40 clone and four metastasis-derived lines. In this latter case, but not the others, metastasis was considered to be random. In the above experiments metastasis-derived lines were passaged in vitro before use.

In contrast, in experiments in which cells were derived directly from metastases and the tumors generating them without going through in vitro culture, Giavazzi et al. (21), Mantovani et al. (22), Weiss et al. (23) and Honn and Sloane (unpublished observation) have been unable to show that spontaneous metastases are as a general rule more metastatic than the primary cancers from which they arose. In our own work, cell suspensions obtained directly from spontaneous pulmonary metastases were injected subcutaneously into non-tumor bearing hosts. Their metastatic behavior was compared with that of cell suspensions obtained directly from the primary tumors which generated them. In the case of B16 melanomas and KHT osteosarcomas, injected minces of metastases gave rise to more pulmonary metastases than minces from their corresponding primary cancers. In contrast, in the case of 3LL and T241 cancers, the primary tumor minces gave rise to more pulmonary

22

metastases than those derived from metastases. When fragments of solid tumors were implanted into animals, no differences were detected between the metastatic behavior of implants taken randomly from several pulmonary metastases and the primary tumors generating them in any of the four tumor types. Due to experimental design, the failure to show differences between the metastatic capabilities of fragments of primary tumors and their metastases were unlikely to have been due to sampling errors of the type discussed by Talmadge and Fidler (20) or Poste and Greig (24).

In view of the difficulties in the interpretation of experiments with cultured cells, it is of interest that the major variation in experimental design between the groups reporting that metastases are in general more metastatic than those that do not is that the former have introduced in vitro culture between sampling metastases and injections into non-tumor bearing hosts. The latter have injected or implanted material directly from one host to another.

The failure to consistently demonstrate different metastatic potentials in metastases and primary tumors is also in accord with earlier conclusions drawn from a critical review of the literature (25). It can be suggested that the evidence for consistent differences between cancer cells in primary cancers and their metastases is sparse with respect to cytogenetics, immunology and differential drug sensitivity and is not as definitive as many seem to assume.

In the absence of immediately identifiable markers it is impossible to determine by direct experiment whether the different behavior of two cancer cell populations is due to different cancer cells (i.e., high and low metastatic phenotypes) or to different numbers of cells with similar metastatic phenotypes. If estimates obtained in mice are relevant to the metastatic process as a whole, then only approximately 1 cancer cell in 100,000 forms a metastasis. It could be argued that this is due on the one hand to random processes with modification by non-random genetic and epigenetic factors. On the other hand, it could be argued that the low efficiency is primarily due to the presence of 1/100,000 "metastatic phenotypes" in the parent cancer, and that metastases arise by an essentially non-random process which can be modified by epigenetic factors and random events. However, studies made by Harris et al. (11) indicate that the generation of metastatic variants is itself a random event! The issue of random or non-random is important with respect to further studies on metastatic mechanisms. Thus, it would seem prudent to address the two non-exclusive problems of not only why the one cancer cell metastasizes, but also why the 99,999 cells do not. The latter problem is important, because even "highly" metastatic clones or subclones of cancer cells of the putative "metastatic phenotype" metastasize with maximum efficiencies of only 0.28%. This indicates that random processes also play an important rate-regulating role in the formation of metastases even from this proposed genetically-determined subpopulation.

D. Conclusions

Attempts to test the concept that metastases arise exclusively or predominantly from a "preexisting metastatic phenotype" have been made in comparatively few tumors. The differences in the metastatic behavior between so-called "low" and "high" metastatic clones are not as significant as proponents of this unproved hypothesis seem to think. First, assay of colonization potential by intravenous injection of cancer cells followed by pulmonary colony counts leads to overestimates of differences in "natural" metastatic potential as indicated in Table 1. Second, even using this assay method, both "low" and "high" metastatic clones form pulmonary colonies albeit in different numbers. In the case of naturally occurring metastasis, cancer cells are not released into the blood in a single pulse as in the assay, but are released continuously. Thus, over a period of time, the "low" metastatic majority could give rise to appreciable numbers of metastases. In addition, even the maximal reported differences between different clones are tiny, compared with the randomly generated metastatic inefficiency of the clones and subclones themselves. Third, realization of the genetic and pathophysiologic dynamism among cancer cell populations makes it understandable that the properties of individual micrometastases may bear temporary and unpredictable relationships to the average properties of their parent primary tumors. This would complicate the interpretation of experimental data.

The present critical review of the experimental data suggests that from an operational viewpoint, metastases and metastatic inefficiency are determined by a series of random processes. Although the presence of metastatic variants could modify the rate or efficiency with which metastasis occurs, they are not expected to produce major modifications in either.

II. RELEASE 1

By definition, a metastasis is a tumor which has lost contiguity with its parent primary lesion. Thus, cell release or detachment is an inherent part of metastasis.

It still appears to be a common misconception that cell detachment is the reverse of cell adhesion. It has been shown in a variety of systems that the plane of detachment is spatially different from adhesion and that the two processes can be modified in different directions by the same agents (26,27). The practical outcome of these differences is that detachment must be measured by detachment experiments and that adhesion must be measured by adhesion experiments.

A. Site

The site of cell detachment from a primary cancer may favor initial dissemination by lymphatic or venous routes. Detachment might occur prior to contact between cancer cells and blood channels, such as situations where the cancer cells are migrating through the host tissues. These cancer cells will have increased opportunity to gain access to lymphatic channels. If contact with blood channels occurs prior to cancer cell detachment, then if the cancer cells can gain access to the channels, venous dissemination will be the preferred initial route. Entry into veins requires an invasive process culminating in exposure of cancer cells to the lumen. They will then be detached by mechanical agitation caused by body movements and trauma (28). In sarcomas (29), where vascular clefts lined by cancer cells are seen, exfoliation is directly into the bloodstream. With the exception of some of the earliest metastatic events, cancer cells are not confined to either the lymphatic or blood systems and appear to move between the two (30). Realization that involved lymph nodes are indicators of general metastatic spread rather than indicators that metastasis is confined to the lymphatic system has led to reappraisal and limitation of radical surgery in the treatment of cancer.

B. Detachment Factors

As tumors often exhibit a supracellular heterogeneity with respect to regions of proliferation, necrosis, blood supply and host-defense reactions, the effects of some of these interrelated variables will be considered.

1. _Growth-rate and detachment_. Quantitative studies on the detachment of cultured cells from protein-coated glass substrata (31) and of parenchymal cells from regenerating, hemihepatectomized mouse livers (26) showed that the faster the growth rate, the more easily the cells detached. Consideration of the whole metastatic cascade indicates the virtual impossibility of definitively assessing the relative importance of any one step in the process. It is therefore interesting that in humans there is an impressive correlation in a group of human epitheliomata between growth rate determined by direct caliper measurements and the incidence of metastatic involvement of local lymph nodes.

2. _Necrosis and detachment_. Necrosis is a common feature of solid tumors (32). For example, Fisher et al. (33) observed varying degrees of tumor necrosis in 60% of sections from 1,539 patients with breast cancer. Experiments in which aliquots of W256 tumors were shaken in vitro revealed that more cancer cells were shaken free from viable, juxta-necrotic regions than from cortical regions of the same tumors. Simple saline extracts of the necrotic regions enhanced the detachment of cortical cancer cells but not those from the juxta-necrotic regions. These results suggested that the facilitation of cancer cell detachment was brought about by agents diffusing from the central necrotic regions. The cells in the juxta-necrotic regions were fully affected by these agents in situ. However, the factors were not normally active in the cancer cortex (34). As discussed below, enzymes can play a major role in cell detachment, and it was therefore of interest that in addition to the viable parts of tumors and the tissues surrounding them (35,36) the necrotic regions also apparently acted as free enzyme pools and were rich in lysosomal enzymes (37).

It was suggested that a major source of free enzymes in the necrotic regions was macrophages (37,38) which were attracted by a combination of chemokinesis (39) and necrotaxis. It is difficult to assess the role in metastasis of naturally occurring necrosis in tumors since unless the detached cells have access to disseminative channels they will not constitute a significant input into the metastatic cascade. However, by creating necrotic regions in tumors inadequate therapy may promote the release of surviving cancer cells.

3. Enzymes and detachment. For many years, enzymes have been used to dissociate tumors into viable cancer cells and to detach cells from culture vessels. In vivo, the effects of enzymes cannot be regarded in all-or-none terms because even if enzymes only reduce the numbers of adhesive or cohesive bonds between cells below the levels of applied distractive forces, then enzyme-facilitated cell detachment will occur. Simple observations of whether or not enzymes cause detachment are of dubious value without reference to measured detachment techniques.

Cell release may be facilitated by enzymatic bond-fission, where the sources of the enzymes are the detached cells themselves or alternatively cancer cells and non-malignant bystanders. Necrotic material promotes cell detachment directly, presumably through its enzyme activity in the region of the cell substratum, and indirectly by promoting lysosomal activation and sublethal autolysis of the target cell periphery (37). In vitro, a number of lysosome-activating agents including antisera (40), endotoxin (41), necrotic extracts and high doses of vitamin A (42) all facilitate detachment. In the case of the first three of these agents, their activity is abrogated by the lysosome stabilizer, hydrocortisone. The cellular levels of lysosomal enzymes are under genetic control and their release is a common event in many pathologic processes including inflammation, tissue destruction, leukocyte infiltrations, tumor growth and regression and response to radiotherapy and chemotherapy. The control of release is coupled to elements of physiologic control including stress. It is therefore of interest that an early event in metastasis, cancer cell release, should be capable of modification by such general biologic mechanisms.

It is also of interest that enzymes should facilitate both cancer cell release and invasion (see Chapters 12, 20 and 21), since invasion of the basement membranes of small blood vessels probably serves to regulate the entry of released cancer cells into the circulation.

III. INVASION

Invasion of the tissues by cancer cells initially involves a "breaking-out" process. This is seen for example, when "in situ" carcinomas penetrate their underlying basement membranes as an essential step in dissemination. After traversing non-vascular tissues, a vascular basement membrane must be breached in order to intravasate. Finally, cancer cells delivered to target organs must extravasate in order to develop into metastases.

Invasive movements of cancer into host tissues can occur through two basic, non-exclusive mechanisms. The first considers that forces associated with expansive tumor growth (vis a tergo) serve to drive the cancer into the surrounding tissues along the pathways of least mechanical resistance. In a mechanically homogenous environment, a benign tumor expands uniformly in the form of an encapsulated sphere. In a non-homogeneous environment more complex configurations are seen, as for example when a benign lipoma meets bone and follows its non-compliant contours. In contrast, the margins of malignant tumors often show a pseudocapsule of compressed normal tissue which is penetrated by single cancer cells or tumor spicules. Thus, even where expansion of a cancer into macroscopically homogenous media is accomplished by expansive growth, penetration appears to require microscopic dissolution of host tissues (43).

The second mechanism of invasive movements involves the active crawling of cancer cells through the tissues. Although active movements of cancer cells have been recognized for over a century, their contribution to invasion has never been quantitated systematically in different cancers. A start in this direction has been made by morphometric analyses of sections of human cutaneous melanomas in which the gradual, centrifugal density patterns from the deep edges of the tumors suggest active invasive movements of the melanoma cells for up to 500 μM in advance of the tumor edge. The presence of higher than average density regions at the tumor periphery suggests that, following phases of limited active movement, the cancer cells stop moving and proliferate. This process of movement followed by proliferation may well be a repetitive cyclic event (44).

Degradation of the intracellular matrix and the basement membrane can play a role in promoting penetration and invasion whether expansive mechanisms or active locomotion of cancer cells are involved. For example, it has been shown in vitro that the degree of active cell movement is increased as the viscosity of the medium is decreased (45). Although it has been known for many years that many tumor fragments exhibit collagenolytic activity, this was usually measured against acid soluble, type I collagen-substrate. This type of collagenolytic activity while facilitating invasion of the connective tissue matrix which is rich in type I collagen would not be expected to degrade the basement membranes of blood vessels since these contain type IV collagen. Thus, on the basis of differential enzyme activity or differential synthesis, a situation could arise where a tumor could invade and destroy local matrix but be incapable of invading blood vessels. In the case of the B16 melanoma series studied by Weiss et al. (6), intravasation was assayed by the increase in pulmonary metastases following massage of a primary cancer. These functional studies indicated that the B16BL6 tumor intravasated, and therefore its natural metastatic behavior matched intravenous injection as shown in Table 1. The failure of intravenous injections of the other tumors to match natural metastasis corresponded to their failure to respond to massage and indicated that for them a major barrier to metastasis was the failure to intravasate, presumably through basement membrane. Discrimination between invasion and metastasis is classically seen in human basal cell carcinomas where massive invasion may be seen in untreated cancers, but where metastasis is exceptionally rare.

Enzymatic degradation has focused attention on its control, particularly in the case of collagenase type I, but also in the case of metallo proteinases, elastases and serine proteinases which degrade type IV collagen. Naturally occurring activators of latent collagenase include plasmin, a serum β_1-globulin (46) and a cathepsin B-like cysteine proteinase (see Chapter 12). The association of plasmin activity with collagenase activation indicates that plasminogen activator (i.e., serine proteinases) which has been associated with cancer and vascular endothelial cells must not be viewed exclusively in terms of fibrinolysis. The production of collagenase by cancer cells can be stimulated by the presence of collagen, endotoxin and heparin (which has been used as an anticoagulant for the prevention of metastases). In vitro, soluble factors obtained from monocytes and lymphocytes such as prostaglandins and proteinases all stimulate collagenase production whereas glucocorticoids and progesterone inhibit production (47). If these in vitro effects occur in vivo, then collagenase-dependent invasion could at least be partially regulated by interactions involving monocytes and lymphocytes and in common with cancer cell release could be coupled to other pathophysiologic factors. It is of interest that in the examples cited regulation of release 1 and invasion is similar since they are sequential steps in the metastatic process.

Details of the biochemistry of invasion are the subject of a number of excellent recent reviews (48,49) and will not be covered here. However, until more data are available it is unwise to make too many generalizations on invasive mechanisms in exclusively biochemical terms of substrates inhibitory to invasion and the abrogation of this inhibition by enzymatic degradation, particularly by collagenases. Thus, the penetration of Walker 256 (W256) and Gardner lymphosarcoma (GL) cells into membrane pores by active movement in vitro is differentially inhibited by fibrin and collagen type I (50). As shown in Table 2, fibrin impregnation partially inhibited the "invasive" movements of W256 cells but totally stopped movement of the GL cells. In contrast, impregnation of membranes with collagen type I gels, partially inhibited the penetration by GL cells but totally prevented W256 movement. In some studies, cancer cells have been seen to actively crawl out of blood vessels where they have been arrested, in a manner resembling diapedesis (51). However, in other cases, cancer cells destroy the blood vessel in a segmental fashion and burst out (52). It appears that different types of arrested cancer cells extravasate through basement membranes in the microvasculature by means of two distinct mechanisms. It would be of obvious interest to determine whether the choice of mechanism depends on enzyme availability.

IV. ARREST

Due to a number of rather ill-defined processes, the bloodstream appears to provide a traumatic environment for cancer cells. Some of

28

the trauma is mechanical, and is probably due to repetitive squeezing
of cancer cells through the microvasculature (53). Some of the
humoral factors have been discussed elsewhere (15). In order to
escape from this trauma, and in order to form metastases, blood-borne
cancer cells must first attach to the endothelium in the
microvasculature of target organs.

Table 2. In Vitro Penetration of Membranes by Walker 256 and Gardner
Lymphosarcoma Cells[a].

8 μM Pore Membranes	Mean Penetration μ M ± S.E. after 4h at 37°C	
	W256	GL
Control	27 ± 2 (25)[b]	91 ± 5 (10)
Fibrin-Filled	13 ± 2 (22)	0 (20)
Collagen I-Filled	0 (35)	22 ± 4 (15)

[a] Data from Turner and Weiss (50).
[b] Number of observations in ( ).

A. Biophysical Aspects of Arrest

All mammalian cells so far examined carry a net negative charge
at their surfaces which generates a mutual electrostatic repulsion
between approaching cells. Thus, contact between cancer cells and the
vascular endothelium is expected to be inhibited by repulsive
interactions. Detailed examination of the physical background to
contact (54,55) has emphasized many of the formidable problems of
correlating cell contact and adhesion with the average physical
parameters of cell surfaces. By the use of appropriate colloid theory
which takes into account both electrostatic and electrodynamic
interactions, average interaction energies between cancer cells and
the vascular endothelium have been computed. It has been calculated
that in order to balance these computed interaction energies, a cancer
cell would have to move in a direction normal to the vascular
endothelium with a kinetic energy corresponding to a velocity of 0.23
cm per second. It is doubtful that such velocities in a direction at
right angles to the axial blood flow can be achieved in the
microvasculature where cancer cell arrest occurs. Using these
computerized maximal total interaction energies, the chances of
contact mediated by thermal (Brownian) agitation may be crudely
estimated for 10 μM radius cancer cells and an idealized flat
vascular endothelium. In this situation, in fewer than one in 10^{1500}
attempts will all of the two opposing surfaces come into contact (15).
The chances of collisions could be increased if contact were regarded
as a non-average phenomenon, involving (initially) only regions of the
involved cell surfaces which carry less than average charge density,

and low radius of curvature macromolecular "hairs" (56). In this situation, collisions are expected to occur between a 10 nm "hair" or probe on a cancer cell and the vascular endothelium (or vice versa) in one attempt out of 100. Laminin, fibronectin, fibrin and/or collagen are among the macromolecular probes which could be used, although of course this type of physical approach gives no clue to the chemical identity of the probes.

Over and above electrostatic repulsion, hydrodynamic interactions play a major role in inhibiting contact between cancer cells and the vascular endothelium. When a cancer cell is carried in the bloodstream, hydrodynamic forces are generated which cause pressure changes and movements of plasma close to the cell surface. When a cancer cell approaches an endothelial surface thus limiting the movement of plasma surrounding the cancer cell, deformation of the hydrodynamic field will occur. This will lead to a significant slowing in the approach rate when the distance separating the two surfaces is of the same magnitude as the cancer cell radius, and the rate of slowing increases with decreasing distance. The approach rates depend on the deformability of the involved cells and the tangential mobility of their surfaces. Deformation of the cancer cells to the macroscopic contours of the endothelium will result in both a decrease in the average distance between their surfaces and an increase in the opposed surface areas, with a consequent increase in their dynamic interactions leading to a slower approach. In contrast, increased tangential mobility at the cell surfaces leads to facilitated movement in the liquid between them and this decrease in viscous friction increases the approach rate. The difficult physical problems associated with hydrodynamic interactions of this type in a biological context are exceptionally well-reviewed by Dimitrov (57).

In the case of clumps of cancer cells, the arrest process appears to involve impaction of cancer cell emboli which are too large to traverse the microvasculature, but for some reason are not directed through large diameter vascular shunts. This simple physical consideration may account for the higher "metastatic" efficiency of multicellular emboli compared with single cancer cells following their intravenous injection. For example, Liotta et al. (58) showed that in the case of T241 fibrosarcomas in C57/Bl mice, intravenous injection of 1,000 cells in clumps containing 6 to 7 cells produced 10 times as many metastases as 100,000 single cancer cells. The multicellular clumps formed pulmonary nodules with an efficiency of approximately 1% compared to a value of 0.01% for single cells. This difference of 2 orders of magnitude due to embolic size difference is at least as impressive as differences between "high" and "low" metastatic clones.

The tentative conclusions to be drawn from biophysical examination of cancer cell arrest at the microvascular endothelium are firstly that it is a non-average phenomenon in terms of the involved cell surfaces. Secondly, the collision-efficiency is probably low, indicating that when arrest occurs it is the result of many attempts. Thirdly, dynamic properties of cancer cells including deformability and tangential mobility can affect arrest. Fourthly, if due to hydrodynamic considerations approach is slow compared to organ microvascular transit time, then an unknown proportion of the cancer cells present in a microvascular bed at any one time will not be arrested at all. Finally, if contact depends on macromolecular "bridges" which may be weak in themselves, particularly sensitive to enzymatic degradation or weakly bound to the cell periphery, then the cancer cell/vascular endothelium associations would have inherent instability leading to release of the attached cells. As discussed later, this process is termed "release 2."

B. The Role of Platelets and Fibrin in Arrest

Numerous reports describe the association of platelet and fibrin deposition around arrested tumor emboli, particularly in areas denuded of endothelium with exposed basement membrane. Observations of this type have provided the underlying rationale for prophylaxis of metastasis by inhibition of platelet interactions and/or fibrino-genesis (see Chapters 10, 11, 14-16, 24 and 25). In reviewing this topic elsewhere (12,59) on the basis of the literature available up to the late 1970's, it appeared that in common with most aspects of metastasis, there is considerable variation between different types of cancer. Thus, Gasic et al. (60) examined a series of murine tumors in vitro and reported a wide spectrum of activity of platelet interactions with 50% showing no interaction at all. It also appeared that at least some of the controversies on fibrin-deposition in relation to arrest originated because different investigators examined material at different times, i.e., either before or after fibrinolysis had occurred (61). Attempts to define mechanisms by interference with fibrinogenesis or platelet interactions have also been controversial, although with the advantage of hindsight, it is now apparent that many of the experiments lacked rigorous pharmacologic design. The apparent controversies on the effects of heparin provide a good example of this in that statements have been made without regard to dose, yet low doses of heparin have anticoagulative effects while high doses sensitize platelets and produce an increase in thromboxane levels (see Chapter 14).

A few generalizations merit consideration. Fibrin deposition could promote or stabilize tumor cell arrest and by withdrawing cancer cells from circulatory trauma could thus promote metastasis. A more direct implication of the metastasis-promoting effects of fibrin comes from a reappraisal of the Revesz (62) phenomenon, in which the addition of large numbers of lethally irradiated cancer cells potentiated the growth of transplants of viable cells. For example, in the case of the "NT" carcinoma in mice, 7,000 viable cells were required for takes in 50% of animals, whereas in the presence of 100,000 lethally irradiated cells, only 4 viable "NT" cells were required (63). It has been suggested by Peters and Hewitt (64) that the effect of the lethally irradiated cells is to produce thromboplastic activity at the injection site, and that local fibrinogenesis prevented the emigration or loss of the viable cancer cells. The fibrin could presumably form a protective cocoon around the injected cells. In contrast to these metastasis-promoting effects, thromboplastic activity could make a significant contribution to the generation of a proliferative thrombophlebitis in those parts of the microvasculature in which cancer cell arrest occurs, leading to vascular occlusion. This may act as a defense mechanism by limiting further intravascular dissemination. However, in total, the impression is gained that local fibrinogenesis has a general metastasis-promoting activity. On the one hand, by its possible role in promoting release 2, fibrinolysis may have an antimetastatic activity, however, on the other hand by activating collagenase systems, plasminogen activator may enhance the invasive extravasation of arrested cancer cells and promote metastasis formation.

C. General Host Effects

Many investigations, including my own, have been made on non-tumor bearing animals. Since metastasis occurs in tumor bearers, it is reasonable to ask whether the sequelae of tumor bearing which include the paraneoplastic "syndromes" affect arrest and other steps in the metastatic process.

The effects of sensitization by prior tumor burden and hyper-immunization by prior injection of lethally radiated cells on pulmonary retention one hour after the tail-vein injections of radiolabeled cells are shown in Table 3. In the three cases studied, tumor burden (sensitization) produced an increase, a decrease or no

Table 3. Retention of Labeled Tumor Cells in the Lungs of Mice.[a]

Animals	TA3 Carcinoma	Gardner Lymphosarcoma	MC-induced Fibrosarcoma
Subcutaneous Tumor Bearers (sensitized)	100	147	58
Hyperimmunized (by injection of x-radiated cells)	N.D.	145	68

[a] 1 hr after tail-vein injection of 4,000,000 cells, expressed as a percentage of non-tumor bearing controls (65).

change in retention (66). Later experiments (67) showed that sensitization to the fibrosarcoma did not modify the retention pattern of injected lymphosarcoma cells and vice versa. Thus, when perturbation of arrest patterns by tumor bearing occurs in these animal tumor systems, it appears to operate through an immunospecific mechanism. It is not my intention to become involved in discussions of the significance of the immune response to cancer in man, and discussions of the precise relevance of immune perturbation to cancer cell arrest patterns would therefore be out of place. However, these experiments serve as an example of altered arrest patterns due to changes in the host, and also of the individuality of the different cancers tested. The results suggest that attention should also be given to perturbations of arrest pattern by other physiologic parameters which may be abnormal in cancer bearers. These include hypercalcemia, autoimmunity, hematologic defects and hypoglycemia. This list is by no means exhaustive.

D. Repetitive Events

Rudenstam (68) has reviewed the enhancing effects of tissue trauma on metastasis formation including mechanical trauma, local ischemia and effects due to chemotherapy, radiotherapy and local irritants. Although for convenience, metastasis is often considered as a cascade of events, it is of course a repetitive process in which pulses of cancer cells continuously enter the cascade. As tumor embolism produces tissue damage, the effects of this damage on succeeding pulses of cancer cells must not be overlooked.

The effects of injury to the microvascular bed on cancer cell retention has been developed into the so-called "Microinjury Hypothesis" (69,70 and Chapter 4). Arterioles either lead through a precapillary sphincter into a capillary bed (microcirculatory unit or modules) which then rejoins arterioles and subsequently venules or alternatively the original arterioles link directly to venules and thus shunt-out the microcirculatory units. The proportion of the blood and contained cancer cells proceeding through the unit or the shunt depends on the tone of the precapillary sphincter. According to the microinjury hypothesis, occlusion of the sphincter by a tumor cell results in injury to the capillary bed downstream and injury to the sphincter. When the occluding cancer cell moves into the capillary bed, it has a higher chance of adhering to the site of microinjury than to the undamaged vascular endothelium. The damaged precapillary sphincter is thought to contract, and thereby direct blood through the arteriolar-venular shunt where the cancer cells have less chance of arrest than in the capillary bed. These expectations are consistent with the direct observations of Zeidman (71) and his colleagues on alternative vascular pathways for tumor emboli, and would constitute one random mechanism for metastatic efficiency.

Experiments were conducted using radiolabeled cancer cells to determine whether a given pulse of cancer cells retained in an organ causes modification in the retention of a second pulse. Rats bearing W256 tumors were given a single tail-vein injection of cancer cells followed after 60 min by an injection of radiolabeled cells. When compared with appropriate controls, no significant change in retention pattern could be detected after 1 hr. However, after 2 hr, more of the second dose was retained in the lungs, and this difference persisted for at least 27 hr. Approximately 25 times more of the second dose than the first was delivered to the extravascular pulmonary tissues (72). These differences which, according to independent evidence, represented increased numbers of extravascular cancer cells, indicated a potential metastatic synergism between the first pulse of cancer cells and the second. While not providing direct evidence to support it, these results are consistent with the microinjury hypothesis.

During natural hematogenous metastasis, cancer cells must be delivered to organs already containing metastases, yet this situation has been largely neglected in most experimental studies. An attempt was therefore made (73) to determine whether the presence of pulmonary metastases from subcutaneous 3LL tumors in mice modified the retention of viable radiolabeled cells given by tail-vein injection. A significantly higher percentage of injected cells was retained over a 6 hr period in the lungs of animals which had carried tumors for 3 wk (100% of mice had overt metastases; mean = 77 metastases) than in those with 1 wk old subcutaneous tumors where only 4/41 animals had overt metastases, and in these there was a mean of 1.5 metastases per animal. In the 3 wk tumor bearers, 4 times as many cancer cells were arrested in the "non-involved" lung tissues than in the metastases themselves. These differences correlated well with the greater relative vascularities of the lungs compared with the tumor tissue. It was also shown that when W256 cells were injected into the portal veins of rats bearing liver tumors, approximately 4 times more cancer cells were arrested in the liver than in the liver tumors on a per gram basis (74). Thus in an organ bearing metastases, it might be expected that these tumors will in fact drive subsequent metastases to progressively decreasing regions of normal tissues, and that metastasis to metastases will be a relatively uncommon event.

It would appear that repetitive events in metastasis are worthy of more attention.

V. RELEASE 2

Other things being equal, and they seldom are, the numbers of metastases developing in a particular organ will depend on some function of the numbers of viable cancer cells delivered to it. However, the number of cells retained is a more operational starting point in comparing the extent of metastasis in different organs then the actual organ dose of cancer cells delivered. In many experiments, when rodents are given tail-vein injections of radiolabeled cells a common pattern of viable cell counts is observed in the lungs as exemplified in Figure 3. Five minutes after the injection, most of the injected cells are retained in the lungs. This provides an index of the arrest phase. This is followed by a release phase during which cells are gradually lost from the lungs so that by 24 hr post-injection most of the cells (counts) have disappeared, and usually between 24 and 48 hr the counts are not significantly different from background. This loss following arrest, which determines the extent of cancer cell retention, could be an obvious rate-regulating step in metastasis. It is termed "release 2" to distinguish it from the detachment of cells from the primary cancer (release 1). Although the same basic mechanisms are thought to operate in both, some of the details are probably different.

As discussed earlier, and in detail elsewhere in this volume (Chapter 8), the arrest of cancer cells at the vascular endothelium is, at least in some cases, associated with fibrin deposition. Plasminogen activator by initiating fibrinolysis may promote the detachment of the temporarily arrested cells, as indeed may other enzymes in the region. It is not suggested that this is a universal mechanism, because treatment of recipient mice with the plasminogen activator inhibitor, ε-aminocaproic acid, did not appreciably affect the organ retention patterns of injected radiolabeled B16 melanoma or lymphosarcoma cells (59).

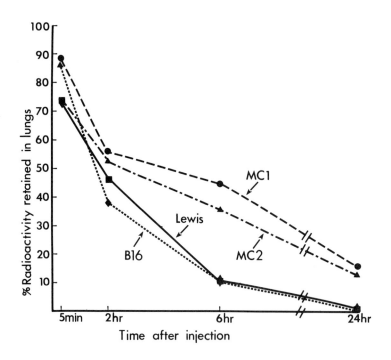

FIGURE 3.   Arrest and Release 2 of Radioactive Cancer Cells from the Lungs of Mice at Specified Time after Tail-Vein Injections (75).

In considering enzyme-enhanced release 2, it must be borne in mind that appropriate enzymes could originate not only in cancer cells, but also in the walls of blood and lymph vessels. The arrest of tumor cells or emboli will induce localized turbulence or obstruction of fluid flow, and this situation leads to localized inflammatory responses including infiltration by polymorphonuclear leukocytes, macrophages and lymphocytes. All of these cells may contribute to local enzyme levels capable of disrupting cancer cell-vascular endothelium-basement membrane associations. In accord with the proposed role of inflammation-coupled enzyme release in release 2, it is of interest that Glaves (76)should have demonstrated that endotoxin-induced stimulation of the reticuloendothelial system promotes the release of previously arrested cancer cells from the lungs of tumor-bearing mice, resulting in a decreased incidence of lung tumors. It was also shown that the potent glucocorticoid triamcinolone acetonide decreases the release of arrested cancer cells from the lungs and increases the incidence of pulmonary tumors, and that in mice treated with both endotoxin and triamcinolone acetonide, the effects of endotoxin were nullified (77). Additional evidence suggesting that proteolytic activity promotes release 2 comes from experiments showing that the antiproteinase aprotinin reduces release 2 and increases the numbers of lung tumors produced by injecting 3LL tumors into mice (78).

This suggestion that release 2 is associated with some sort of host defense reaction has been studied with respect to the traffic of W256 cancer cells over 27 hr periods in the rat (14). Following tail vein injection, most of the W256 cells were temporarily arrested in the lungs and then slowly released. Some of the cells released from the lungs were temporarily arrested in the liver. Although only 2% of radiolabeled cells present in the lungs at any time were non-viable, approximately half of those temporarily arrested in the liver were dead. These measurements were in accord with the observation that following intravenous injection of W256 cells, tumors were ten times more frequent in the lungs than the livers. Direct injection of cancer cells into the liver indicates that the reduced viability of cancer cells at this site is not due to an inherently hostile hepatic environment. Injections into and sampling from other points in the vasculature indicated that only small proportions of the cancer cells were killed on their way to the lungs, during their arrest in the pulmonary microcirculation or between the left ventricle, aorta, hepatic artery and liver. By a process of elimination, it was concluded that a significant amount of trauma resulting in cancer cell death occurs during the events culminating in their release from temporary arrest sites at the pulmonary vascular endothelium. Whatever mechanism is responsible, this "first organ processing" supports the view that release 2 may be a significant rate-regulator in metastasis.

VI. THE FORMATION OF METASTASES FROM MICROMETASTASES

A proportion of that fraction of cancer cells retained in the microvasculature succeeds in extravasating into the target organ. However, not all of these cancer cells progress into overt metastases. Autopsies often reveal microscopic metastases not diagnosed during life, and investigators have observed that many organs in which cancer cells have not been detected in random sections from tumor-bearing animals contain, in fact, covert malignant cells whose presence can only be revealed when the tissues are transplanted into tumor-free animals.

There is much to commend the concept of the dormant state in which tumors remain in a small micrometastasis-state and do not progress into overt metastases. Two mechanisms have been proposed to

account for dormancy: the first is that cells remain for a protracted
if not indefinite time in a G stage of the cell cycle. However,
direct evidence for this is lacking. The second possibility is that a
pseudodormant state exists in which cell replication is matched by
cell loss. This would require a low rate of replication and could be
brought about in the absence of tumor vascularization when nutrition
would be dependent on diffusion. The neovascularization of tumors
occurs by their invasion with sprouts from nearby capillaries.
Folkman (79) has described a number of factors inducing endothelial
mitosis in adjacent host vasculature. Folkman's original concept of a
specific "tumor angiogenic factor" has now been widened to include
other angiogenic factors which include prostaglandins and whose source
is not exclusively cancer cells. Much research is currently directed
at controlling metastasis by means of agents inhibiting the
neovascularization of micrometastases.

Host homeostatic controls may contribute to the restraint of
subclinical metastases. Metastatic "explosions" are well-recognized
following the surgical removal of primary cancers or psychological
stress. I have no idea how common this phenomenon is, but a single
example creates a lasting impression! The ultimate expression of
control, namely tumor regression, is well-documented but is very rare.
Control, involving host-defense reactions which include the ubiquitous
natural killer cells and macrophages, also includes growth limitations
imposed by blood supply. Perhaps a quantitative approach to the ratio
of micrometastases to metastases will result from studies of various
tumor markers, but as yet this is an ill-defined field. This is
disappointing because the whole question of micrometastases is
exceptionally important in the planning of adjuvant therapy.

VII. CONCLUSIONS

Any brief overview of metastasis will of necessity omit
discussion of major issues, this is no exception! However, some of
these omissions will be covered in other chapters.

The salient feature of the natural history of metastasis is in my
view its inefficiency. It is therefore of great interest that a
number of the therapeutic and pretherapeutic studies described in this
volume are based on exploitation of facets of the natural history of
metastasis that account for some aspects of inefficiency.

REFERENCES

1. Fidler IJ and Kripke ML. Science 197:893-895, 1977.
2. Weiss L. Am. J. Pathol. 97:601-608, 1979.
3. Fidler IJ. Nature (London) 242:148-149, 1973.
4. Fidler IJ, Gersten DM and Budmen MB. Cancer Res. 36:3160-3165, 1976.
5. Hart IR. Am. J. Pathol. 97:587-600, 1979.
6. Weiss L, Mayhew E, Rapp DG and Holmes JC. Br. J. Cancer 45:44-53, 1982.

7. Chambers AF, Hill RP and Ling V. Cancer Res. 41:1368-1372, 1981.
8. Williams JC, Gusterson BA and Coombes RC. Br. J. Cancer 45:588-597, 1982.
9. Foulds L. Neoplastic Development, Academic Press, London, Vol. 1, 1969.
10. Cifone MA and Fidler IJ. Proc. Natl. Acad. Sci. USA 77:6949-6952, 1981.
11. Harris, JF, Chambers AF, Hill RP and Ling V. Proc. Natl. Acad. Sci. USA 79:5547-5551, 1982.
12. Weiss L. In: Liver Metastasis (Eds. Weiss L and Gilbert HA), G.K. Hall, Boston, pp. 126-157, 1982.
13. Poste G, Doll J and Fidler IJ. Proc. Natl. Acad. Sci. USA 78:6226-6230, 1981.
14. Weiss L. Int. J. Cancer 25:385-392, 1980.
15. Weiss L. In: Tumor Invasion and Metastasis (Eds. Liotta LA and Hart IR), Martinus Nijhoff, The Hague, pp. 81-98, 1982.
16. Onuigbo WI. In: Bone Metastasis (Eds. Weiss L and Gilbert HA), G.K. Hall, Boston, pp. 1-10, 1981.
17. Viadana E, Bross IDJ and Pickren JW. In: Pulmonary Metastasis (Eds. Weiss L and Gilbert HA), G.K. Hall, Boston, pp. 142-167, 1978.
18. Fidler IJ and Hart IR. Science 217:998-1003, 1982.
19. Raz A, Hanna N and Fidler IJ. J. Natl. Cancer Inst. 66:183-189, 1981.
20. Talmadge JE and Fidler IJ. J. Natl. Cancer Inst. 69:975-980, 1982.
21. Giavazzi R, Allessandri G, Spreafico F, Garattini S and Mantovani A. Cancer (Philadelphia) 42:462-472, 1980.
22. Mantovani A, Giavazzi R, Allessandri G, Spreafico F and Garattini S. Eur. J. Cancer 17:71-76, 1981.
23. Weiss L, Holmes JC and Ward PM. Br. J. Cancer, in press, 1983.
24. Poste G and Grieg R. Invasion and Metastasis 2:137-176, 1982.
25. Weiss L. Pathobiol. Annu. 10:51-81, 1980.
26. Weiss L. Gann Monogr. Cancer Res. 20:292-315, 1977.
27. Weiss L and Ward PM. Cancer Metastasis Rev., in press, 1983.
28. Cole WH, McDonald GO, Roberts SS and Southwick HW. Dissemination of Cancer. Appleton-Century-Crofts, New York, 1961.
29. Willis RA. The Spread of Tumors in the Human Body. London, 1952.
30. Weiss L. In: Lymphatic System Metastasis (Eds. Weiss L, Gilbert HA and Ballon SC), G.K. Hall, Boston, pp. 1-40, 1980.
31. Weiss L. Exp. Cell Res. 33:277-288, 1964,
32. Weiss L and Holmes JC. In: Proteinases and Tumor Invasion (Eds. Strauli P, Barrett AJ and Baici A), Raven Press, New York, pp. 181-200, 1980.
33. Fisher ER, Palekav AS, Gregorio RM, Redmond C and Fisher B. Hum. Pathol. 9:523-530, 1978.
34. Weiss L. Int. J. Cancer 20:87-92, 1977.
35. Gullino PM. Prog. Exp. Tumor Res. 81:1-40, 1966.
36. Sylven B. Eur. J. Cancer 4:463-474, 1968.
37. Weiss L. Int. J. Cancer 22:196-203, 1978.
38. Pantalone RM and Page RC. Proc. Natl. Acad. Sci. USA 72:2091-2094, 1975.
39. Turner GA and Weiss L. Int. J. Cancer 26:247-254, 1980.
40. Weiss L. Exp. Cell Res. 37:540-551, 1965.
41. Neiders ME and Weiss L. Arch. Oral Biol. 18:499-504, 1973.
42. Weiss L. J. Theor. Biol. 2:236-250, 1962.
43. Dingemans KP and Roos E. In: Liver Metastasis (Eds. Weiss L and Gilbert HA), G.K. Hall, Boston, pp. 51-76, 1982.
44. Weiss L and Suh O. In: Basic Mechanisms and Clinical Treatments of Tumor Metastasis. Academic Press, New York, in press, 1983.
45. Folger R, Weiss L, Glaves D, Subjeck JR and Harlos JP. J. Cell Sci. 31:245-257, 1978.
46. Woolley DE, Roberts DR and Evanson JM. Nature (London) 261:325-327, 1976.

47. Biswas C. In: Tumor Invasion and Metastasis (Eds. Liotta L and Hart IR), Martinus Nijhoff, The Hague, pp. 413-425, 1982.
48. Recklies AD and Poole AR. In: Liver Metastasis (Eds. Weiss L and Gilbert HA), G.K. Hall, Boston, pp. 77-95, 1982.
49. Liotta LA and Hart IR. Tumor Invasion and Metastasis. Martinus Nijhoff, The Hague, 1982.
50. Turner GA and Weiss L. Invasion Metastasis, in press, 1983.
51. Wood S, Holyoke ED and Yardley JM. Proc. Can. Cancer Res. Conf. 4:167-223, 1961.
52. Wallace AC, Chew E-C and Jones DS. In: Lung Metastasis (Eds. Weiss L and Gilbert HA), G.K. Hall, Boston, pp. 26-42, 1978.
53. Sato H and Suzuki M. In: Fundamental Aspects of Metastasis (Ed. Weiss L), American Elsevier, New York, pp. 311-318, 1976.
54. Weiss L. Fed. Proc. Fed. Am. Soc. Exp. Biol. 30:1649-1657, 1971.
55. Weiss L and Harlos JP. In: Intercellular Communication (Ed. DeMello WC), Plenum Press, New York, pp. 33-59, 1977.
56. Weiss L, Nir S, Harlos JP and Subjeck JR. J. Theor. Biol. 51:439-454, 1975.
57. Dimitrov DS. Prog. Surf. Sci., in press, 1983.
58. Liotta LA, Kleinerman J and Saidel GM. Cancer Res. 36:889-894, 1976.
59. Glaves D and Weiss L. In: The Handbook of Cancer Immunology (Ed. Waters H), Garland STPM Press, New York, Vol. 6, pp. 1-31, 1981.
60. Gasic GJ, Gasic TB, Galanti N, Johnson T and Murphy S. Int. J. Cancer 11:704-718, 1973.
61. Chew E-C and Wallace AC. Cancer Res. 36:1904-1909, 1976.
62. Revesz L. Nature (London) 178:1391-1392, 1956.
63. Hewitt HB, Blake ER and Porter EH. Br. J. Cancer 28:123-135, 1973.
64. Peters LJ and Hewitt HB. Br. J. Cancer 29:279-291, 1974.
65. Weiss L. In: Pulmonary Metastasis (Eds. Weiss L and Gilbert HA), G.K. Hall, Boston, pp. 5-25, 1978.
66. Weiss L, Glaves D and Waite DA. Int. J. Cancer 13:850-862, 1974.
67. Weiss L and Glaves D. Int. J. Cancer 18:774-777, 1976.
68. Rudenstam CM. Acta Chir. Scand. Suppl. 391:1-83, 1968.
69. Kawaguchi T and Nakamura K. Gann 68:65-71, 1977.
70. Warren BA. In: Brain Metastasis (Eds. Weiss L, Gilbert HA and Posner JB), G.K. Hall, Boston, pp. 81-99, 1980.
71. Zeidman I. Cytologia 9:136-138, 1965.
72. Weiss L, Holmes J and Crispe IN. Br. J. Cancer 40:483-488, 1979.
73. Weiss L and Ward PM. Cancer Res. 42:1898-1903, 1982.
74. Weiss L. Med. Biol. 56:398-402, 1978.
75. Weiss L. and Glaves D. Ann. N.Y. Acad. Sci., in press, 1983.
76. Glaves D. Int. J. Cancer 26:115-122, 1981.
77. Glaves D and Weiss L. Int. J. Cancer 27:475-479, 1981.
78. Turner GA and Weiss L. Cancer Res. 41:2576-2580, 1981.
79. Folkman J. Adv. Cancer Res. 19:331-358, 1974.

CHAPTER 3. OVERVIEW ON BLOOD COAGULATION PROTEINS

JOYCE E. GARDINER AND JOHN H. GRIFFIN

I. INTRODUCTION

Coagulation of blood results from the conversion of a soluble plasma protein, fibrinogen, into fibrin monomers which undergo spontaneous polymerization to form an isoluble network of fibers. Under normal circumstances clotting is brought about by a sequence of reactions which can be likened to a cascade, in which the activation of one coagulation factor triggers a change in the next coagulation factor to its active form (Figure 1). This zymogen-to-enzyme conversion sequence allows for linear and nonlinear amplification as well as feedback regulation of the system. Blood platelets participate in coagulation by providing phospholipid or lipoprotein surfaces upon which the coagulation proteins are brought into contact with one another. Mammalian blood also contains an enzyme system, termed the fibrinolytic enzyme system, which is capable of dissolving blood clots. This chapter will provide a summary of these basic features of the blood coagulation system.

II. STRUCTURAL CHARACTERISTICS OF SERINE PROTEINASES

Most of the plasma proteins participating in blood coagulation have been isolated and characterized. Table 1 lists these proteins together with their Roman numeral designations and common names. A number of serine proteinases are found in the clotting cascade, namely factors IIa, VIIa, IXa, Xa, XIa, XIIa and activated protein C. These enzymes, by definition, contain a unique, unusually reactive serine side chain which forms a transient covalent linkage with the carbonyl carbon atom in the susceptible peptide or ester bond of substrates (1). An important feature of the serine proteinases is the "charge relay" system in the active site of the enzyme. This system was first recognized by Blow et al. (2) in chymotrypsin. According to their proposal, Ser-195, His-57 and Asp-102 are linked in a hydrogen bond network and the hydroxyl oxygen atom of Ser-195 participates as a strong nucleophile during catalysis.

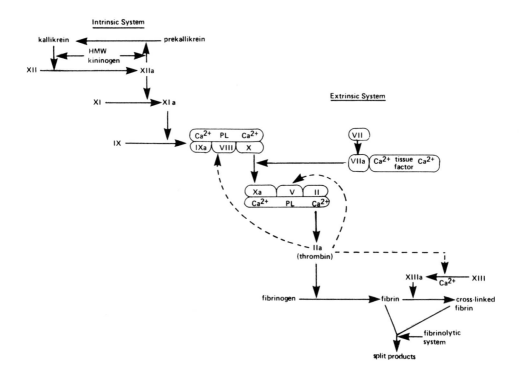

FIGURE 1. A Simplified Scheme of the Coagulation Sequences. For the sake of simplicity important control systems such as feedback mechanisms and humoral inhibitors (for example, antithrombin III) are omitted. The "extrinsic" and "intrinsic" systems are separated for descriptive purposes and their many possible points of interaction are omitted. The dashed lines indicate some procoagulant activities of thrombin considered to be the most important at the present time (127).

The reaction sequence shown in Figure 2 is generally applicable to the serine proteinases which participate in blood coagulation. The amino acid sequence surrounding the active site serine residue of these proteinases shows a very high degree of sequence homology with the pancreatic serine proteinases, tryspin, chymotrypsin and elastase (3), suggesting that the various blood coagulation enzymes hydrolyze their respective peptide or ester substrates by way of tetrahedral and acyl intermediates in the same way as the pancreatic serine proteinases.

Table 1. The Blood Coagulation Factors and Some of their Properties.

Roman Numeral Designation	Common Synonyms	Functions
I	Fibrinogen	Final Substrate
II	Prothrombin	Serine Proteinase
III	Thromboplastin, Tissue Factor	Cofactor
IV	Calcium ions	
V	Proaccelerin	Cofactor
VII	Proconvertin	Serine Proteinase
VIII	Antihemophilic Factor	Cofactor
IX	Christmas Factor	Serine Proteinase
X	Stuart-Prower Factor	Serine Proteinase
XI	Plasma Thromboplastin antecedent	Serine Proteinase
XII	Hagemen Factor	Serine Proteinase
XIII	Fibrin-stabilizing Factor	Transamidase
	Plasma Prekallikrein (Fletcher Factor)	Serine Proteinase
	High MW Kininogen	Cofactor

Activation of the zymogen forms of serine proteinases is brought about by a limited protelysis which results in the generation of a new amino terminal amino acid, e.g., isoleucine-16 in the case of chymotrypsin (4). The new terminal α-amino group is then able to form an ion pair with the carboxyl group of an aspartic acid adjacent to the active serine. This leads to a conformational change in the protein and a marked increase in its enzymatic activity (3,5). Proteolytic activation of the coagulation zymogens may occur with no decrease in molecular weight as in the case of factor VII (6-9), factor XI (10,11) and factor XII (12). In comparison, the activation of prothrombin leads to a 50% decrease in its molecular weight (13-16).

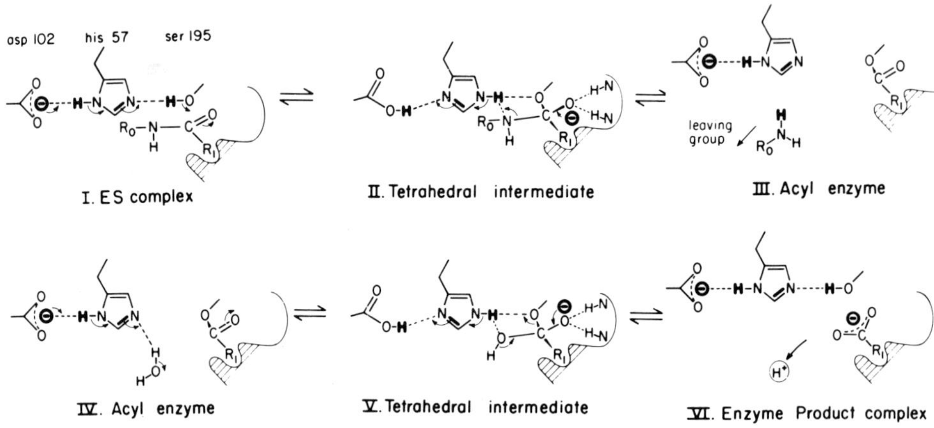

FIGURE 2. A Mechanism for Serine Proteinase Hydrolysis of Peptides or Amides (124).

The similarities in structure of the coagulation zymogens are illustrated in Figure 3 (17). The active site serine, histidine and aspartate residues are all located in polypeptide chains derived from the carboxyl-terminal end of the zymogens and are approximately 250 amino acid residues long. The amino-terminal portions of the zymogens are retained after activation by all the proteins except prothrombin. These amino-terminal regions of the clotting zymogens possess the surface-binding properties which make possible the 10,000 to 100,000-fold amplification of the proteolytic activations.

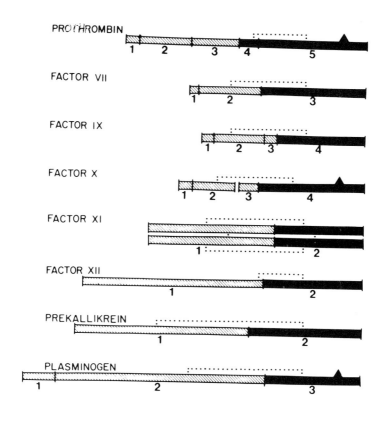

FIGURE 3. Schematic Structures for the Coagulation Proteinase Zymogens (17). Each proteinase zymogen may be divided into a carboxyl terminal region of approximately 250 residues which contains the active site residues (shown in solid black) and an amino-terminal region (shown by the cross-hatched zone) which varies from approximately 150 residues to 582 residues. The presence of such large, amino-terminal regions most clearly distinguishes the coagulation proteinase zymogens from the related pancreatic serine proteinase zymogens. In the four vitamin K-dependent proteins (prothrombin and Factors VII, IX and X), the amino-terminal ends are highly homologous and contains Gla residues (shown by the clear zones and numbered 1 on the diagrams). Factor XI appears to be exceptional among the proteinase zymogens in that it is apparently "dimeric" with two disulfide-linked chains each of which fits the general model independently. The dotted line represents disulfide bonding.

III. THE ROLE OF VITAMIN K

Vitamin K was discovered in 1929 when Dam noticed that chicks developed bleeding problems when fed on diets extracted with polar solvents (18-22). This led to the discovery of a new lipid-soluble vitamin named vitamin K. Dam and coworkers also noted that the defect in coagulation was due to a decrease in the amount of prothrombin in plasma of the deficient chicks. Similar effects in humans and cows were then reported for reduced plasma levels of factor VII, factor IX and factor X following the administration of vitamin-K antagonists such as dicoumarol (22-26). More recently three additional vitamin K-dependent plasma proteins have been isolated, namely protein C, protein S and protein Z (27-29). Protein C, when activated by thrombin, has potent anticoagulant and profibrinolytic properties (30-35) and it has been suggested that protein S may function as a cofactor of activated protein C (36,37).

A number of proposals have been advanced over the years for the mechanism of action of vitamin K. For example, several investigators reported the presence of an inactive prothrombin molecule in humans and cows treated with vitamin K antagonists (38-43). Although the abnormal prothrombin had a molecular weight and amino acid composition which was essentially identical to normal prothrombin, the abnormal prothrombin did not bind to $BaSO_4$ and it also had an abnormality in its Ca^{++}-dependent electrophoretic mobility. These data indicated that prothrombin was synthesized in humans and cows in the absence of vitamin K but it had little biological activity. Furthermore, the lack of biological activity was suggested to be related to the inability of the abnormal protein to bind Ca^{++}.

A major advance in defining the role of vitamin K came with the discovery of γ-carboxyglutamic acid by Stenflo and coworkers in 1974 (45). This new amino acid was initially shown to be present in positions 7 and 8 of prothrombin. The γ-carboxyglutamic acid content has now been determined for prothrombin, factor IX, factor X, protein C and protein S from human and bovine plasma. The γ-carboxyglutamic acid has been shown to occur in nearly the same ten to twelve positions in the amino terminal portions of all of these proteins. A relationship between Ca^{++} binding by normal prothrombin and the conversion of prothrombin to thrombin was suggested from the demonstration that the portion of the prothrombin molecule that is responsible for the Ca^{++}-mediated binding of prothrombin to phospholipids was the same region of the prothrombin molecule that contained the γ-carboxyglutamic acid residues (45). The anticoagulant effect of the vitamin K antagonists was thus deduced to be due to the inability of prothrombin which lacks γ-carboxyglutamic acid residues to bind to phospholipid bilayers or cell membranes. This proposal was shown to be correct when it was demonstrated that abnormal or descarboxyprothrombin does not bind to phospholipids. Thus its activation is not accelerated by phospholipids as is that of normal prothrombin (46). The same requirement for Ca^{++}-mediated binding of factor Xa to phospholipid for phospholipid acceleration of prothrombin activation has been shown (47).

Vitamin K is necessary to bring about the final step in the biosynthesis of factors II, VII, IX and X. The normal mechanism of protein synthesis in the liver produces individual precursor proteins for each of these factors and a vitamin K-dependent mechanism converts glutamic acid groups in these proteins to γ-carboxyglutamic acid residues. Oral anticoagulants like dicoumarol interfere with this carboxylation and reduce the level of γ-carboxylation of coagulation factors II, VII, IX and X.

IV. FIBRINOGEN

The central event in the coagulation of vertebrate blood is the thrombin catalyzed conversion of fibrinogen into fibrin. The vertebrate fibrinogen molecule is unusual in that it has properties characteristic of both a globular and a fibrous protein. The molecule consists of three pairs of disulfide-linked polypeptide chains designated $(A\alpha)_2$, $(B\beta)_2$ and γ_2. A and B represent the two fibrinopeptides cleaved from fibrinogen in the transformation of soluble fibrinogen into the spontaneously polymerizing fibrin polymer (48,49). Covalent structural changes resulting from thrombin proteolysis reduce the molecular mass by a very small amount, approximately 6,000 out of 340,000 daltons, but expose the polymerization sites of the fibrin monomer and permit gelation to occur (49). The fibrin gel can be strengthened by the introduction of covalent bonds between neighboring molecules in the polymer. This stabilization is brought about by an enzyme, factor XIIIa. The zymogen of this enzyme, factor XIII, is present in plasma and also in mammalian platelets. Factor XIII has a molecular weight of 320,000 (50) and is composed of four noncovalently associated subunits a_2 b_2 (51). The platelet enzyme is smaller and is composed of only two a subunits (52). In both cases, activation of factor XIII is initiated by the thrombin-catalyzed removal of a peptide from the amino terminus of the a chains which appear to be identical in the plasma and platelet forms of this enzyme. The active enzyme is a Ca^{++}-dependent, sulfhydryl type transglutaminase (53). During physiological fibrin formation factor XIIIa joins together neighboring molecules in the fibrin polymer by the formation of peptide bonds between the side chains of lysine and glutamine residues, leading to the formation of γ-glutamyl-lysine cross-links (54). Covalently stabilized fibrin is mechanically stronger than non-cross-linked fibrin (55) and also is possibly more resistant to fibrinolysis.

V. REGULATION OF BLOOD COAGUALTION

Two important pathways exist for the formation of fibrin and these have been designated the intrinsic and the extrinsic coagulation pathways.

A. The Intrinsic Pathway

The intrinsic pathway is initiated by the contact of blood with a "foreign" surface. The details of the sequence have been modified as new information was obtained but the overall scheme has remained unaltered for the past decade. The intrinsic pathway of coagulation as it is known today is illustrated in Figure 1. The term "intrinsic" is used because the factors involved in this pathway are found intrinsically in blood.

Exposure of human plasma to a variety of negatively-charged surfaces such as glass, celite, sulfatides or collagen results in the activation of the zymogen, factor XII, to the serine proteinase, factor XIIa (56). Factor XIIa then converts the zymogen prekallikrein to kallikrein and factor XI to factor XIa by limited proteolysis (57,58). These reactions are greatly enhanced by a plasma protein, high molecular weight (HMW) kininogen, which appears to act as a cofactor (59,60). The small quantities of the serine proteinase kallikrein which are formed in this fashion then serve to convert more factor XII to factor XIIa. This reaction is also enhanced by HMW-kininogen which constitutes a positive feedback mechanism. Furthermore, factor XIIa formed by kallikrein activation will then activate more prekallikrein to kallikrein in the presence of HMW-kininogen (59). HMW-kininogen serves not only as a precursor to kinins, but also promotes the binding of factor XI and prekallikrein to negative surfaces where they are activated by surface-bound factor XIIa (61).

Factor XIa is then able to activate the factor IX zymogen, a vitamin K-dependent glycoprotein, which forms a complex with the cofactor factor VIII, phospholipids and Ca^{++} ions before converting factor X to factor Xa (62). Factor Xa complexes with the cofactors, factor Va, calcium and phospholipids and activates prothrombin to thrombin (63).

Although considerable progress has been made during the past decade in elucidating the molecular events involved in the initiation of the intrinsic pathway, there are many questions which remain unanswered. Perhaps the most obvious deficit is the lack of knowledge of the normal function of this pathway or the identifcation of the surface which is required for its initial activation. Attention has recently been directed towards endothelial cells as potential activators of the contact system and the kinin-forming pathway since homogenates of cultured rabbit endothelial cells contain enzyme activity capable of cleaving rabbit factor XII (64). The endothelial activation is associated with membrane fragments, suggesting that it may remain localized when endothelial cells are injured (56). Certain collagen preparations can also provide a surface which is capable of initiating the intrinsic pathway (65,66). Therefore it has been proposed that in an area of damaged endothelium structural elements of the subendothelium may be available to localize factor XII and HMW-kininogen, with endothelial cells then providing proteinases for contact activation.

Patients deficient in factor XII, HMW-kininogen or prekallikrein rarely present with a bleeding diathesis. Patients with factor XI deficiency do present with variable bleeding problems and it has been speculated that platelet-dependent activation of factor XI initiates a physiologically important pathway.

B. The Extrinsic Pathway

Clot formation via the extrinsic system requires an extrinsic
factor, tissue factor, from outside the blood plasma for its
initiation. This may be provided by injury to the plasma membranes of
endothelial cells allowing the release of membrane-bound tissue factor
into the circulation where it is able to recognize and activate factor
VII. Tissue factor may also be derived from white cells and may
appear in response to both immunological and nonimmunological stimuli
(e.g., endotoxin). Elevated levels of tissue factor are notably
present in patients with promyelocytic leukemia.

Factor VIIa enzymatically converts factor X to its active form,
factor Xa, by cleaving a specific arginyl-isoleucine peptide bond in
the heavy chain of factor X (67). In addition to initiating a
preliminary attack on prothrombin, factor Xa can also amplify the
initial response further by activating factor VII in a positive
feedback mechanism designed to increase rapidly the overall level of
factor VIIa.

C. The Relationship between the Intrinsic and Extrinsic Pathways

In the widely recognized formulation of the coagulation pathways,
factor X is the converging point of both the extrinsic and intrinsic
systems and all subsequent reactions involving factor V, prothrombin
and fibrinogen are common to both pathways. However, evidence has
accumulated for more complicated interrelationships between the two
pathways. Biggs and Nossel (68) observed that diluted tissue factor
does not generate normal amounts of thrombin in factor VIII or factor
IX deficient plasmas. Josso and Prou-Wartelle (69) confirmed these
results and reported that factor VIII was essential for the
procoagulant activity of diluted thromboplastin. Osterud and Rapaport
(70) showed that a mixture of partially purified factor VIII and
tissue factor could activate purified factor IX and Zur et al. (71)
described similar findings using purified bovine clotting factors.
Thus, factor VII plus tissue factor can activate factor IX. Recently,
Marlar et al. (72) studied the interrelationships between the
intrinsic and extrinsic coagulation pathways by evaluating factor X
activation in normal and various deficient human plasmas when clotting
was triggered by dilute rabbit or human thromboplastin. They reported
that at high concentrations of tissue factor the rate of factor X
activation was similar in normal plasma and factor IX and factor VIII
deficient plasmas. However, at low concentrations of tissue factor,
the rate and extent of factor X activation was proportionately lower
in factor VIII and factor IX deficient plasmas as compared to normal
plasma. Reconstitution of factor VIII or factor IX deficient plasmas
with their respective missing proteins restored normal factor X
activation. These results suggest that there is an "alternative"
extrinsic pathway in human blood coagulation involving factors VIII
and IX.

VI. INHIBITORS OF BLOOD COAGULATION

Protein C is a vitamin K-dependent serine proteinase zymogen (23,73) that is activated by thrombin (74). This reaction is catalyzed by an endothelial cell surface cofactor, thrombomodulin (75). Activated protein C is highly anticoagulant in vitro because it inactivates factors V and VIII in plasma (76). The recent discovery of protein C deficiency associated with familial thromboembolic disease indicates that this protein may be a physiologically important inhibitor of blood coagulation (77,78). Human plasma contains several well-characterized proteinase inhibitors which form stoichiometric complexes with proteinases.

Inherited deficiencies of antithrombin III are associated with thromboembolic disease (79,80). Antithrombin III is most probably the main physiological inhibitor of thrombin and factor Xa (81). Its inhibitory effects on factor IXa, factor XIa and factor XIIa have also been demonstrated.

Recently a second heparin-dependent inhibitor of thrombin, named heparin cofactor II, has been isolated from human plasma (82). Tollefson and Blank (82) demonstrated that at relatively high heparin concentrations in vitro heparin cofactor II reacts with thrombin more rapidly than does antithrombin III. Dermatan sulfate also stimulates the inhibition of thrombin by heparin cofactor II but not by antithrombin III.

Plasma contains several other proteinase inhibitors of the blood coagulation factors. The glycoprotein, α_2-macroglobulin, forms complexes with plasmin and thrombin (83). Analysis of the thrombin-inhibiting activity of plasma has indicated that antithrombin III accounts for about 75% and α_2-macroglobulin for about 25% inhibition (84,85). $\overline{C1}$ inactivator, a glycoprotein with a molecular weight of 104,000 inhibits $\overline{C1}$, plasma kallikrein, factor XIIa and factor XIa (86). Alpha$_1$-antitrypsin does not seem to play a role in the inhibition of thrombin under physiological conditions (87), but has been shown to inhibit factor XIa (88).

VII. ROLE OF PLATELETS IN BLOOD COAGULATION

In 1972 Walsh (89) proposed the hypothesis that platelets play a crucial role in all phases of the intrinsic blood coagulation pathway. The platelet membrane carries specific receptors for several coagulation factors and both specific and non-specific adsorption of factors to the platelet surface may generate high local concentrations of clotting factors as well as protect them from coagulation inhibitors. Thrombin formed by the coagulation cascade may activate platelets to cause release of platelet activators such as ADP and promote further thrombin generation.

Phospholipids have been shown to substitute for platelets in several coagulation reactions. These include the formation of thrombin from prothrombin and factors Xa and Va in the presence of Ca^{++} (90) as well as in the activation of factor X by factors IXa and

VIII in the presence of Ca^{++} (91). The passive coagulant property of platelets which stimulates prothrombin activation has been termed platelet factor 3. This activity is released following damage to the platelet membrane and becomes available when platelets adhere together at a site of injury (92,93).

There are several proteins present in the α-granules of platelets which have heparin-neutralizing activities. These proteins include platelet factor 4 , low affinity platelet factor 4 and β-thromboglobulin. It has been suggested that the role of these proteins is to control hemostasis through removal of endogenous heparin. While their physiological functions are not known, it has been shown that increased levels of antigenic activity appear in plasmas of patients with various pathological conditions (94).

A number of coagulation proteins referred to as the platelet forms of these proteins cannot be removed from platelet suspensions even after extensive washing. Platelet fibrinogen is localized in the α-granules (95). Factor V activity is also present within the platelet α-granules (96) and this activity has been reported to be released from bovine platelets in the activated form (97). von Willebrand factor (factor VIII-related antigen) is present in the α-granules and is released upon platelet stimulation (98). Platelet cytoplasm contains a form of factor XIII which differs from the plasma form in consisting of a dimer of enzymatically active α-chains and in lacking the β-chains present in the plasma form (99). Factor XI-like activity (100) and antigen (101) have been reported to be firmly attached to the platelet membrane although this has been controversial (102). Recently the presence of HMW-kininogen antigen in platelets has been reported (103).

Although the physiological significance of the platelet-associated coagulation factors is not clear, platelets bind prothrombinase components and greatly accelerate prothrombin activation (90). Factor V released from platelets or taken up from plasma may serve, at least in part, as the factor Xa receptor on platelets (104,105). There is evidence to suggest that platelets participate in the initiation of intrinsic coagulation. Walsh (106) initially suggested that nonaggregated stimulated platelets enhance the activation of factor XII and factor XI in the absence of Ca^{++}, and recent studies using purified proteins and platelets have confirmed this (107). Moreover, stimulated platelets exhibit high affinity receptors for factor XI although the functional signficance of this is not known (108).

VIII. FIBRINOLYSIS

The fibrinolytic enzyme system of blood is capable of dissolving blood clots. Liquefaction of the fibrin clot is caused by the splitting of only a few peptide bonds and this specific splitting is effected by the blood serine proteinase, plasmin, which is formed by activation of the zymogen, plasminogen.

As illustrated in Figure 4, plasminogen activation may occur by three different pathways: an intrinsic pathway in which all compoents involved are present in precursor form in the blood, an extrinsic pathway in which the activator originates from tissues or from the vessel wall and is released into the blood by certain stimuli or trauma and an exogenous pathway in which an activating substance like streptokinase participates. Streptokinase and urokinase are two plasminogen activators currently used therapeutically for thromboembolic disorders, and tissue-type plasminogen activator is in the earliest stages of clinical trials. All plasminogen activators studied so far exert their action through hydrolysis of the Arg-560-Val-561 bond in plasminogen.

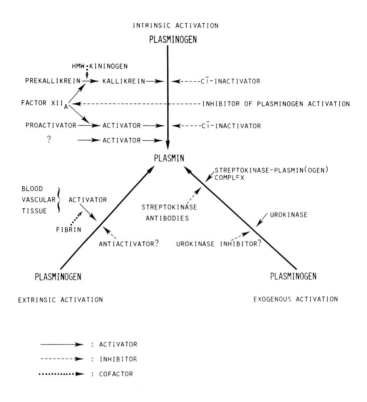

FIGURE 4. Schematic Representation of Activation Pathways of Plasminogen (111).

Intrinsic activation of plasminogen may occur by one or more pathways involving factor XII, prekallikrein, HMW-kininogen and possibly other components. The exact mechanism of this activation as well as its biological role is presently unknown. The present knowledge on the pathways of intrinsic fibrinolysis has been reviewed elsewhere (109,110).

Urokinase is the most extensively studied plasminogen activator of human origin. However, the principal endogenous activator of plasminogen in blood, tissue activator (111), is presumed to be present in the endothelium of blood vessels and is released "on demand" by exercise, hypercoagulability, pharmacological or other stimuli (112). In contrast to urokinase, tissue activator is adsorbed onto fibrin clots (113) and, in a purified system, plasmin formation is greatly enhanced by the presence of fibrin (111,114,115).

It has been postulated that inhibitors of extrinsic plasminogen activators are present in the plasma in the form of a complex with plasminogen activators, a complex which dissociates in the presence of fibrin (116). The formation of such a reversible activator-inhibitor complex has been invoked to explain the rapid lysis of fibrin in plasma and the resistance of fibrinogen to degradation by plasmin (117). However, the most likely explanation for the enhancing effect of fibrin on plasminogen activation may involve the specific adsorption of both activator and plasminogen to its surface thereby facilitating activation (114,115,118). Evidence for the existence of a specific inhibitor of extrinsic plasminogen activators in plasma in the form of a reversible complex is presently preliminary. There is evidence that a significant amount of extrinsic plasminogen activator released in the blood is cleared in vivo by mechanisms other than neutralization by plasma inhibitors (119,120).

Human plasma contains a fast-acting and physiologically important inhibitor of plasmin called α_2-antiplasmin (121-123). In plasma, plasmin is very rapidly neutralized by α_2-antiplasmin and this inhibitor is responsible for all of the fast acting plasmin-neutralizing activity of plasma. An inherited deficiency of α_2-antiplasmin is associated with a notable bleeding diathesis characterized by delayed bleeding that is probably due to untimely fibrinolysis (124-126).

REFERENCES

1. Matthews DA, Alden RA, Birktoft JJ, Freer ST and Kraut J. J. Biol. Chem. 250:7120-7126, 1975.
2. Blow DM, Birktoft JJ and Hartley BS. Nature (London) 221:337-340, 1969.
3. Davie EW, Fujikawa K, Kurachi K and Kisiel W. Methods Enzymol. 48:227-318, 1979.
4. Stroud RM, Kreger M, Koeppe RE, Kossiakoff AA and Chambers JL. In: Proteases and Biological Control (Eds. Reich E, Rifkin DB and Shaw E), Cold Spring Harbor Laboratory, New York, pp. 13-32, 1975.
5. Stroud RM. Sci. Am. 231:74-88, 1974.

6. Radcliffe R and Nemerson Y. J. Biol. Chem. 251:4797-4802, 1976.
7. Radcliffe R and Nemerson Y. J. Biol. Chem. 250:388-395, 1975.
8. Silverberg SA, Ostapchuk P and Nemerson Y. Blood 48:976, 1976.
9. Kisiel W, Fujikawa K and Davie EW. Biochemistry 16:4189-4194, 1977.
10. Bouma B and Griffin JH. J. Biol. Chem. 252:6432-6437, 1977.
11. Kurachi K and Davie EW. Biochemistry 16:5831-5839, 1977.
12. Revak SD, Cochrane CG and Griffin JH. J. Clin. Invest. 59:1167-1175, 1977.
13. Suttie JW and Jackson CM. Physiol. Rev. 57:1-70, 1977.
14. Magnusson S, Sottrup-Jensen L, Petersen TE and Claeys H. In: Prothrombin and Related Coagulation Factors (Eds. Hemker HC and Veltkamp JJ), Leiden University Press, Leiden, pp. 25-46, 1975.
15. Jackson CM. Br. J. Haematol. 39:1-8, 1978.
16. Seegers WH, Hassouna HI, Hewett-Emmett D, Walz DA and Andary TJ. Semin. Thromb. Hemostasis, pp. 211-283, 1975.
17. Jackson CM and Nemerson Y. Annu. Rev. Biochem. 49:765-781, 1980.
18. Dam H. Biochem. Z. 215:468, 1929.
19. Dam H. Biochem. Z. 215:475, 1929.
20. Dam H. Biochem. Z. 220:158, 1930.
21. Dam H. Nature (London) 135:652, 1935.
22. Dam H. Biochem. J. 29:1273, 1935.
23. Owen CA, Jr., Magath TB and Bollman JL. Am. J. Physiol. 166:1-11, 1951.
24. Koller F, Loeliger A and Duckert F. Acta Haematol. 6:1-18, 1951.
25. Aggeler PM, White SG, Glendering MB, Page EW, Leake TB and Bates G. Proc. Soc. Exp. Biol. Med. 79:692-694, 1952.
26. Biggs R, Douglas AS, Macfarlane RG, Dacie JV, Pitney WR, Merskey C and O'Brien JR. Br. Med. J. 2:1378-1382, 1952.
27. Hougie C, Barrow EM and Graham JB. J. Clin. Invest. 36:485-496, 1957.
28. Stenflo J. J. Biol. Chem. 251:355-363, 1976.
29. DiScipio RG, Hermodson MA, Yates SG and Davie EW. Biochemistry 16:698-706, 1977.
30. Prowse CV and Esnouf MP. Biochem. Soc. Trans. 5:255-256, 1977.
31. Marciniak E. J. Lab. Clin. Med. 79:924-934, 1972.
32. Marciniak E. Science 170:452, 1970.
33. Kisiel W, Canfield WM, Ericsson LH and Davie EW. Biochemistry 16:5824-5831, 1979.
34. Kisiel W. J. Clin. Invest. 64:761-769, 1979.
35. Seegers WH, McCoy LE, Groben HD, Sakuragawa N and Agrawal BL. Thromb. Res. 1:443-460, 1972.
36. Esmon CT, Comp PC and Walker FJ. In: Vitamin K Metabolism and Vitamin K-Dependent Proteins (Ed. Suttie JW), University Park Press, pp. 72-83, 1980.
37. Walker FJ. J. Biol. Chem. 255:5521-5524, 1980.
38. Walker FJ. J. Biol. Chem. 256:11128-11131, 1981.
39. Hemker HC, Veltkamp JJ, Hensen A and Loeliger EA. Nature (London) 200:589-590, 1963.
40. Ganrot PO and Nilehn JE. Scand. J. Clin. Lab. Invest. 22:23-28, 1968.
41. Stenflo J. Acta Chem. Scand. 24:3762-3763, 1970.
42. Nelsestuen GL and Suttie JW. J. Biol. Chem. 247:8176-8182, 1972.
43. Reekers PP, Lindout MJ, Kop-Klaassen BHM and Hemker HC. Biochim. Biophys. Acta 317:559-562, 1973.
44. Suttie JW. In: Handbook of Lipid Research. Plenum Press, New York, 2:211-277, 1978.
45. Stenflo J, Fernlund P, Eagan W and Roepstorff P. Proc. Natl. Acad. Sci. USA 71:2730-2733, 1974.
46. Gitel SN, Owen WG, Esmon CT and Jackson CM. Proc. Natl. Acad. Sci. USA 70:1344-1348, 1973.

47. Esmon CT, Suttie JW and Jackson CM. J. Biol. Chem. 250:4095-4099, 1975.
48. Lindhout MH, Kop-Klaassen BHM and Hemker HC. Biochim. Biophys. Acta 533:342-345, 1978.
49. Doolittle RF. Horiz. Biochem. Biophys. 3:164-191, 1977.
50. Doolittle RF. In: The Plasma Proteins (Ed. Putnam FW), Academic Press, New York, 2:109-161, 1975.
51. Loewy AG, Dahlberg A, Dunathan D, Kreil R and Wolfinger HL, Jr. J. Biol. Chem. 236:2634-2643, 1961.
52. Schwartz ML, Pizzo SV, Hill RL and McKee PA. J. Biol. Chem. 248:1395-1407, 1973.
53. Bohn H, Haupt H and Kranz T. Blut 25:235-248, 1972.
54. Folk JE and Chung SI. Adv. Enzymol. Relat. Areas Mol. Biol. 38:109-191, 1973.
55. Folk JE and Finlayson JS. Adv. Protein Chem. 31:1-133, 1977.
56. Gerth C, Roberts WW and Ferry JD. Biophys. Chem. 2:208-217, 1974.
57. Griffin JH and Cochrane CG. Semin. Thromb. Hemostasis 5:254-273, 1979.
58. Bouma BN and Griffin JH. J. Biol. Chem. 252:6432-6437, 1977.
59. Bouma BN and Griffin JH. Thromb. Haemostasis 38:136, 1977.
60. Griffin JH and Cochrane CG. Proc. Natl. Acad. Sci. USA 73:2554-2558, 1976.
61. Meier HK, Webster ME, Mandle T, Colman RW and Kaplan AP. J. Clin. Invest. 60:18-31, 1977.
62. Revak SD, Cochrane CG, Bouma BN and Griffin JH. J. Exp. Med. 147:719-729, 1978.
63. Fujikawa K, Legaz ME, Kato H and Davie EW. Biochemistry 13:4508-4516, 1974.
64. Suttie JW and Jackson CM. Physiol. Rev. 57:1-70, 1977.
65. Wiggins RC, Loskutoff DJ, Cochrane CG, Griffin JH and Edgington TS. J. Clin. Invest. 65:197-206, 1980.
66. Niewiarowski S, Bankowski L and Fiedoreck T. Experientia 20:367, 1964.
67. Wilner GD, Nossel HL and Leroy EC. J. Clin. Invest. 47:2608-2615, 1968.
68. Biggs R and Nossel HL. Thromb. Diath. Haemorrh. 6:1-4, 1961.
69. Josso F and Prou-Wartelle O. Thromb. Diath. Haemorrh. 17:35-44, 1965.
70. Osterud B and Rapaport SI. Proc. Natl. Acad. Sci. USA 74:5250-5264, 1977.
71. Zur M, Shastri K and Nemerson Y. Blood 52:198, 1978.
72. Marlar RA, Kleiss AJ and Griffin JH. Blood 60:1353-1358, 1982.
73. Esmon CT, Stenflo J, Suttie JW and Jackson CM. J. Biol. Chem. 251:3052-3056, 1976.
74. Kisiel W, Ericsson LH and Davie EW. Biochemistry 15:4893-4900, 1976.
75. Esmon NL, Owen WG and Esmon CT. J. Biol. Chem. 257:859-864, 1982.
76. Marlar RA, Kleiss AJ and Griffin JH. Blood 59:1064-1072, 1982.
77. Griffin JH, Evatt B, Zimmerman TS, Kleiss AJ and Wideman C. J. Clin. Invest. 68:1370-1373, 1981.
78. Bertina RM, Broekmans AW, van der Linden IK and Mertens K. Thromb. Haemostasis 48:1-5, 1982.
79. Egeberg O. Thromb. Diath. Haemorrh. 13:516-530, 1965.
80. Marciniak E, Farley CH and DeSimone PA. Blood 43:219-231, 1974.
81. Abildgaard U. In: The Physiological Inhibitors of Coagulation and Fibrinolysis (Eds. Collen D, Wiman B and Verstraete M), Elsevier/North Holland, Amsterdam, pp. 19-29, 1979.
82. Tollefson DM and Blank MK. J. Clin. Invest. 68:589-596, 1981.
83. Abildgaard U. In: The Physiological Inhibitors of Blood Coagulation and Fibrinolysis (Eds. Collen D, Wiman B, Verstraete M), Elsevier/North Holland, Amsterdam, pp. 239-241, 1979.
84. Abildgaard U. Scand. J. Clin. Lab. Invest. 19:190-195, 1967.
85. Shapiro SS and Anderson DB. In: Chemistry and Biology of Thrombin (Eds. Lundbland RL, Fenton JW and Mann KG), Ann Arbor Science, Ann Arbor, MI, pp. 1361-1374, 1977.

86. Harpel PC. Methods Enzymol. 45:751-760, 1976.
87. Learned LA, Bloom JW and Hunter MJ. Thromb. Res. 8:99-109, 1976.
88. Heck LW and Kaplan AL. J. Exp. Med. 140:1615-1630, 1974.
89. Walsh PN. Br. J. Haematol. 22:205-217, 1972.
90. Milstone JH. Fed. Proc. Fed. Am. Soc. Exp. Biol. 23:742-748, 1964.
91. Schiffman S, Rapaport SI and Chong MMY. Proc. Soc. Exp. Biol. Med. 123:736-742, 1966.
92. Joist JH, Dolezel G, Lloyd JV, Kinlough-Rathbone RL and Mustard JF. J. Lab. Clin. Med. 84:474-482, 1974.
93. Mustard JF, Moore S, Packham MA and Kinlough-Rathbone RL. Prog. Biochem. Pharmacol. 14:312-325, 1977.
94. Brown TR, Ho-Li TTS and Walz DA. Clin. Chim. Acta 101:225-233, 1980.
95. James HL, Ganguly P and Jackson CW. Thromb. Haemostasis 38:939, 1977.
96. Chesney CM, Pifer D and Colman RW. Proc. Natl. Acad. Sci. USA 78:5180-5184, 1981.
97. Ittyerah TR, Rawala R and Colman RW. Thromb. Haemostasis 42:324, 1979.
98. Slot JW, Bouma BN, Montgomery R and Zimmerman TS. Thromb. Res. 13:871-881, 1978.
99. Schwartz ML, Pizzo V, Hill RL and McKee PA. J. Biol. Chem. 248:1395-1407, 1973.
100. Lipscomb MA and Walsh PN. J. Clin. Invest. 63:1006-1014, 1979.
101. Connelan JM, Bowden DS, Smith I and Castaldi PA. Thromb. Res. 17:225-238, 1980.
102. Schiffman S, Rimon A and Rapaport SI. Br. J. Haematol. 35:429-436, 1977.
103. Schmaier AH, Tuszynski GP, Walsh PN and Colman RW. Clin. Res. 28:323, 1980.
104. Miletich JP, Jackson CM and Majerus PW. J. Biol. Chem. 253:6908-6916, 1978.
105. Miletich JP, Majerus DW and Majerus PW. J. Clin. Invest. 62:824-831, 1978.
106. Walsh PN. Br. J. Haematol. 22:237-254, 1972.
107. Walsh PN and Griffin JH. Blood 57:106-118, 1981.
108. Greengard JS, Walsh PN and Griffin JH. Blood 58:194, 1981.
109. Ratnoff OD. In: Haemostasis: Biochemistry, Physiology and Pathology (Eds. Ogston D and Bennett B), John Wiley and Sons, London, pp. 25-35, 1977.
110. Ogston D and Bennett B. Br. Med. Bull. 34:107-112, 1978.
111. Collen D. Thromb. Haemostasis 43:77, 1980.
112. Todd AS. J. Pathol. Bacteriol. 78:281-283, 1959.
113. Thorsen S, Glas-Greenwalt P and Astrup T. Thromb. Diath. Haemorrh. 28:65-73, 1972.
114. Camiolo SM, Thorsen S and Astrup T. Proc. Soc. Exp. Biol. Med. 138:277-280, 1971.
115. Wallen P. In: Thrombosis and Urokinase (Eds. Paoletti R and Sherry S), Academic Press, London, pp. 91-102, 1977.
116. Gurewich V, Hyde E and Lipinski B. Blood 46:555-556, 1975.
117. Mullertz S. Ph.D. Thesis, Eijnar Munksgaard, Copenhagen, 1956.
118. Wiman B and Collen D. Nature (London) 272:549-550, 1978.
119. Fletcher AP, Biederman O, Moore D, Alkjersign N and Sherry S. J. Clin. Invest. 43:681-695, 1964.
120. Tytgat G, Collen D and DeVreker RA. Acta Haematol. 40:265-274, 1968.
121. Collen D. Eur. J. Biochem. 69:209-216, 1976.
122. Moroi M and Aoki N. J. Biol. Chem. 251:5956-5965, 1976.
123. Mullertz S and Clemmensen I. Biochem. J. 159:545-553, 1976.
124. Aoki N, Saito H, Kamiya T, Koie K, Sakata Y and Masarami K. J. Clin. Invest. 63:877-884, 1979.
125. Kluft C, Vellenga E and Brommer EJP. Lancet 2:206, 1979.

126. Miles LA, Plow EF, Donnelly KJ, Hougie C and Griffin JH.   Blood $\underline{59}$:1240–1251, 1982.

127. Bloom A.L. $\underline{In}$:   Haemostasis and Thrombosis (Eds. Bloom AL and Thomas DP), Churchill Livingstone, Edinburgh, pp. 321–370, 1981.

CHAPTER 4. THE MICROINJURY HYPOTHESIS AND METASTASIS

BRUCE A. WARREN

I. THE SILENT SECTOR OF THE METASTATIC CASCADE

Metastatic deposits are, of course, a major problem in the treatment of the patient with malignant disease. The known biological nature, frequency and growth vary enormously depending upon the specific type of tumor under consideration. As the biology of specific tumors is studied in detail there probably will be found to be major differences among tumors in factors operative in the metastatic cascade.

From the work of Folkman (1) and others it is evident that beyond a certain number of tumor cells successful growth in the extravascular site requires the elaboration of a tumor angiogenesis factor. The growth of a micrometastasis into a sizable metastatic deposit visible to the naked eye is dependent on a number of factors released by the tumor cells and the appropriate response by the host tissues. In delineating steps in the metastatic cascade it is useful to provide points which may later be keyed into clinical observations, during surgery or post mortem, of the spread of malignancies in man. Minimal visible metastatic deposit is one such point. I use the term micrometastasis here to mean a group of viable and multiplying tumor cells which is outside the vascular or lymphatic channels and in parenchymal tissue.

The step in the metastatic cascade which seems to be a necessary antecedent to blood borne metastatic deposits is the blood borne embolus (Figure 1). The characteristics of the blood borne tumor embolus which is successful in producing a viable micrometastasis are probably numerous and certainly greatly dependent on the type of host tissue in which the embolus arrests. The features of such an embolus include: 1. There must be a proportion of the population of cells present that are viable cells of the primary tumor. 2. Some of these must be capable of dividing. 3. The cells must show resistance to the defense mechanisms of the host. 4. The cells must be capable of extravasation from the vasculature.

Metastasis is a highly inefficient process (see Chapter 2). The presence of circulating tumor cells or tumor cell-platelet thrombi is not indicative of a poor prognosis. However, tumor cell emboli which may not themselves produce a micrometastatic lesion may still participate in the metastatic process. Showers of these emboli may result in vessel damage as discussed below.

FIGURE 1.   The Development of a Major Metastatic Deposit and the
Silent Sector of the Metastatic Cascade.

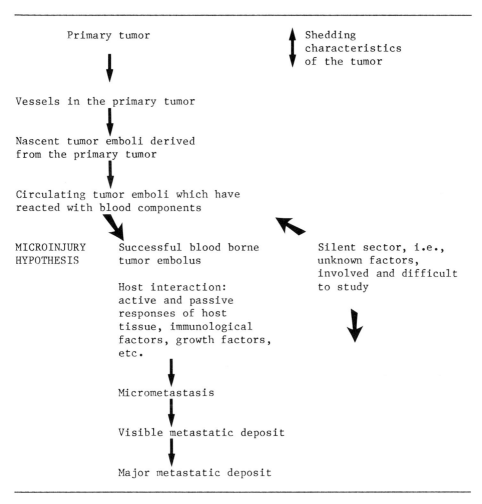

The term silent sector of the metastatic cascade is used to
indicate the difficulty in studying the factors involved in this part
of the overall process.   The shedding characteristics of tumors and
the number and type of tumor cell emboli released into the blood
vessels of the tumor and subsequently into circulation are amenable to
experimental design.   However, it has not been possible to design
experiments predictive of which emboli will successfully metastasize.
The microinjury hypothesis is an attempt to explain the silent sector
of the metastatic cascade.

II. THE MICROINJURY HYPOTHESIS

This hypothesis suggests that showers of tumor emboli discharged into a capillary system repeatedly plug the entrance to capillary beds. Anoxic degeneration of the endothelium of portions of the capillary network then ensues and such areas provide preferential adhesion sites for circulating tumor emboli (2). The variations in structure in different organs of the smallest units of the microcirculation (the microcirculatory modules) are vital determinants in the development of metastases within the framework of this hypothesis.

These are diverse local injuries to tissues which result in an increase in the number of metastases from circulating tumor cells at the site of injury (for review see 3,4) and our earlier work is highly supportive of the concept that an injured vessel wall allows a more ready attachment at that site for circulating tumor cells (4-7). It is apparent that the progress through the vessel wall and the arrest of tumor cells within the lumen depends upon the interaction of tumor cells and the endothelial lining (with its adjacent basement membrane) together with the intervention of constituents of the bloodstream.

How these multiple forms of injury are translated into increased metastatic deposits is not clear although the suggestion that endothelial injury is involved as a common factor has been made. Direct local injury in vitro to endothelial cells results in the exposure of bare basement membrane to which malignant cells will adhere (4 and Chapters 20 and 21). Indirect local injury in vivo, especially where the endothelium shows intracellular fenestrations, aids in attachment of tumor cells.

Tumor cells may pass without hindrance through the capillary bed if they are small and single or they may obstruct the capillary bed for a prolonged time if they are large. It is suggested that the site of obstruction would occur at the precapillary sphincter and that the site of microinjury due to hypoxia following stasis would be at the venular end of the capillary bed (Figure 2).

Occasionally, in vivo, in thin preparations one can see leukocytes blocking the entrances to capillary beds. In the case of tumor emboli this plugging may result in significant damage or microinjury to some sites of the capillary bed.

On unplugging, the blood flows again through the area and brings to the injured area fresh tumor emboli. These new emboli adhere to the site of the microinjury and because of the injury the damaged wall readily allows transit of tumor cells from the lumen to the extravascular position (see Chapter 21).

The shedding characteristics of the malignant tumor are important from the viewpoint both of the number of tumor cells shed, whether or not they are in clumps and the number of cells in each clump. The possible fates of the tumor cell emboli are transit, disintegration and finally blockage with penetration of the endothelium or impaction with attrition of the endothelium.

The microinjury hypothesis is consistent with present information regarding the release into the circulation of showers of tumor cells from primary or secondary deposits of malignant tumors. In the study by Kawaguchi and Nakamura (2) they found that:

1. "Island-forming" strains of tumors (AH-130, AH-272 and AH-7974) resulted in low cerebral passage rate and metastatic foci.

2. Single cell strains (Yoshida sarcoma, AH-7974F, AH-66F and AH-13) showed high rates of transcerebral passage and no metastases.

They concluded that the incidence of metastases corresponds directly to the frequency of arrested tumor cells in some models (2). The microinjury hypothesis was based on their work and the following pertinent observations by Sato and others (8) and Fujikura (9): a. transient circulating tumor cells in arterioles and metarterioles may result in functional disturbance of the microcirculation, and b. tissue injury can occur from tumor embolism (9). The microinjury hypothesis is summarized in Figure 2.

III. CONCLUSION

Arrest of the tumor embolus in the microcirculation following detachment from the primary tumor is closely connected with micrometastasis formation. Damage to tissues and to the microcirculation results in preferential location of metastases to those sites which are damaged when tumor cells are circulating. The microinjury hypothesis of metastasis formation is based on the following premise: showering of the microcirculatory bed by emboli impedes blood flow and results in regions of stagnation and hypoxia. Damage to endothelium occurs in such regions. Intermittent flow will bring viable tumor emboli to such sites. These sites favor adhesion of tumor emboli and easy passage through what remains of the vessel wall. Supporting in vitro and in vivo evidence for this is available and it can be shown that tumor cells can react in the way suggested by the microinjury hypothesis.

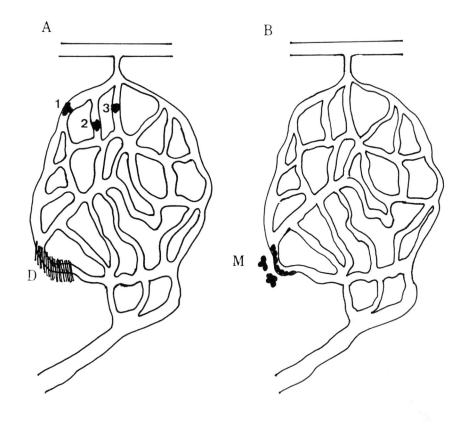

FIGURE 2. Diagramatic Representation of the Microinjury Hypotheis.
Both Figures 2A and B represent the same capillary bed at different
times. An arteriole is indicated at the top and a draining venule at
the bottom of the diagrams. Figure 2A illustrates the initial or
primary event during which circulating tumor cell emboli first come in
contact with the capillary bed and impact within several of the
vascular branches (1,2,3). This impaction results in hypoxic damage
(D) to capillaries distal to these sites. Eventually such emboli are
destroyed or disintegrate allowing blood flow through the capillary.
With circulation restored a fresh wave of tumor emboli enter. These
preferentially adhere to sites of damage such as the regions injured
by the earlier hypoxia. Arrest and adhesion occurs at these sites
with the possible subsequent progression to formation of a
micrometastasis (M).

REFERENCES

1. Folkman J. Cancer Res. $\underline{34}$:2109–2113, 1974.
2. Kawaguchi T and Nakamura K. Gann $\underline{68}$:65–71, 1977.
3. Rudenstam CM. Acta Chir. Scand. Suppl. 391, 1968.
4. Warren BA and Guldner FH. Angiologica $\underline{6}$:32–53, 1969.
5. Warren BA. J. Med. $\underline{4}$:150, 1973.
6. Warren BA. Z. Krebsforsch Klin. Onkol. $\underline{87}$:1–15, 1976.
7. Warren BA and Vales O. Br. J. Exp. Pathol. $\underline{53}$:301–313, 1972.
8. Sato H, Suzuki M and Kurokawa Y. Kosankinbyo Kenkyu Zasshi $\underline{19}$:2, 1967.
9. Fujikura T, Isomura S and Kawaai S. Nippon Byori Gakkai Kaishi $\underline{61}$:141, 1972.

CHAPTER 5. HEMOSTATIC ABNORMALITIES IN TUMOR-BEARING ANIMALS

MARIA BENEDETTA DONATI

I. INTRODUCTION

Although the first description of vascular thrombosis in cancer patients is more than one century old (1), several unresolved questions still remain on the involvement of the hemostatic system in malignancy. First, clinical studies have repeatedly demonstrated that malignant disease is associated with a high incidence of hemostatic disorders, ranging from isolated abnormalities of laboratory tests to vascular thrombosis, hemorrhage or overt disseminated intravascular coagulation (DIC). On the other hand, using different techniques, several investigators have shown the presence of fibrin deposits in and around tumors as a sign of the activation of clotting in malignancy (2-4).

The mechanisms by which malignant cells (or their products or secretions) interact with the various components of the hemostatic system - thus leading to fibrin deposition - is still a matter of debate. These mechanisms cannot be studied in patients due to a number of interfering factors. Indeed, the different stages of the disease, the different extents of metastatic involvement and the possible presence of concomitant infections in patients at the time of study make it very difficult to establish correlations and to investigate mechanisms under relatively standardized conditions. Moreover, chemotherapeutic agents, immunomodulators and radiotherapy have per se so many effects on the hemostatic system that it may be impossible to evaluate any cancer-associated disturbances of the hemostatic system in patients. The use of animal models is therefore particularly helpful in this context. In the present survey, we shall consider the relatively limited amount of information available on hemostatic changes in animal tumor models and some possible mechanisms responsible for these changes.

II. ANIMAL MODELS OF DISSEMINATION

The observation of blood coagulation changes after the injection of tumor cells into a healthy host has been considered an argument in favor of the involvement of platelets and fibrin during cancer cell spread. However, the choice of models for these studies needs careful consideration.

Indeed, most in vivo data on cancer cell interactions with the hemostatic system have been obtained in artificial models of tumor growth, such as hematogenous dissemination after intravenous injection of large numbers of cancer cells. In these conditions the pulmonary filter may be overloaded by cells which can form lung emboli rather than metastases; this type of dissemination process bypasses the first steps of local tumor invasion, such as development of cell proteolytic and/or migratory properties, detachment from the primary site and penetration through the vascular wall into the bloodstream. This is a condition of tumor spread which appears far removed from the dissemination process occurring in patients bearing solid tumors, particularly if one considers that tumor cells are injected abruptly into healthy recipients in the absence of the complex metabolic and immunological changes generally induced in the host by the growing tumor.

In contrast, the metastatic involvement of lung and other organs after the intramuscular or subcutaneous injection of tumor cells is a model which more closely mimics the condition in patients with disseminating solid tumors. In the latter system, the effects on the host of both the primary tumor and the metastases can be monitored (5).

New tools to evaluate the changes of the hemostatic system during tumor and metastasis growth have been provided recently. It has been suggested that metastases do not result from random survival of cells released from the primary tumor, but from the selective growth of specialized subpopulations of highly metastatic cells with specific properties which could affect their pattern of arrest (6). This concept has been developed from the study of so-called metastatic variants. These are cell sublines derived from isolated lung nodules of the same primary tumor which consistently exhibit different metastatic capacity when reinjected in syngeneic animals. These sublines have been very useful in investigating the correlations between patterns of metastasis and behavior of the hemostatic components.

III. LUNG COLONY MODELS

Ten years ago, Hilgard and coworkers (7,8) showed that the intravenous injection of Walker 256 carcinosarcoma cells triggered the acute onset of intravascular coagulation with marked thrombocytopenia, hypofibrinogenemia, increase in fibrin(ogen) degradation products and hypocoagulability. However, injection, under the same conditions, of dead cells or of particulate, inert material of a similar size provoked similar effects (8). This coagulopathy was presumably due to activation of the coagulation cascade through the contact phase or to entry into the circulation of tissue-derived thromboplastic material.

On the other hand, the intravenous injection of Lewis lung carcinoma (3LL) cells into syngeneic C57BL/6 mice induced a rapid fall in blood platelet count and fibrinogen level within a few minutes and, during the following hour, an increase in serum fibrin(ogen) degradation products (9). This syndrome depended on the size of the inoculum and was rapidly reversible (within less than two hours). No hemostatic changes could be measured in the subsequent hours and days during lodgment and growth of metastatic cells in the lungs (Table 1).

Table 1. Development of Hemostatic Changes following the Intravenous Injection of 3LL Cells (9). Note the discrepancy between acute and delayed effects.

| | Time after cancer cell injection | |
	15 min	15 da
Thrombocytopenia	+	−
Hyperfibrinogenemia	+	−
Increase in fibrinogen degradation products	+	−
Lung colonies		+

The intravasuclar coagulation triggered by cancer cell injection could be prevented by treating the animals either with platelet aggregation inhibitors (aspirin, ditazole, dipyridamole and congeners) or with anticoagulants (warfarin, heparin) (5,10). The observation that in these animals inhibitors of platelet aggregation also prevented the defibrination syndrome, suggests that platelets may play an important role in the activation of clotting subsequent to tumor cell injection. On the other hand, we have repeatedly found that treatment with an anticoagulant, such as warfarin, prevented not only the drop in fibrinogen level but also the associated thrombocytopenia (11,12). It is thus possible that thrombin generation would, at least partially, contribute to platelet activation following injection of some types of tumor cells. Preliminary experiments indicate that thrombocytopenia occurs when cancer cells with high procoagulant activity (3LL) are injected into mice, whereas no decrease in platelets follows the injection of cells deprived of procoagulant effect, such as those taken from warfarin-treated animals (13).

Cancer cell-induced acute thrombocytopenia was also significantly reduced in bg/bg C57BL/6 mice with a congenital defect of platelet serotonin storage. These animals had a markedly disturbed hemostasis, as indicated by the excessively prolonged bleeding time and the impaired response of platelets to the intravenous injection of ADP or collagen. With two different types of cancer cells, 3LL and murine fibrosarcoma cells (M_4, subline of mFS6, see below) no thrombocytopenia in bg/bg mice was observed (14). It thus appears that integrity of platelet function or, at least, of the "release reaction" is required for platelets to interact in vivo with cancer cells.

IV. SPONTANEOUS METASTASIS MODELS

The involvement of the hemostatic system during the growth of experimental tumors has only been considered in a few models. Microangiopathic hemolytic anemia, associated with chronic intravascular coagulation, has been shown to occur in rats bearing the non-disseminating Walker 256 carcinosarcoma implanted i.m. (7). Interestingly enough, the laboratory picture also included hypercalcemia, possibly important in triggering the intravascular activation of clotting. The development of thrombocytopenia during tumor growth was a common feature in several murine tumors. These include 3LL, JW sarcoma (JWS), B16 melanoma and mFS6, a benzopyrene-induced fibrosarcoma (12).

In the 3LL spontaneous metastasis model, kinetic studies with labeled platelets indicated that progressive thrombocytopenia was associated with normal platelet survival and there was no evidence for an increased splenic pool (9). Bone marrow examination indicated a reduced number of megakaryocytes, thus suggesting an impaired platelet production rather than an increased platelet consumption. This was confirmed by the observation that neither chronic anticoagulant treatment nor antiaggregation corrected the thrombocytopenia (5). In the 3LL system, progressive thrombocytopenia was accompanied by microangiopathic hemolytic anemia and increased fibrinogen survival and radioactive fibrin accumulation within the tumor. Occasionally, an increase in serum fibrinogen degradation products was measured. Whole blood fibrinolytic activity, prothrombin and partial thromboplastin times, as well as platelet aggregation response to ADP, were unchanged throughout the observation period (9,15). The laboratory picture thus observed in this model appears very similar to that of patients with solid, disseminating tumors who may often suffer from low grade, compensated intravascular clotting; this syndrome does not induce marked changes in conventional laboratory tests and is sometimes difficult to detect and monitor (16).

Other murine tumors may mimic different aspects of the hematological disturbances occurring in cancer patients. JW sarcoma (JWS) arose spontaneously in the lung of a mouse (Balb/c) (17). It may be of interest to mention some peculiarities of JWS-induced hemostatic changes in relation to those already summarized for the 3LL. Both tumors can produce spontaneous metastases in the lungs upon i.m. or s.c. implantation; however, 3LL secondary nodules are encapsulated and can be easily enucleated from the lungs, whereas JWS metastases are infiltrating and difficult to distinguish from the surrounding tissue. Thrombocytopenia and hyperfibrinogenemia were found in both models; however, the survival of radiolabeled fibrinogen was decreased in 3LL, whereas it was normal in JWS and the fibrinolytic activity, normal in 3LL, was markedly depressed in JWS (Table 2). Fibrin accumulated at the tumor site in 3LL but not in JWS (9,17). Despite these differences, the fraction of cardiac output distributed per gram of tumoral tissue (measured by a radiolabeled microsphere technique) was very similar in both tumors (18). When tested in vitro, 3LL cells had higher procoagulant and lower fibrinolytic activity than JWS cells (19,20). It is tempting to

Table 2. Discrepancies between 3LL- and JWS-Induced Changes in the Host's Hemostatic System (5,9,17,19,20).

	JWS	3LL
Thrombocytopenia	+	+
Anemia	–	+
Hyperfibrinogenemia	+	+
Shortened fibrinogen survival	–	+
Hypofibrinolysis	+	–
Fibrin accumulation	–	+
Cell procoagulant activity	+	++
Cell fibrinolytic activity	++	+

speculate that these peculiarities would influence the different fibrin deposition patterns observed in the two models. The presence of fibrin around 3LL cells would contribute to its encapsulated appearance, in contrast to the infiltrating and locally invading behavior of JWS cells.

V. PATHOPHYSIOLOGICAL MECHANISMS

In patients with various types of solid tumors, marked hemostatic changes may be present concomitantly with widespread metastases (4). In the 3LL model, the observed hemostatic changes, although appearing mainly during the phase of metastasis growth, do not show any clear pathogenetic link with metastasis formation. Indeed, if one considers different conditions of 3LL growth, the hemostatic changes in 3LL appeared closely related to the presence of the primary tumor. Indeed no changes were detected when lung metastases grew in the absence of the primary as in the artificial lung colony model or in the spontaneous model after surgical removal of the primary (5,12). Moreover, the same hemostatic changes were still found when animals were subjected to antimetastatic therapy with warfarin or a vitamin K-deficient diet (5,11,13). These data suggest that the presence of the primary tumor uniquely influences the host's hemostatic system.

From available experimental models, it appears that neither tumor-associated necrosis nor immunogenic characteristics of the tumor cells play a major role in these changes. Indeed, the latter occurred in models which grew accompanied by completely different extents of necrosis or which had different immunogenic potential (3LL, JWS, mFS6). Despite these considerations, it must be recognized that, in the 3LL, the above mentioned hemostatic changes appeared in parallel with the development of necrosis (Table 3). The latter was documented histologically, macroscopically and on the basis of the dramatic drop in the relative blood supply (per gram of tumor tissue) during the second and third week after tumor cell implantation (18).

Table 3. Appearance of Hemostatic Changes[a] in 3LL-Bearing Mice in Relation to the Development of Tumor Necrosis (18).

	Time after tumor implantation		
	1 wk	2 wk	3 wk
Primary tumor weight (g)	0.48 ± 0.03[b]	5.09 ± 0.36	8.53 ± 0.42
Necrotic tissue (g)	undetectable	1.62 ± 0.58	4.37 ± 0.20
Cardiac output fraction (%/g of tumor)	2.30 ± 0.20	0.81 ± 0.02	0.78 ± 0.01
Platelet count (% of controls)	105 ± 6	68 ± 11	24 ± 8

[a] Represented by the platelet count
[b] Means $\pm$ S.E. of 7-12 values per group

It has been suggested that the primary tumor exerts an inhibitory effect on the growth of metastatic nodules through a still undefined mediator (21). It would be worth investigating whether a similar mechanism operates in depressing platelet production.

The concept of hemostatic changes being linked to the presence of the primary tumor, not of metastases, is further supported by observations made on metastatic variants of the mFS6 fibrosarcoma. Sublines developed from isolated lung nodules of this tumor gave rise when implanted i.m. to primary tumors of the same weight but to completely different types of metastatic growth, ranging from 0 to 100% metastatic incidence (22). When any of these sublines was implanted into syngeneic hosts, the same type of hemostatic changes were observed, irrespective of the extent of metastatic involvement (23). Similarly to the 3LL model, progressive thrombocytopenia and hyperfibrinogenemia were found in the second half of the observation period of mFS6-bearing animals.

This model also allows investigation of the mechanisms of the observed hemostatic changes. As indicated in Table 4, the tumors derived from the various sublines induced the same degree of thrombocytopenia and hyperfibrinogenemia, despite completely different characteristics of the corresponding tumor cells. Indeed, M_4 and M_7 cells, which aggregated mouse blood platelets in vitro (12),[4] did not induce a more marked thrombocytopenia than the two other sublines. M_8 and M_9, which had a many-fold higher "tissue factor" procoagulant activity (24), did not induce intravascular clotting activation, as one could expect. This may be explained in several ways: first of all, the cancer cell properties, such as procoagulant, fibrinolytic and platelet aggregating activity measured in vitro may be expressed somewhat artifactually in respect to the in vivo conditions; on the other hand, the cell number during hematogenous dissemination and/or their lifespan might not be sufficient to influence the host's hemostatic components at least at the systemic level. Most probably, the correlation between cancer cell activities and the activation of blood clotting components would be closer if it was possible to monitor local phenomena, such as the presence of activated coagulation factors in blood draining from a tumor vascular bed. In patients with ovarian carcinomas, a urokinase-like fibrinolytic activity of the cells could in fact be detected in blood from veins draining the tumor, whereas no activity was seen in peripheral blood (25).

On the other hand, there may be conditions where the presence of a growing tumor influences both locally and systemically the host's clotting system. In rabbits bearing the V_2 carcinoma, macrophages harvested from either intraperitoneal or subcutaneous implants expressed a very strong procoagulant activity as compared to peritoneal macrophages in the same animals; circulating mononuclear cells produced higher tissue thromboplastin activity upon endotoxin stimulation (26). This suggests that, in tumor-bearing individuals, mononuclear phagocytes might play an important role in systemic activation of clotting and in fibrin deposition at the host-tumor interface.

VI. CONCLUSIONS

During the development of solid tumors in animals a number of changes may occur in the host's hemostatic system. Most of these changes are linked to the presence of the primary tumor and, presumably, to other factors such as acute phase reaction, release of toxic material from necrotic tissue and circulation of blood through abnormal, neovascularized beds. It is not known whether some more specific factor released from the tumor would affect the hemostatic components of the host. A closer correlation between cancer cell activities and the host's hemostatic disturbances can be observed in acute experiments on the defibrination syndrome induced by the intravenous injection of cancer cells.

Table 4. Cancer Cell Activities and Hemostatic Changes in Tumor-Bearing Animals Implanted i.m. with mFS6 Metastatic Variants (12,22-24).

Tumor Subline	Metastasis Incidence %	IN VITRO CELL PROPERTIES		IN VIVO HEMOSTATIC CHANGES	
		Platelet Aggregation	Procoagulant Activity	Thrombocytopenia	Hypercoagulation
mFS6	55	-	+	+	-
M4	95	++	+	+	-
M7	100	++	+	+	-
M8	5	-	++	+	-
M9	0	-	++	+	-

ACKNOWLEDGEMENTS

The author's work reviewed in this survey has been supported by the Italian National Research Council (Contract 82.01403.96), the National Institutes of Health, National Cancer Institute, Bethesda, MD, USA (Grant RO1CA 26824) and by the Italian Association for Cancer Research, Milano, Italy. Vanna Pistotti and Anna Mancini helped prepare the manuscript.

REFERENCES

1. Trousseau A. Clinique Medicale de l'Hotel-Dieu de Paris J.B. Bailliere et Fils, Paris, 5th Edition, 3:94, 1865.
2. Donati MB, Davidson JF and Garrattini S. Malignancy and the Hemostatic System. Raven Press, New York, 1981.
3. Donati MB and Poggi A. Br. J. Haematol. 44:173-182, 1980.
4. Donati MB, Poggi A and Semeraro N. In: Recent Advances in Blood Coagulation (Ed. Poller L), Churchill Livingstone, Edinburgh, pp. 227-259, 1981.
5. Poggi A, Donati MB and Garrattini S. In: Malignancy and the Hemostatic System (Eds. Donati MB, Davidson JF and Garattini S), Raven Press, New York, pp. 89-101, 1981.
6. Poste G and Fidler IJ. Nature (London) 283:139-146, 1980.
7. Hilgard P, Hohage R, Schmitt W and Kohle W. Br. J. Haematol. 24:245-254, 1973.
8. Hilgard P and Gordon-Smith EC. Br. J. Haematol. 26:651-659, 1974.
9. Poggi A, Polentarutti N, Donati MB, de Gaetano G and Garattini S. Cancer Res. 37:272-277, 1977.
10. Mussoni L, Poggi A, Donati MB and de Gaetano G. Haemostasis 6:260-265, 1977.
11. Poggi A, Mussoni L, Kornblihtt L, Ballabio E, de Gaetano G and Donati MB. Lancet 1:163-164, 1978.
12. Donati MB, Rotilio D, Delaini F, Giavazzi R, Mantovani A and Poggi A. In: Interaction of Platelets and Tumor Cells (Ed. Jamieson GA), Alan R. Liss, New York, pp. 159-176, 1982.
13. Delaini F, Colucci M, De Bellis Vitti G, Locati D, Poggi A, Semeraro N and Donati MB. Thromb. Res. 24:263-266, 1981.
14. Valori VM, Buczko W, Delaini F, Lampugnani MG, Di Palo L, Herberman RB and Donati MB. Thromb. Haemostasis 50:214, 1983.
15. Giraldi T, Sava G, Mitri E and Cherubino R. Eur. J. Cancer Clin. Oncol. (in press), 1983.
16. Donati MB. In: Blood Coagulation and Haemostasis. A Practical Guide. (Ed. Thomson JM), Churchill Livingstone, Edinburgh, pp. 158-199, 1980.
17. Chmielweska J, Poggi A, Mussoni L, Donati MB and Garattini S. Eur. J. Cancer 16:1399-1407, 1980.
18. Raczka E, Quintana A, Poggi A and Donati MB. Eur. J. Cancer Clin. Oncol. (in press), 1983.
19. Curatolo L, Colucci M, Cambini AL, Poggi A, Morasca L, Donati MB and Semeraro N. Br. J. Cancer 40:228-233, 1979.
20. Latallo ZS, Kowalski-Loth B, Chmielewska J, Teisseyre E, Raczka E and Kopec M. In: Progress in Chemical Fibrinolysis and Thrombolysis (Eds. Davidson JF, Cepelak V, Samama MM and Desnoyers PC), Churchill Livingstone, Edinburgh, Vol. 4, pp. 411-415, 1979.
21. Yuhas JM and Pazmino NH. Cancer Res. 34:2005-2010, 1974.

22. Giavazzi R, Alessandri G, Spreafico R, Garattini S and Mantovani A. Br. J. Cancer 42:462-472, 1980.
23. Delaini F, Giavazzi R, De Bellis Vitti G, Alessandri G, Mantovani A and Donati MB. Br. J. Cancer 43:100-104, 1981.
24. Colucci M, Giavazzi R, Alessandri G, Semeraro N, Mantovani A and Donati MB. Blood 57:733-735, 1981.
25. Astedt B. In: Malignancy and the Hemostatic System (Eds. Donati MB, Davidson JF and Garattini S), Raven Press, New York, pp. 83-88, 1981.
26. Lorenzet R, Peri G, Locati D, Allavena P, Colucci M, Semeraro N, Mantovani A and Donati MB. Blood (in press), 1983.

CHAPTER 6. EVIDENCE FOR A TUMOR PROTEINASE IN BLOOD COAGULATION

I. INTRODUCTION

There is a large amount of experimental evidence that supports the concept of an association between blood coagulation and malignant disease. Since several chapters within this volume describe detailed historical and recent evidence for this association, I will only summarize this information to provide perspective about the evidence that led investigators to look for procoagulants associated with malignant tissue. The following discussion will review tumor-derived procoagulants with emphasis on evidence for a unique tumor-derived proteolytic enzyme that initiates blood coagulation (for further evidence see Chapter 12).

Disseminated intravascular coagulation (1-3) and other abnormalities of the coagulation system (4-6) have been repeatedly identified as pathological features of malignant disease (see also Chapters 22 and 24). There is increased removal of fibrinogen from the circulation of animals and humans with cancer (7,8), and much of the resulting fibrin is deposited in and around solid tumors (9,10 and Chapter 8). This deposition of fibrin is thought to promote tumor growth by providing a supporting network or "cocoon" of fibrin at the advancing margin of the tumor (11,12), by promoting tumor vascularization (10,13) and possibly by limiting access of the host defense system to tumor cells (10,14). Fibrin is also associated with blood-borne malignant cells and is thought to promote metastasis by facilitating the clumping of these malignant cells with platelets or other blood cells (15-17). These events may promote the lodging of tumor cell-platelet aggregates in small capillaries of organs susceptible to metastatic invasion. Furthermore, it has been suggested that fibrin associated with malignant cells in the hematologic phase of metastasis may protect the malignant cells from the host defense system (10,14). Tumor growth and metastasis are decreased by inhibition of fibrin formation in the host by anticoagulant therapy with heparin (18,19) or warfarin (18,20-24), by proteinase inhibitors that prevent thrombus formation (25), by therapy with fibrinolysin (15,20,26,27) or by defibrination of the host (28,29). This evidence suggests that fibrin may play an important role in the growth and metastasis of tumors and led investigators to look for tumor specific substances that might cause the abnormal initiation of coagulation.

The first efforts to identify and characterize a tumor-derived procoagulant were undertaken by O'Meara and his associates (11,30-38). During more than a decade of published research, they demonstrated that a wide variety of tumor tissues and extracts of tumor cells possessed greater ability to initiate coagulation than normal tissues. This coagulation was presumed to be due to the presence of a tumor procoagulant or "cancer coagulative factor." They found that tumor procoagulant was a heat and acid labile lipoprotein that was qualitatively different from normal tissue factor. This procoagulant factor was tentatively identified as a long-chain free fatty acid associated with serum proteins such as albumin (38,39). In light of current observations, their conclusion about the nature of the procoagulant may have been incorrect. However, they clearly established the presence of a substance from malignant cells that induces coagulation. These studies provided the essential foundation for the further development of research on tumor-derived procoagulants.

Pineo et al. (40) isolated a heat- and acid-stable glycoprotein from the mucus of nonmalignant tissues (bronchial secretions, ovarian cyst fluid and saliva). They demonstrated that this glycoprotein initiated coagulation by activating factor X nonproteolytically and suggested that this substance may be responsible for the hyper-coagulable state associated with mucus-secreting adenocarcinomas.

Other investigators have identified a clot stabilizing enzyme, factor XIII, which facilitates coagulation (41). Recently, Dvorak and his associates (42,43) have provided good evidence for the presence of a factor V-like activity associated with tumors. This substance does not initiate coagulation but rather accelerates the rate of prothrombin activation by factor Xa (44). All of these are possible mechanisms for the activity of tumor-derived coagulants. However, the discussion in this chapter will focus on the initiation of blood coagulation by a tumor proteinase and tissue factor. Other suggested tumor-derived substances that participate in blood coagulation will not be considered further.

The majority of the evidence that has been compiled during the past 10 yrs points to the activity of two systems in the initiation of coagulation by malignant cells -- a proteinase that directly activates factor X (cancer procoagulant) and tissue factor (factor III), the lipoprotein procoagulant associated with normal tissue (45,46).

II. PURIFICATION OF CANCER PROCOAGULANT

For the past 10 yrs, we have studied a tumor-derived proteolytic procoagulant, termed cancer procoagulant, which initiates coagulation by directly activating factor X. As an essential first phase of this research it was necessary to purify this protein and characterize its physical, chemical and enzymatic properties. Sumner Wood (15,20) first demonstrated that rabbit V2 carcinoma was associated with active fibrin deposition. We purified the procoagulant from this tumor because we could obtain large quantities of the tumor in a simple and reproducible fashion. We subsequently purified cancer procoagulant to homogeneity by a series of column chromatographic steps including gel filtration over a 1.5 agarose resin, p-chloromercurialbenzoate affinity chromatography, benzamidineSepharose affinity chromatography and phenyl-Sepharose hydrophobic chromatography (47,48). An antibody was developed to the purified antigen by immunization in a goat. Antibody partially purified from the goat antisera and coupled to cyanogen bromide-activated Sepharose has been used in subsequent purification procedures. The purification of cancer procoagulant by immunoaffinity chromatography was carried out by extracting V2 carcinoma tumors in three changes of 20 mM veronal buffer (pH 7.8) (47-49); the extract was concentrated approximately 10-fold by Amicon PM-10 ultrafiltration and precipitated with 50% ethanol. The redissolved precipitate was then reprecipitated with 40% ammonium sulfate saturation. The precipitate (redissolved) was applied to an immunoaffinity column, the column washed thoroughly with veronal buffer to remove unbound protein, and the bound protein eluted with 3 M KSCN. The KSCN was dialyzed from the eluate, and the sample was analyzed for procoagulant activity by measuring the recalcification clotting time of citrated normal plasma. The properties of the procoagulant were determined, as described below, to confirm that it was cancer procoagulant. The purity of the sample was assessed by SDS-polyacrylamide gel electrophoresis (Figure 1).

Not only has this purification procedure provided rapid, easy and reproducible purification of cancer procoagulant from V2 carcinoma and from other tumor sources, but it has demonstrated the specificity of the antibody. Recently, an IgM monoclonal antibody has been developed with the mouse hybridoma system (unpublished observations), and its specificity has been demonstrated in a similar manner by selectively removing the procoagulant from a crude tumor extract by immunoaffinity chromatography.

III. CHARACTERIZATION OF CANCER PROCOAGULANT

There are several types of substances in tissue extracts that will initiate coagulation in normal citrated plasma including tissue factor and other types of proteinases such as those present in the coagulation cascade. Therefore, it was important to establish specific properties of cancer procoagulant that would allow us to distinguish this enzyme from other procoagulants. In early studies, we found that diisopropylfluorophosphate (DFP) would block the activity of cancer procoagulant but had no effect on tissue factor (49). In addition, while cancer procoagulant initiates the coagulation of factor VII-deficient human plasma (50) or factor VII-depleted bovine plasma (51), normal tissue factor requires factor VII for its procoagulant activity (45). Inhibition by DFP and activity in factor VII-deficient plasmas provided necessary criteria to distinguish cancer procoagulant from tissue factor but not from other proteinases in the coagulation cascade. Subsequently, we demonstrated that cancer procoagulant was a cysteine proteinase that was reversibly inhibited by 0.1 mM $HgCl_2$ and was irreversibly inhibited by 1 mM iodoacetamide (48) and by 10 μM carbobenzyloxy lysyl diazomethyl ketone (manuscript in preparation).

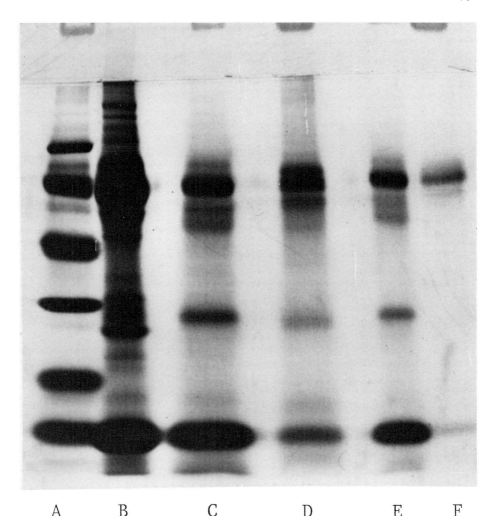

FIGURE 1. SDS Polyacrylamide Gel Electrophoretic Analysis of Samples from the Immunoaffinity Purification of Cancer Procoagulant. An antibody to purified cancer procoagulant was raised in a goat, the partially purified goat antibody was coupled to cyanogen bromide-activated Sepharose. A crude tumor extract (column B) was partially purified by the precipitation steps (column C) described in the text and applied to immunoaffinity resin. After washing unbound protein from the resin (column D is wash 1, column E is wash 2), the bound protein was eluted with 3 M KSCN (column F). The purified protein shown in column F contained procoagulant activity with characteristics of cancer procoagulant. Molecular weight standards (column A) include phosphorylase b (94,000 daltons), bovine serum albumin (68,000 daltons), ovalbumin (43,000 daltons), carbonic anhydrase (30,000 daltons), soybean trypsin inhibitor (20,000 daltons) and α lact-albumin (14,000 daltons).

The active-site sulfhydryl group of many cysteine proteinases, including cancer procoagulant, can be oxidized during the course of biochemical manipulation (52). We used 10 µM KCN to facilitate reductive reactivation of cancer procoagulant (53). There is no evidence that these cysteine proteinase properties of cancer procoagulant are common to the serine proteinases of the coagulation cascade. Furthermore, cancer procoagulant has a molecular weight of 68,000, a molecular weight that is different from the other clotting factors. These characteristics have provided a means to clearly distinguish cancer procoagulant from tissue factor. For example, tissue factor is inactive in factor VII-deficient plasma, it is not inhibited by DFP, Hg^{++} or iodoacetamide, and the active lipoprotein has a substantially higher molecular weight than 68,000 (45). The activated clotting factors (factors VIIa, IXa and Xa) which are most likely to directly activate factor X are serine proteinases that are not inhibited by Hg^{++} or iodoacetamide, are probably not reactivated by KCN and have a molecular weight of 53,000 (54), 45,000 (55) and 42,000 daltons (56), respectively. Based on these observations, cancer procoagulant appears to be different from the other known clotting factors that could initiate coagulation and might be present in tumor extracts.

Cancer procoagulant initiates coagulation of factor VIII-deficient plasma (49) and factor VII-deficient plasma (49,50) suggesting that in the coagulation cascade it is activating either factor X or prothrombin (factor II) directly (49). To determine the site of activity of cancer procoagulant, we performed a two-stage assay in which we incubated purified prothrombin or factor X with purified cancer procoagulant in the first stage of the assay. Aliquots of the stage 1 reaction mixture were removed at timed intervals and assayed for the level of activated clotting factor (thrombin or Xa) in the second stage of the assay. Cancer procoagulant did not activate prothrombin in this two-stage assay system under conditions in which Typain snake venom actively initiated coagulation (49). In contrast, cancer procoagulant activated factor X in this assay system in a fashion similar to the Russell's viper venom control (47,49). The activation of bovine factor X involves the proteolytic cleavage of the proenzyme [(Factor Xα) molecular weight = 55,000] to either factor Xβ, a proteolytically inactive precursor with a molecular weight of 52,000 or to factor Xaα, a coagulant enzyme with a molecular weight of 45,000. Both factor Xβ and Xaα are eventually converted to factor Xaβ, a coagulant proteinase with a molecular weight of 42,000 (56). To demonstrate that the activation of factor X by cancer procoagulant was due to proteolytic activity we incubated purified factor X with purified cancer procoagulant. Timed aliquots were removed and mixed with SDS-polyacrylamide gel sample buffer and electrophoresed on a 10% polyacrylamide gel to separate the distinct molecular weight forms of factor X and Xa (47). Activation of factor X was similar to that of the Russell's viper venom control. These data demonstrate that cancer procoagulant activates factor X in the coagulation cascade by proteolytic activation, a mechanism that is similar to that of other factor X activating enzymes including Russell's viper venom, factor VIIa and factor IXa.

Work from several other laboratories has confirmed the presence of a factor X-activating substance from malignant cells which initiates coagulation. Sakuragawa et al. (57,58) found a substance that appeared to activate factor X in extracts of promyelocytic leukemia cells and gastric tumors. Curatolo et al. (59), Colucci et al. (60), Hilgard and Whur (61) and Catlan and Bresson (62) have demonstrated that extracts and cell suspensions of Lewis lung carcinoma (3LL) contain a procoagulant that will initiate coagulation in the absence of factor VII. Lewis lung carcinoma cells will directly activate factor X as measured with a chromogenic substrate for Xa (60). Furthermore, treatment of tumor-bearing animals with warfarin diminishes this procoagulant activity, suggesting that this X activator may contain γ-carboxyglutamic acid (23,24).

In summary, a cysteine proteinase has been purified from malignant tissue. This cysteine proteinase initiates coagulation by directly activating factor X in the coagulation cascade and has physical, chemical and enzymatic properties that are different than known coagulation proteins.

IV. DISTRIBUTION OF CANCER PROCOAGULANT

Is cancer procoagulant unique to malignant tissue and what is its distribution among various kinds of malignant tissues? To answer these questions, we obtained samples of normal and malignant tissue from surgical specimens, extracted the tissue and assayed the extract for procoagulant activity, inhibition by DFP and activity in factor VII-depleted bovine plasma (51). All of the procoagulant activity in approximately 75% of the malignant tissue extracts had the characteristics of cancer procoagulant. The remaining 25% of the extracts had procoagulant activity consistent with both tissue factor and cancer procoagulant. The procoagulant activity was partially inhibited by 5 mM DFP and was partially active in factor VII-depleted plasma. None of the normal tissue extracts contained procoagulant that was inhibited by DFP and was active in factor VII-depleted plasma suggesting that normal procoagulant is tissue factor (45). In a second study (50), we evaluated the distribution of cancer procoagulant in normal and transformed hamster fibroblasts. Serum-free medium from all of the transformed fibroblasts contained procoagulant activity that was inhibited by DFP and was active in factor VII-deficient human plasma. Serum-free medium from the normal fibroblasts contained procoagulant activity which was insensitive to DFP and required factor VII. In a third study (63), we determined the level and characteristics of the procoagulant activity of intact, viable normal and malignant cell suspensions. In this study we found that the procoagulant associated with normal cells was insensitive to DFP while that associated with the malignant cells was inhibited by DFP. Table 1 summarizes the data from our laboratory on the presence of cancer procoagulant in samples from normal and malignant cells and tissues. These data support the hypothesis that cancer procoagulant is derived from neoplastic cells and not from normal cells. Studies from other laboratories have demonstrated the presence of cancer procoagulant-like enzyme in 3LL cells (59-62), Ca 755 cells (62), gastric cancers (58) and promyelocytic leukemia cells (57).

Table 1. Measurement and Characterization of Cancer Procoagulant in Tumor Extracts (Ext), Suspensions of Intact Viable Cells (CS) and in Serum-Free Tissue Culture Medium (TCM).[a]

Source of Procoagulant	Species	Type of Sample	Number
Adenocarcinoma--colon, kidney	human	Ext	9
Carcinoma--breast, liver, kidney, lung	human	Ext	8
Neuroblastoma--liver	human	Ext	1
Sarcoma--abdomen	human	Ext	1
Liposarcoma--abdomen, leg	human	Ext	2
V2 Carcinoma	rabbit	Ext/CS/TCM	1
Parietal Yolk Sac Carcinoma	mouse	Ext/TCM	1
SV-40 Transformed Fibroblasts	hamster	TCM	5
Chemically Transformed Fibroblasts	hamster	TCM	2
B16 Melanoma	mouse	Ext/CS/TCM	2
HT-29 Carcinoma	human	CS/TCM	1
LVP Hepatoma	human	TCM	1

[a]Details of these studies are described in references 50, 51 and 63.

V. TISSUE FACTOR AS THE TUMOR PROCOAGULANT

In normal cells, tissue factor is the lipoprotein cofactor that is exposed during cellular injury and facilitates the activity of factor VII (VIIa) (45). Factor X is activated by the factor VIIa-tissue factor complex (45). There is evidence that tissue factor activity may be expressed on malignant cells (42,43,64-72). The events that facilitate the expression of this lipoprotein on malignant cells are not known but may be due to necrosis of tumor cells (73) or due to the host immune system and blood cells that infiltrate the tumor (73-78). A variety of studies prior to 1975 demonstrated thromboplastin activity in ovarian tumors (65), rat hepatoma cells (64), T-241 Lewis sarcoma cells (67) and other types of malignant tissue (66,67). However, in general there was no effort to distinguish between tissue factor and cancer procoagulant in these studies because the distinguishing characteristics of the latter procoagulant had not been established. More recently, several investigators have demonstrated tissue factor as a property of malignant cells and have performed the appropriate studies to characterize tissue factor or its site of activation of the coagulation cascade (69-72). These investigators have demonstrated activity that required factor VII to initiate coagulation, was insensitive to serine or cysteine proteinase inhibitors and cross-reacted with an antibody to tissue factor. In these studies it must be pointed out that tissue factor may be derived from blood monocytes that infiltrate and accumulate within the tumor and therefore provide the necessary ingredients to initiate coagulation (74-78). Thus, tissue factor-initiated coagulation by malignant cells appears to play a role in the activation of the coagulation system in several types of malignancy.

Throughout the search for an explanation for the hyper-coagulability and fibrin deposition associated with malignant tissue, investigators have been faced with a variety of technical problems that have influenced the experimental results and the conclusions they have drawn from their research. I would like to consider some of these problems at this point because it is clear that efforts to elucidate the role of tissue factor, cancer procoagulant and other coagulants in tumor-induced coagulation have been influenced by some of the problems. Some tumors produce tissue factor (69-72,79) while others produce cancer procoagulant (50,51,59-63); so the selection of the tumor type studied is important when procoagulants from malignant tissue are being analyzed. The procedure for extracting tissue factor from cells has been well established (45,46) and use of this method yields quantitative recovery of this stable lipoprotein. Investigators have looked at activity of intact malignant cells in an effort to extrapolate the in vitro measurements to determine the level of tissue factor expressed by the malignant cell in vivo. This is very difficult because almost any type of manipulation such as treatment with dilute proteolytic enzyme solutions (80) or physical manipulation of cells (81,82) will facilitate the expression of tissue factor on cell surfaces (70,72). This is also true of most blood cells including monocytes (74-79). Thus, it is difficult to evaluate the relative contribution of tissue factor in the in vivo generation of tumor-induced coagulation because artifacts are easily generated by slight perturbation of the experimental system.

In a similar fashion, the expression of cancer procoagulant by malignant cells is subject to experimental problems. Cancer procoagulant is a labile enzyme that can be denatured under a variety of experimental conditions, as discussed above, including oxidation of its active site sulfhydryl resulting in loss of activity. In addition, there are probably a spectrum of naturally occurring plasma and cellular inhibitors that influence the expression of its cysteine proteinase activity (unpublished observations). Thus, the problems with cancer procoagulant appear to be the opposite of those of tissue factor, i.e., there are a variety of experimental manipulations that will facilitate loss of cancer procoagulant activity whereas similar experimental manipulations may facilitate the expression of the more stable tissue factor activity.

VI. RATIONALE FOR CANCER PROCOAGULANT

Much of our experimental data suggests that cancer procoagulant is not associated with normal cells but is produced by neoplastic cells. What is the explanation for the production of a new enzymatic activity by tumor cells when it wasn't produced by the normal cell before malignant transformation? There are several possible explanations. A precursor enzyme may be present in normal cells and become activated in neoplasia. An inhibitor may be produced by normal cells and its production cease in neoplasia, allowing the expression of the enzyme activity. A third explanation is the presence of the genetic code for this enzyme in normal cells but the expression of the gene does not occur in the absence of malignant transformation. Although all three explanations may prevail, we have data that supports the third explanation. Recently, we have obtained evidence for the presence of a factor X activator in extracts of amnion and chorion tissue from normal human placenta (83). This procoagulant crossreacts with the antibody to cancer procoagulant from V2 carcinoma, is active in factor VII-deficient human plasma, is inhibited by $HgCl_2$ and iodoacetamide and has a molecular weight of 68,000 daltons. These are the same properties as cancer procoagulant. Other investigators have identified a similar procoagulant activity in amniotic fluid (84). Since amnion is poorly differentiated tissue from fetal origin and malignant tissue is dedifferentiated normal tissue, our data suggest that this factor X activator may be expressed in undifferentiated or dedifferentiated tissue. The genetic code for this protein may exist in normal cells but its expression is repressed in the normal differentiated state.

Currently, there is a renewed interest in the role of blood coagulation and fibrin formation in malignant disease. The relative importance of cancer procoagulant in tumor-induced coagulation is not clear. Both cancer procoagulant-induced and tissue factor-induced coagulation are probably subject to a variety of coagulation control mechanisms, so that the net effect of either or both of these activities in a tumor-bearing animal is difficult to establish. Moreover, the microenvironment around the malignant cell in a solid tumor or around a blood-borne malignant cell may be more important in the expression of tumor-initiated activity than the macroenvironment expressed in the whole tumor or in the blood of the tumor-bearing animal. Regardless, it seems clear that initiation of coagulation in cancer probably plays an important role in the pathophysiology of this disease.

ACKNOWLEDGEMENTS

This work was supported by NIH Grant CA-14408, DRR Grant RR-00051, the Colorado Heart Association, an American Cancer Society Grant PF1789, a donation from Mrs. L.G. Hickey and a grant from Western Biomedical Development Corporation.

REFERENCES

1. Trousseau A. Clinique Medicale de l'Hotel-dieu de Paris. J.B. Bailliere et Fils, Paris, 5th Edition 3:94, 1865.
2. Gore JM, Appelbaum JS, Greene HL, Dexter L and Dalen JE. Ann. Intern. Med. 96:556-560, 1982.
3. Nusbacher J. N.Y. State J. Med. 64:2166-2173, 1964.
4. Miller SP, Sanchez-Avalos J, Stefanski T and Zuckerman L. Cancer (Philadelphia) 20:1452-1465, 1967.
5. Pochedly C, Miller SP and Mehta A. Oncology 28:517-522, 1973.
6. Van der Walt JA, Gomperts ED and Kew MC. Cancer (Philadelphia) 40:1593-1603, 1977.
7. Franks JJ, Gordon SG, Kao B, Sullivan T and Kirch D. In: Plasma Protein Turnover (Eds. Bianchi R, Mariani G and McFarlane AS), MacMillan Press, Denver, pp. 423-440, 1976.
8. Lyman GH, Bettigde RE, Robson E, Ambrus JL and Urban H. Cancer (Philadelphia) 41:1113-1122, 1978.
9. Ogura T, Tsubura E and Yamamura Y. Gann 61:443-449, 1970.
10. Dvorak HF, Dvorak AM, Manseau EJ, Wilberg L and Churchill WH. J. Natl. Cancer Inst. 62:(6)1459-1472, 1979.
11. O'Meara RAQ and Jackson RD. Ir. J. Med. Sci. 391:327-328, 1958.
12. Day ED, Planinsek JA and Pressman D. J. Natl. Cancer Inst. 22:413-426, 1959.
13. Goodall CM, Saunders AG and Shubik P. J. Natl. Cancer Inst. 35:495-521, 1965.
14. Donati MB, Poggi A and Semeraro N. In: Recent Advances in Blood Coagulation (Ed. Poller L), Churchill Livingstone, Edinburgh, pp. 227-259, 1982.
15. Wood S Jr. Bull. Schweiz. Akad. Med. Wiss. 20:92-121, 1964.
16. Kinjo M. Br. J. Cancer 38:293-301, 1978.
17. Gasic GJ, Boettiger D, Catalafamo JL, Gasic TD and Stewart GJ. Cancer Res. 38:2950-2954, 1978.
18. Millar RC and Ketcham AS. J. Med. 5:23-31, 1974.
19. Hilgard P and Thornes RD. Eur. J. Cancer 12:755-762, 1976.
20. Wood S Jr. J. Med. 5:7-22, 1974.
21. Zacharski LR, Henderson WG, Rickles FR, Forman WB, Cornell CJ Jr, Forcier RJ, Edwards R, Headley E, Kim S-H, O'Donnell JR, O'Dell R, Tornyos K and Kwaan HC. J. Am. Med. Assoc. 245:831-835, 1981.
22. Brown JM. Cancer Res. 33:1217-1224, 1973.
23. Poggi A, Colucci M, Delaini F, Semeraro N and Donati MB. Eur. J. Cancer 16:1641-1642, 1980.
24. Colucci M, Delaini F, Vitti G, Locati D, Poggi A, Semeraro N and Donati MB. In: Metastasis: Clinical and Experimental Aspects (Eds. Hellman K, Hilgard P and Eccles S), Martinus Nijhoff, The Hague, pp. 90-94, 1980.
25. Saito D, Sawamura M, Umezawa K, Kanai Y, Furihata C, Matsushima T and Sugimura T. Cancer Res. 40:2539-2542, 1980.
26. Kodama Y and Tanaka K. Gann 69:9-18, 1978.
27. Ambrus JL, Ambrus CM, Pickern J, Slodes S and Bross I. J. Med. 6:433-458, 1975.
28. Wood S Jr. and Hilgard PH. Johns Hopkins Med. J. 133:207-213, 1973.
29. Donati MB, Mussoni L, Poggi A, de Gaetano G and Garattini S. Eur. J. Cancer 14:343-347, 1978.
30. O'Meara RAQ. Ir. J. Med. Sci. 394:474-479, 1958.
31. O'Meara RAQ. Arch. "De Vecchi" Anat. Patol. Med. Clin. 31:365-384, 1960.
32. O'Meara RAQ. In: The Morphological Precursors of Cancer (Ed. Severi L), Perugia, pp. 21-34, 1962.
33. O'Meara RAQ. Bull. Soc. Int. Chir. 23:24-29, 1964.
34. O'Meara RAQ and Thornes RD. Ir. J. Med. Sci. 424:106-112, 1961.

82

35. O'Meara RAQ. Thromb. Diath. Haemorrh. Suppl. 28:137-142, 1968.
36. Boggust WA, O'Brien DJ, O'Meara RAQ and Thornes RD. Ir. J. Med. Sci. 447:131-144, 1963.
37. Boggust WA and O'Meara RAQ Ir. J. Med. Sci. 481:11-21, 1966.
38. Boggust WA, O'Meara RAQ and Fullerton WW. Eur. J. Cancer 3:467-473, 1968.
39. Fullerton WW, Boggust WA and O'Meara RAQ. J. Clin. Pathol. 20:624-628, 1967.
40. Pineo GF, Rogoeczi E, Hatton MWC and Brian MC. J. Lab. Clin. Med. 82:255-266, 1973.
41. Laki K, Tyler HM and Yancey ST. Biochem. Biophys. Res. Commun. 24:776-781, 1966.
42. Dvorak HF, Orenstein NS, Carvalho AC, Churchill WH, Dvorak AM, Galli SJ, Feder J, Bitzer AM, Rypysc J and Giovinco P. J. Immunol. 122:166-174, 1979.
43. Dvorak HF, Quay SC, Orenstein NS, Dvorak AM. Hahn P, Bitzer AM and Carvalho AC. Science 212:923-924, 1981.
44. Nesheim ME, Taswell JB and Mann KG. J. Biol. Chem. 254:10952-10962, 1962.
45. Nemerson Y and Bach R. Prog. Hemostasis Thromb. 6, 237-261, 1982.
46. Bach R, Nemerson Y and Konigsberg W J. Biol. Chem. 256:8324-8331, 1981.
47. Gordon SG. J. Histochem. Cytochem. 29:457-463, 1981.
48. Gordon SG and Cross BA. J. Clin. Invest. 67:1665-1671, 1981.
49. Gordon SG, Franks JJ and Lewis B. Thromb. Res. 6:127-137, 1975.
50. Gordon SG and Lewis B. Cancer Res. 38:2467-2472, 1978.
51. Gordon SG, Franks JJ and Lewis BJ. J. Natl. Cancer Inst. 62:773-776, 1979.
52. Kezdy FJ and Kaiser ET. Methods Enzymol. 45:3-12, 1976.
53. Gould NR and Liener IE. Biochemistry 4:90-98, 1965.
54. Bajaj SP, Rapaport SI and Brown SF. J. Biol. Chem. 256:253-259, 1981.
55. Osterud B, Bouma BN and Griffin JH. J. Biol. Chem. 253:5946-5951, 1978.
56. Fujikawa K, Titani K and Davie EW. Proc. Natl. Acad. Sci. USA 72:3359-3363, 1975.
57. Sakuragawa N, Takahashi K, Hoshiyama M, Jimbo C, Matsuoka M and Onishi Y. Thromb. Res. 8:263-273, 1976.
58. Sakuragawa N, Takahashi K, Hoshiyama M, Jimbo C, Ashizawa K, Matsuoka M and Ohnishi Y. Thromb. Res. 10:457-463, 1977.
59. Curatolo L, Colucci M, Cambini AL, Poggi A, Morasca L, Donati MB and Semeraro N. Br. J. Cancer 40:228-233, 1979.
60. Colucci M, Curatolo L, Donati MB and Semeraro N. Thromb. Res. 18:589-595, 1980.
61. Hilgard P and Whur P. Br. J. Cancer 41:642-643, 1980.
62. Cattan A and Bresson ML. Biomedicine 25:252-254, 1976.
63. Gordon SG, Gilbert LC and Lewis BJ. Thromb. Res. 26:379-387, 1982.
64. Khato J, Suzuki M and Sato H. Gann 65:289-294, 1974.
65. Svanberg L. Thromb. Res. 6:307-313, 1975.
66. Peterson H-I and Zettergren L. Acta. Chir. Scand. 136:365-368, 1970.
67. Frank AL and Holyoke ED. Int. J. Cancer 3:677-682, 1968.
68. Holyoke ED, Frank AL and Weiss L. Int. J. Cancer 9:258-263, 1972.
69. Gouault-Heilmann M, Chardon E, Sultan C and Josso F. Br. J. Haematol. 30:151-158, 1975.
70. Kinjo M, Oka K, Naito S, Kohga S, Tanaka K, Oboshi S, Hayata Y. and Yasumoto K. Br. J. Cancer 39:15-23, 1979.
71. Matsuda M and Aoki N. Thromb. Res. 13:311-324, 1978.
72. Kohga S. Gann 69:461-470, 1978.
73. Edgington,TS. J. Lab. Clin. Med. 96:1-4, 1980.
74. Hiller E, Saal JG and Riethmuller G. Haemostasis 6:347-350, 1977.
75. Edwards RL, Rickles FR and Cronlund M. J. Lab. Clin. Med. 98:917-928, 1981.
76. Osterud B and Bjorklid E. Scand. J. Haematol. 29:175-184, 1982.
77. Osterud B and Bjorklid E. Biochem. Biophys. Res. Commun. 108:620-626, 1982.

78. Hudig D and Bajaj SP. Thromb. Res. 27:321-332, 1982.
79. Colucci M, Giavazzi R, Alessandri G, Semeraro N, Mantovani A and Donati MB. Blood 57:733-735, 1981.
80. Maynard JR, Heckman CA, Pitlick FA and Nemerson Y. J. Clin. Invest. 55:814-824, 1975.
81. Zeldis S, Nemerson Y and Pitlick FA. Science 175:766-768, 1972.
82. Maynard JR, Fintel DJ, Pitlick FA and Nemerson Y. Lab. Invest. 35:542-549, 1976.
83. Hasiba U, Poole M, Cross B and Gordon SG. Clin. Res. 31:39A, 1983.
84. Salem HH, Walters WA, Perkin JL, Handley CJ and Firkin BG. Br. J. Obstet. Gynaecol. 89:733-737, 1982.

CHAPTER 7. RELATIONSHIP BETWEEN PROCOAGULANT ACTIVITY AND METASTATIC CAPACITY OF TUMOR CELLS

MARIA BENEDETTA DONATI, NICOLA SEMERARO AND STUART G. GORDON

I. INTRODUCTION

The involvement of blood coagulation in cancer cell growth and dissemination has been suggested on the basis of a variety of clinical and laboratory observations. Malignant disease is associated with a high incidence of vascular thrombosis, as recognized by Trousseau more than a century ago (1), and this has been repeatedly demonstrated in many clinical studies by other investigators (2-6). Disseminated intravascular coagulation (DIC), probably the most complex and severe acquired coagulopathy, frequently occurs in patients bearing solid, metastatic tumors and several types of leukemias (4,7). Moreover, malignancy is one of the main risk factors which potentiate the incidence of thrombosis during post-operative or post-trauma periods (7). Clinical laboratory findings have demonstrated a number of hemostatic abnormalities indicating an overt or low grade activation of the clotting system in malignant disease, even in the absence of hemorrhagic or thrombotic signs (8-13). These laboratory changes include shortened partial thromboplastin time, elevated levels of one or more clotting factors, increased levels of soluble fibrin monomers and of fibrinopeptide A, reduced levels of antithrombin and depressed fibrinolysis. As an _in vivo_ sign of activation of the coagulation system, the turnover of radiolabeled platelets and/or fibrinogen is significantly enhanced in cancer patients with otherwise normal coagulation parameters (14-16). Studies in laboratory animals bearing different types of experimental tumors have confirmed the clinical observations by documenting the activation of blood clotting during the development of a tumor and growth of metastatic nodules (17-20).

Using histochemical, immunological or radioisotopic techniques, several investigators demonstrated fibrin deposition in and around tumors in both human and experimental malignancies (19,21-25). In experimental models, not only were primary tumors surrounded by a fibrin coat, but disseminated tumor cells were associated with platelets and fibrin threads to form clumps that occluded the microcirculation (25,26). These animal model studies, discussed later in this chapter, have offered the opportunity to analyze the possible correlations between tumor cell-induced hemostatic changes and the development of metastases (27-30).

II. FIBRIN AND TUMORS

Several hypotheses have been formulated about the possible role
of fibrin in the metastatic process. It has been proposed that fibrin
in and around primary tumors might provide a suitable stroma for tumor
cell invasion into normal tissues and serve as a stimulus for
neovascularization (31-33). In powerfully immunogenic tumors the
presence of a fibrin coat would represent a biological barrier against
the host's immunologic defense system (34). Moreover, the presence of
fibrin within tumor tissues could impair or delay the access of
chemotherapeutic agents to target cancer cells (35). On the basis of
pharmacological data with fibrinolysis inhibitors, other investigators
have postulated that fibrin deposition in tumors would impair
detachment of cells from primary tumors and might be part of a host
defense reaction against cancer cell invasion (26,34). Once tumor
cells have entered the circulation, the presence of fibrin and
platelet aggregates is unequivocally considered to favor the
initiation of metastatic growth by obstruction of the microcirculation
and extravasation of tumor cells (36-38).

The wide spectrum of hypotheses and suggestions about the role of
fibrin in cancer growth is due to differences in the animal models and
tumors studied, including the histological type of the tumor, the
route of cancer cell inoculation, the animal species used and the
immunological status of the host (17,39). As a general comment, most
of the assumptions present in the literature on this problem are
derived indirectly from pharmacological studies in which the
hemostatic system of the host has been altered by anticoagulants,
anti- or pro-fibrinolytic agents or platelet inhibiting drugs. A more
precise knowledge of the mechanisms leading to clotting inactivation
in malignancy would probably clarify the postulated role of fibrin in
tumor growth and metastasis formation.

There are numerous potential mechanisms by which blood
coagulation may be triggered in malignancy. Blood platelets may be
activated by contact with cancer cells (37) and this may lead to
unmasking or enhancement of platelet coagulant activities.
Alternatively, mononuclear cells (monocytes or macrophages) could play
a similar role since they can produce a procoagulant activity in
response to various stimuli (40-42). These cells are an integral part
of the lymphoreticular infiltrate of many experimental and human
tumors (43,44). Whether they do indeed contribute to fibrin
deposition within tumors is still a matter of controversy. Recently,
we demonstrated that mononuclear cells isolated from rabbit V2
carcinoma tissue had a much higher tissue factor activity than
circulating monocytes or peritoneal macrophages harvested from the
same animal (45). In contrast, macrophage infiltrate of four
different types of murine tumors was not only devoid of spontaneous
procoagulant activity but was even insensitive to in vitro stimulation
by endotoxin (46). Since most tumors undergo neovascularization, the
potentially abnormal endothelial lining of the neoformed vessels might
be responsible for activation of the contact system, thus triggering
blood clotting through the intrinsic pathway. Furthermore, the
destruction of normal tissues and subsequent liberation of tissue
enzymes and tissue factor during the natural course of tumor

development is another possible mechanism to trigger blood coagulation via the extrinsic pathway. Besides these relatively poorly defined mechanisms, the most probable cause of the initiation of blood coagulation in malignancy is the production of clot-promoting substances by cancer cells themselves. We shall discuss here the mechanisms of the best known cancer cell procoagulants and critically review the current status of evidence suggesting a link between the procoagulant activity of cancer cells and their metastatic capacity.

III. CANCER CELL PROCOAGULANTS

The existence of a procoagulant activity in cancer cells was first proposed by O'Meara and his associates on the basis of observations made on tumor tissue homogenates or extracts; they found a "cancer coagulative factor" in several human cancers (47,48) and subsequently in various types of experimental tumors. Some studies emphasized that greater amounts of thromboplastic activity were produced by malignant tissue than by benign or normal tissues (47,49,50), whereas in other studies no quantitative differences were found (51,52). More recent investigations have centered on the question of qualitative differences with respect to the mechanism(s) of activation of blood clotting between procoagulants from normal and malignant tissues or from different malignancies (51-56). Essentially two types of procoagulants have been described in tumor cells: tissue factor (tissue thromboplastin), a lipoprotein requiring coagulation factor VII for its expression, and cancer procoagulant, a proteolytic enzyme that directly activates factor X.

Tissue factor promotes clotting through the extrinsic pathway and is the procoagulant in some malignant cells from both solid tumors and leukemias. The promyelocyte represents the paradigmatic example in this context. Isolated leukemic promyelocytes have potent clot promoting activity which is antigenically related to brain tissue factor (57); this activity is mainly confined to the cell granular fraction. The presence of tissue factor in leukemic promyelocytes is compatible with the high incidence of the DIC syndrome in this type of leukemia. Tissue factor activity has been described in many experimental tumors. Evidence that this procoagulant influences the localization of fibrin in tumor tissue is supported by a study in which tumor tissue from a mouse mammary carcinoma with high thromboplastic activity had greater uptake of intravenously administered labeled fibrinogen than that of a mouse sarcoma with low thrombplastic activity (58).

Pineo et al. (59) reported a factor X activating procoagulant in extracts of mucus from nonpurulent chronic bronchitis secretions and suggested this procoagulant may be responsible for coagulation problems associated with mucus-producing adenocarcinomas. Subsequently, a procoagulant was purified and partially characterized from extracts of rabbit V2 carcinoma (60). This procoagulant, called cancer procoagulant, is discussed in more detail in Chapter 6 of this volume. It is a cysteine proteinase with a molecular weight of 68,000 daltons that initiates coagulation by directly activating factor X in the coagulation cascade (61). It has been identified enzymatically and immunologically in extracts of several human and animal tumors, in culture media from several transformed cells in tissue culture and associated with intact malignant cells, but not in normal tissue and cell counterparts of these malignant samples (51,52,62,63). Of particular importance to this discussion is the identification of this procoagulant in B16 mouse melanoma cells (62), Lewis lung carcinoma (3LL) cells (54,55), JW sarcoma cells and Ehrlich carcinoma (64) since some of these cells have been employed in the metastasis studies described below.

IV. ROLE OF PROCOAGULANTS IN METASTASIS

It is still relatively difficult, with the knowledge available, to establish the importance of tumor procoagulants in cancer invasion. As mentioned in our studies on murine tumors, we found the same degree of procoagulant activity in cells from both the primary tumor and metastatic nodules of 3LL and the same type of procoagulant in two metastasizing tumors (3LL and JW sarcoma) and in a non-metastasizing one, Ehrlich carcinoma. Gordon and Lewis (52) found no apparent correlation between the specific activity of cancer procoagulant and tumorigenicity of transformed fibroblasts. Thus, there is no evidence of a relationship between tumor cell procoagulant activity and invasive growth of the tumor.

In contrast, recent studies to identify properties of cancer cells that promote their metastatic capacity suggest a possible relationship to tumor cell procoagulants. The studies have generally utilized systems of cells derived from the same parental tumor but endowed with different metastatic potential. Such metastatic variants were selected either biologically (through in vitro/in vivo passages) or pharmacologically. There are two metastasis models that have been used in this type of study and, in this context, deserve some comments since they may significantly influence the type of results that were obtained. In the hematologic phase model, metastatic formation is monitored after intravenous injection of cancer cells. In this condition, cancer cells or tumor emboli are usually arrested in the lungs, the first capillary bed with which they come in contact. This artificial model reflects events in the final steps of the metastatic process including transport in the blood and arrest, invasion and growth in the target organ (Table 1). Thus, any pharmacological manipulation that enhances (or decreases) coagulation will probably promote (or diminish) metastasis by increasing (or decreasing) cell aggregation that may directly affect the arrest of the cells in the pulmonary capillaries (17). Furthermore, animals do not show any of the usual biological changes associated with the growth of the primary tumor such as changes in the plasma protein pattern or changes in the components of the hemostatic system (27,65). However, this model may mimic the dissemination process that occurs in selected clinical conditions, such as following surgical removal of solid tumors.

More authentic information on the metastatic process can be obtained from models where spontaneous metastases form through dissemination from a primary implantation site. This model reflects all the phases of tumor dissemination including detachment from the primary tumor, entry into the bloodstream, transport in blood and uptake by target organs (17; Table 1). The major disadvantage of this model is the inability to characterize the biochemical and molecular biological properties of the potentially metastatic cells shed from the primary tumor into the circulation.

Table 1. List of the Steps in the Metastatic Process.

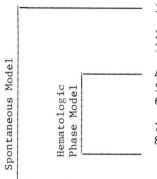

1. Tumor growth and invasion of normal tissue
2. Penetration of vascular basement membrane
3. Shedding of viable cells from the primary tumor into the bloodstream
4. Transport in circulation
5. Arrest of blood-borne tumor cells
6. Attachment to capillary subendothelium basement membrane
7. Migration into target tissues
8. Growth and vascularization of metastatic tumor

A. Hematologic Phase Model

Cellular procoagulant activity in metastasis formation was studied in the "hematologic phase" metastasis model. Two metastatic variants of B16 mouse melanoma were used, B16F1, with a low incidence of lung colonization, and B16F10, with a high incidence of lung colonization. B16 melanoma cells produce cancer procoagulant (62). The cellular procoagulant of the intact B16 cells was higher in the cells with higher metastatic potential. When both F1 and F10 cells were cultured for different periods of time (1-4 da) there was a progressive decrease in both procoagulant activity and metastatic potential (30). Regression analysis of the level of procoagulant activity and the number of lung tumor colonies gave a strong positive correlation (r = 0.9) (Figure 1). These results suggest that the cellular procoagulant activity and, therefore, the ability of the tumor cells to form fibrin is an important requirement for the steps of the metastatic process which follow the entry of tumor cells into the circulatory system.

B. Spontaneous Models

In a "spontaneous" metastasis model using 3LL, chronic vitamin K deficiency, induced either dietarily or pharmacologically, was able to depress both the cancer cell procoagulant activity and lung metastasis growth (66,67). In animals treated continuously with warfarin from

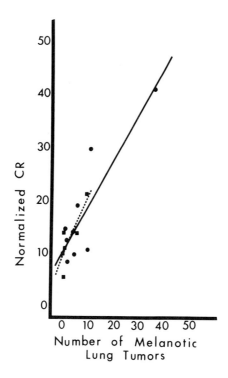

FIGURE 1. The Relationship between Cellular Procoagulant Activity and Metastatic Capacity. Cell suspensions of 50,000 viable B16F1 (■) or B16F10 (●) cells were assayed for procoagulant activity (Normalized CR) in a recalcification clotting time assay and injected into the tail vein of mice for analysis of metastatic capacity by counting the number of lung tumors 3 wk later. Each point represents the average of 2-4 values for procoagulant activity and the median of 4-5 values for metastatic capacity for the same cell suspension. The regression line for the B16F1 cells (----) is y = 1.26x + 9.11 (correlation coefficient r = 0.8) and for the B16F10 cells (———) is y = 1.07x + 9.84 (r = 0.9); these regression lines are not statistically different. Regression analysis of additional experiments (not shown) with B16F1 cells had r = 0.78 and with B16F10 had r = 0.66 and 0.99 (30).

da 7 after tumor implantation until death and animals fed a vitamin K-deficient diet starting 7 da before implantation, there was a significant reduction in the number and weight of lung metastases concomitant with a significant reduction in tumor cell procoagulant activity (Table 2). Administration of vitamin K to animals with pharmacologically induced or a dietary deficiency of vitamin K completely restored both the metastatic capacity and the procoagulant activity of tumor cells (Table 2). It should be mentioned that in the

Table 2. Effect of Dietary and Pharmacological Induction of Vitamin K-Deficiency on Prothrombin Complex Levels in Plasma Measured by Thrombotest and on Lewis Lung Carcinoma Cell Procoagulant Activity and Metastatic Potential[a].

Experimental Group	Thrombotest	Cell Procoagulant	Lung Metastasis Weight
Control	100[b]	100	100
Control + vit K	98-106	95-110	102-121
Dietary vit K def.	<5	10-15	10-18
Dietary vit K def. + vit K	90-110	100-108	98-109
Warfarin	<5	10-15	5-15
Warfarin + vit K	95-105	98-105	92-110

[a]For details see 66,67.

[b]Data are expressed as percent of controls (ranges of 10-12 values per group).

3LL bearing mice treated with another coumarin drug, phenprocoumon, the procoagulant activity of tumor extracts was also reduced as compared to extracts from untreated mice (68). The mechanism by which vitamin K deficiency exerts its antimetastatic activity has not been defined. Vitamin K is required for post-ribosomal γ-carboxylation of certain glutamic acid residues in different proteins to form the structural moiety responsible for their specific calcium binding activity (69). Among these proteins, the four clotting factors of the prothrombin complex are included. However, plasma anticoagulation resulting from impaired synthesis of these factors does not necessarily account for the antimetastatic effect of vitamin K deficiency. Indeed it is worth mentioning that hypocoagulability induced by other means (heparin or defibrinating enzymes) does not affect the metastatic behavior of the same cells (67,70). The case of heparin deserves some comment. As shown in Table 3, heparin treatment at doses inducing marked hypocoagulability (activated partial thromboplastin time of 2-3 fold the control values) did not affect either the procoagulant activity or the metastatic potential of 3LL cells. Thus, both warfarin and heparin induce systemic hypocoagulability but differ mainly in the fact that only warfarin affects a cellular procoagulant. This does not seem to be due to low plasma levels of vitamin K-dependent clotting factors since

Table 3. Effect of Warfarin and Heparin Anticoagulation on Lewis Lung Carcinoma Cell Procoagulant and Metastatic Potential[a].

Experimental Group	Plasma Anti-Coagulation		Cell Procoagulant (arbitrary units)	Lung Metastasis Weight (mg)
Control	Thrombotest (%)	98 ± 2[b]	102 ± 5	53 ± 9
Warfarin	Thrombotest (%)	<5	16 ± 1	7 ± 1
Control	APTT[c] (sec)	32 ± 4	100 ± 5	60 ± 7
Heparin	APTT (sec)	79 ± 11	104 ± 3	68 ± 8

[a]For details see 67,70.
[b]Means $\pm$ SE of 10-12 values per group.
[c]Activated partial thromboplastin time, APTT.

administration of a concentrate of mouse prothrombin complex normalized the activity of the plasma prothrombin complex without correcting cancer cell procoagulant activity (67). It is not yet known whether the antimetastatic activity of warfarin can be ascribed only to the inhibition by warfarin of the above mentioned cancer procoagulant or to the inhibition of some other vitamin K-dependent calcium-binding protein, which is still unknown but which could play an important role in cancer cell invasiveness (see also Chapter 17). Further evidence supporting the link between the antimetastatic effect of warfarin and its ability to reduce cancer cell procoagulant comes from the study of three other murine tumor models (Table 4). Both the JW sarcoma (29) and the B16 melanoma are susceptible to the antimetastatic effect of warfarin and both have a cancer procoagulant (the same as that found in 3LL cells).

Table 4. Type of Cancer Cell Procoagulant and Response to Warfarin in Different Murine Tumors. Warfarin effects plasma hypocoagulability, inhibition of cellular coagulation and inhibition of metastatic potential.

Tumor	Type of Procoagulant	Response to Warfarin		
		Plasma Prothrombin Complex Activity	Cell Procoagulant	Metastatic Potential
3LL	Factor X activator	↓	↓	↓
JWS	Factor X activator	↓	↓	↓
B16	Factor X activator	↓	↓	↓
mFS6	Tissue factor	↓	→	→

In contrast, we have studied the procoagulant activity and metastatic capacity of different sublines from a benzopyrene-induced fibrosarcoma, mFS6. Lung nodules isolated from animals with the same primary tumor weight and growth kinetics (28) had different metastatic capacities when reinjected into syngeneic hosts. The procoagulant activity of both the parent line and the sublines was identified as tissue factor. When compared to the parent line, the two sublines with the lowest metastatic capacity had 6-8 times greater procoagulant activity (72). Furthermore, neither metastatic growth nor tissue factor activity were affected by warfarin (71). In this model, it is tempting to speculate that fibrin deposition at the tumor site impairs detachment of cells from the primary tumor, reducing the number of tumor cells in the circulation of animals bearing the poorly metastatic line as compared to the highly metastatic line and thus reducing metastasis formation.

Two studies on the B16 melanoma (using both the "hematologic phase" model and the "spontaneous" model) and the pharmacological data in Lewis lung carcinoma support the concept that there is a direct association between the level of cellular cancer procoagulant activity and the metastatic capacity of these cancer cells. This appears to be true for both metastatic models indicating that the "arrest" of the blood-borne tumor cells appears to be an important (rate limiting) step in the final development of metastasis. Indeed, arrest is known to be favored by factors that increase blood coagulability and platelet aggregation or decrease fibrinolysis. However, in another model of spontaneous metastasis where tissue factor is the tumor cell procoagulant, the process of detachment (shedding) of cells from the primary tumor may be more influential in governing the metastatic capacity and importance of the cell procoagulant in the "arrest" step may be substantially less significant.

V. CLINICAL RELEVANCE

Although different types of technical procedures have allowed detection of fibrin in human tumors, it is still difficult to establish a clear correlation between cell procoagulant, fibrin deposition and metastases in patients. Recently, Zacharski and coworkers (73 and Chapter 24) have reported the occurrence of both fibrin and of the putative initiator of clot formation, tissue factor, in small cell carcinoma of the lung. The progression of the disease and the survival of patients with small cell carcinoma responded to warfarin anticoagulant therapy (74). It is not yet known whether warfarin would reduce both fibrin deposition and small cell carcinoma procoagulant activity.

In conclusion, there is now sufficient experimental evidence that fibrin interacts with cancer cells in vitro and that hemostatic changes occur during tumor growth and dissemination. There is also some indication that cancer cell procoagulants, by promoting fibrin deposition, play a role in metastasis formation. All of this, however, stems from observations made exclusively in experimental animals. Further basic and clinical research is warranted to support the concept that cancer procoagulant plays a role in the dissemination of human malignancies.

REFERENCES

1. Trousseau A. Clinique Medicale de l'Hotel-Dieu de Paris. J.B. Bailliere et Fils, Paris, 5th Edition 3:94, 1865.
2. Lieberman JS, Borrero J, Urdanetta E and Wright IS. J. Am Med. Assoc. 177:542-545, 1961.
3. Nusbacher J. N.Y. State J. Med. 64:2166, 1964.
4. Sack GH, Jr., Levin J and Bell W. Medicine 56:1-37, 1977.
5. Rickles FR and Edwards RL. Blood 62:14-31, 1983.
6. Gore JM, Appelbaum JS, Greene HL, Dexter L and Dalen JE. Ann. Intern. Med. 96:556-560, 1982.
7. Bick RL. Semin. Thromb. Hemostasis 5:1-26, 1978.
8. Donati MB, Poggi A and Semeraro N. In: Recent Advances in Blood Coagulation (Ed. Poller L), Churchill Livingstone, Edinburgh, pp. 227-259, 1981.
9. Sun NC, McAfee WM, Hum GJ and Weiner JM. Am. J. Clin. Pathol. 71:10-16, 1979.
10. Miller SP, Sanchez-Avalos J, Stefanski T and Zuckerman L. Cancer (Philadelphia) 20:1452-1465, 1967.
11. Hagedorn AB, Bowie EJW, Elveback LR and Owen CA. Mayo Clin. Proc. 49:649-653, 1974.
12. Rickles FR, Edwards RL, Barb C and Cronlund M. Cancer (Philadelphia) 51:301-307, 1983.
13. Myers TJ, Rickles FR, Barb C and Cronlund M. Blood 57:518-525, 1981.
14. Slichter SJ and Harker LA. Ann. N.Y. Acad. Sci. 230:252-261, 1974.
15. Lyman GH, Bettigole RE, Robson E, Ambrus JL and Urban H. Cancer (Philadelphia) 1:1113-1122, 1978.
16. Harker LA and Slichter SJ. N. Engl. J. Med. 287:999-1005, 1972.
17. Poggi A, Donati MB and Garattini S. In: Malignancy and the Hemostatic System (Eds. Donati MB, Davidson JF and Garattini S), Raven Press, New York, pp. 89-102, 1981.
18. Wood S, Jr. Bull Schweiz. Akad. Med. Wiss. 20:92-121, 1964.
19. Jones DS, Wallace AC and Fraser EE. J. Natl. Cancer Inst. 46:493-504, 1971.
20. Chew E and Wallace AC. Cancer Res. 36:1904-1909, 1976.
21. Robson EB, Murawski GF and Bettigole RE. Thromb. Haemostasis 37:484-508, 1977.
22. Day ED, Planinsek JA and Pressman D. J. Natl. Cancer Inst. 22:413-426, 1959.
23. Ogura T, Tsubura E and Yamamura Y. Gann 61:443, 1970.
24. Dewey WC, Bale WF, Rose RB and Marrack D. Acta Unio. Int. Cancrum 19:185, 1963.
25. Hiramoto R, Bernecky J, Jurandouski J and Pressman D. Cancer Res. 20:592-593, 1960.
26. Peterson HI. Cancer Treat. Rev. 4:213-217, 1977.
27. Poggi A, Polentarutti N, Donati MB, de Gaetano G and Garattini S. Cancer Res. 37:272-277, 1977.
28. Delaini F, Giavazzi R, De Bellis Vitti G, Alessandri G, Mantovani A and Donati MB. Br. J. Cancer 43:100-105, 1981.
29. Chmielevska J, Poggi A, Mussoni L, Donati MB and Garattini S. Eur. J. Cancer 16:1399-1407, 1980.
30. Gilbert LC and Gordon SG. Cancer Res. 43:536-540, 1983.
31. O'Meara RAQ. Thromb. Diath. Haemorrh. Suppl. 28:137-146, 1968.
32. Ambrus JL, Ambrus CM, Pickern J, Soldes S and Bross I. J. Med. 6:433-458, 1975.

33. Day Ed, Planinsek JA and Pressman D. J. Natl. Cancer Inst. 22:413–426, 1959.
34. Dvorak HF, Dvorak AM, Marseau FJ, Wiberg L and Churchill WH. J. Natl. Cancer Inst. 62:1459–1472, 1979.
35. Hilgard P and Thornes RD. Eur. J. Cancer 12:755–762, 1976.
36. Tanaka N, Ogawa H, Tanaka K, Kinjo M and Kohga S. Invasion Metastasis 1:149–157, 1981.
37. Gasic GJ, Boettiger D, Catalfamo JL, Gasic TB and Stewart GJ. In: Platelets: A Multidisciplinary Approach (Eds. de Gaetano G and Garattini S), Raven Press, New York, pp. 447–456, 1978.
38. Kinjo M. Br. J. Cancer 38:293–301, 1978.
39. Donati MB, Rotilio D, Delaini F, Giavazzi R, Mantovani A and Poggi A. In: Interaction of Platelets and Tumor Cells (Ed. Jamieson G), Alan R. Liss, New York, pp. 159–176, 1982.
40. Edwards RL and Rickles FR. Lymphokine Rep. 1:181–210, 1980.
41. Edgington TS, Levy GA, Schwartz BS and Fair DS. In: Advances in Immunopathology (Ed. Weigle), Elsevier North Holland, Amsterdam, pp. 173–196, 1981.
42. Edwards RL, Rickles FR and Cronlund M. J. Lab. Clin. Med. 98:917–928, 1981.
43. Evans R. Transplantation 14:468–473, 1972.
44. Hayry P and Totterman TH. Eur. J. Immunol. 8:866–871, 1978.
45. Lorenzet R, Peri G, Locati D, Allavena P, Colucci M, Semeraro N, Mantovani A and Donati MB. Blood (in press), 1983.
46. Guarini A, Acero R, Lorenzet R, Mantovani A, Semeraro N and Donati MB. Thromb. Haemostasis 50:148, 1983.
47. O'Meara RAQ. Ir. J. Med. Sci. 394:474–479, 1958.
48. Boggust WA, O'Brein DJ, O'Meara RAQ and Thornes RD. Ir. J. Med. Sci. 477:131, 1967.
49. Svanberg L. Thromb. Res. 6:307, 1975.
50. Frank AL and Holyoke ED. Int. J. Cancer 3:677, 1968.
51. Gordon SG, Franks JJ and Lewis BJ. J. Natl. Cancer Inst. 62:773–776, 1979.
52. Gordon SG and Lewis BJ. Cancer Res. 38:2467–2472, 1978.
53. Dvorak HF, Quay SC, Orenstein NS, Dvorak AM, Hahn P, Bitzer AM and Carvalho AC. Science 212:923–924, 1981.
54. Curatolo L, Colucci M, Cambini AL, Poggi A, Morasca L, Donati MB and Semeraro N. Br. J. Cancer 40:228–233, 1979.
55. Hilgard P and Whur P. Br. J. Cancer 41:642–643, 1980.
56. Colucci M, Giavazzi R, Alessandri G, Semeraro N, Mantovani A and Donati MB. Blood 57:733–735, 1981.
57. Gouault–Heilmann M, Chardon E, Sultan C and Josso F. Br. J. Haematol. 30:151–158, 1975.
58. Peterson HI, Appelgren KL and Rosengren BHO. Eur. J. Cancer 5:535–542, 1969.
59. Pineo GF, Regoeczi E, Hatton MWC and Brain MC. J. Lab. Clin. Med. 82:255–266, 1973.
60. Gordon SG, Franks JJ and Lewis BJ. Thromb. Res. 6:127–137, 1975.
61. Gordon SG and Cross BA. J. Clin. Invest. 67:1665–1671, 1981.
62. Gordon SG, Gilbert LC and Lewis BJ. Thromb. Res. 26:379–387, 1982.
63. Gordon SG. J. Histochem. Cytochem. 29:457–463, 1981.
64. Curatolo L, Colucci M, Cambini AL, Poggi A, Morasca L, Donati MB and Semeraro N. Br. J. Cancer 40:228–233, 1979.
65. Donati MB and Poggi A. Br. J. Haematol. 44:173–182, 1980.
66. Delaini F, Colucci M, De Bellis Vitti G, Locati D, Poggi A, Semeraro N and Donati MB. Thromb. Res. 24:263–267, 1981.
67. Colucci M, Delaini F, De Bellis Vitti G, Locati D, Poggi A, Semeraro N and Donati MB. Biochem. Pharmacol. 32:1689–1691, 1983.

68. Hilgard P. In: Malignancy and the Hemostatic System (Eds. Donati MB, Davidson JF and Garattini S), Raven Press, New York, pp. 103–112, 1981.
69. Stenflo J and Suttie JW. Annu. Rev. Biochem. 46:157–172, 1977.
70. Donati MB, Mussoni L, Poggi A, de Gaetano G and Garattini S. Eur. J. Cancer 14:343–347, 1978.
71. Lorenzet R, Bottazzi B, Locati D, Colucci M, Mantovani A, Semeraro N and Donati MB. Eur. J. Cancer (in press), 1983.
72. Colucci M, Giavazzi R, Alessandri G, Semeraro N, Mantovani A and Donati MB. Blood 57:733–735, 1981.
73. Zacharski LR, Schned AR and Sorenson GD. Cancer Res. (in press), 1983.
74. Zacharski LR, Henderson WG, Rickles FR, Forman WB, Cornell CJ, Jr., Jackson Forcier R, Edwards R, Headly E, Kim SH, O'Donnell JR, O'Dell R, Tornyos K and Kwaan HC. J. Am. Med. Assoc. 245:831–835, 1981.

CHAPTER 8. FIBRIN FORMATION: IMPLICATIONS FOR TUMOR GROWTH AND METASTASIS

HAROLD F. DVORAK, DONALD R. SENGER AND ANN M. DVORAK

I. INTRODUCTION AND HISTORICAL BACKGROUND

Whether undertaken by pathologists, immunologist, or biochemists, studies of tumor biology have traditionally concentrated on the malignant cells themselves, their abnormal morphology, their altered metabolism and more recently, their panoply of surface antigens. Yet, tumors are comprised not only of malignant cells but also of stroma. In the case of many solid tumors stroma may actually comprise the bulk of the mass perceived as tumor with the naked eye. In any event, tumors are dependent on stroma for nutrient supply and removal of metabolic wastes. Tumor stroma is not a homogeneous entity but rather consists of several connective tissue elements including collagen of several types, elastin, fibronectin, glycosaminoglycans, interstitial fluid, new blood vessels and, as we shall discuss in this chapter, fibrin.

Fibrin occupies a somewhat enigmatic position among tumor stromal elements. Although a relationship between malignancy and coagulation was suggested by Trousseau (1) more than a century ago, the first reports of fibrin deposits in and around tumors date back only about 25 years (2,3). One major reason for this delay is the fact that fibrin is not readily visualized in tissues by routine histological methods unless it is present in relatively large amounts, amounts much larger than are present in most tumors. Furthermore, so-called "special stains" for fibrins, such as phosphotungstic acid, lead to variable and often unreproducible results and frequently do not stain tumor-associated fibrin. As a result, the original claims of fibrin deposition in tumors, based on routine light microscopy (4), were not convincing, particularly in the absence of photomicrographs illustrating such deposits. The first satisfactory evidence for the presence of fibrin in tumor stroma was indirect, coming from the studies of Pressman and his colleagues who showed that both radiolabeled fibrinogen and antibodies directed against fibrinogen/fibrin were selectively localized in tumors when injected systemically into experimental animals (5,6). Direct demonstration of fibrin in tumor stroma required the development of new immunohisto-chemical approaches and once again Pressman's group led the way by demonstrating fibrin in several animal and human tumors with antibodies to fibrinogen/fibrin by the immunofluorescence technique (7,8). To date, immunohistochemistry (immunofluorescence or more recently immunoperoxidase) and transmission electron microscopy remain the most reliable and sensitive methods for definitively demonstrating fibrin in tissues, benign or malignant.

Although fibrin had been demonstrated in only a handful of tumors in these early studies, a number of investigators jumped to the conclusion that fibrin must be important to tumor biology and made extensive attempts to treat tumors with anticoagulant drugs, notably coumarin derivatives and heparin. The results obtained were quite variable and even contradictory, varying from reports of dramatic cures to enhanced solid tumor growth (for review see 9 and 10). Unfortunately, the scientific quality of this work was uneven and at least four fundamental conceptual problems were overlooked. 1) It is relatively easy to inhibit intravascular coagulation with drugs such as warfarin or heparin; it is quite another matter to prevent the clotting of extravasated plasma proteins in tissues outside the circulation at sites of solid tumor growth. 2) Monitoring the status of plasma anticoagulation provides little information about clotting in tissues. 3) The studies assumed that any effects observed on tumor growth or metastasis reflected the action of the drugs tested on the coagulation system. However, both warfarin and heparin may have diverse effects unrelated to clotting on a wide variety of cell systems, especially in the high doses that were employed (11,12). 4) Finally, all of these studies neglected to monitor the variable actually being tested, i.e., they failed to determine whether the solid tumors under study in fact contained fibrin in their stroma and, if so, whether the anticoagulant drugs employed reduced this fibrin or altered its nature.

In addition, several investigations pointed specifically to a role for fibrin in tumor metastasis (10,12-16). Following intravenous injection of tumor cells in experimental animals, fibrin was observed by immunohistochemistry and by electron microscopy associated with tumor cell clumps that lodged in lung capillaries prior to implantation. These findings were in agreement with reports suggesting that: 1) tumor cells possess potent procoagulant activity (see below) and 2) anticoagulant therapy may reduce the incidence of colonization in the lung following intravenous tumor cell injection (16). This type of study is open to criticism. Foreign particles of many types, not just tumor cells, may become coated with fibrin when injected into the blood and the possibility that normal cells become similarly coated was not examined. Thus, existing evidence does not exclude the possibility that fibrin deposits in relation to metastasizing tumor cells in the circulation represent only an epiphenomenon or even an experimental artifact. Whether fibrin deposition characterizes and/or abets metastatic tumor implantation, therefore, is open to question and can be settled only by study of spontaneous models of tumor metastasis. Here the results are mixed and in some instances heparin, for example, may actually enhance spontaneous metastasis (12). Reassuringly, it can be stated that fibrin deposition is a feature of spontaneous metastasis in at least one such tumor model, the murine Lewis lung carcinoma. This tumor metastasizes to the lungs several weeks after implantation in the footpad and both metastases and primary tumor are characterized by abundant fibrin deposits (I. Goldberg and H.F. Dvorak, unpublished data). Taken together, it is fair to state that at present there is no overwhelming evidence to implicate fibrin in tumor metastasis. On the other hand, there is evidence, as this chapter will develop, that fibrin is present in many growing tumors and that tumor cells are responsible for its deposition. It follows, therefore, that students of tumor biology will want to learn as much as possible about fibrin, as about any other component of the tumor microenvironment, because such studies may open important new avenues to controlling both malignant growth and metastasis.

II. THE NATURE OF FIBRIN DEPOSITS IN TISSUE

The term fibrin is often used imprecisely and indeed does not describe a single chemical entity. Fibrinogen, the precursor of fibrin, is a 340 K dalton hexamer, composed of three pairs of nonidentical polypeptide chains (A α, B β and γ chains) covalently bound together in a dimeric structure by disulfide bonds (17). In normal clotting (18,19) thrombin splits off, in sequence, fibrinopeptides A and B from fibrinogen leading to the formation of soluble fibrin monomers which join together to form insoluble, non-crosslinked fibrin polymers. Non-crosslinked fibrin is held together only by noncovalent bonds. Only with the further action of clotting factor XIII$_a$, a transglutaminase also activated by thrombin, does such fibrin become covalently crosslinked via the gamma and alpha chains to yield the urea insoluble molecule commonly referred to as fibrin (20,21). However, factor XIII$_a$, if present in the absence of thrombin, may itself polymerize fibrinogen to form a gel, a product that retains fibrinopeptides A and B (20). Also, fibrinogen and both crosslinked and non-crosslinked forms of fibrin are readily degraded by proteolytic enzymes and particularly by plasmin. Plasmin is a serine proteinase that is generated from the circulating plasma protein zymogen, plasminogen, by limited proteolytic cleavage (22-24). The several enzymes generating plasmin, collectively termed plasminogen activators, are also serine proteinases. Plasmin digests fibrinogen in a well-defined series of steps generating sequentially X, Y, D and E fragments as well as smaller peptides (25). Certain of these degradation fragments, as well as the fibrinopeptides released during clotting, have known biological activities including the capacity to inhibit coagulation, to contract smooth muscle, to serve a chemotactic function, to suppress the immune response and to increase microvascular permeability (25-36).

Which of these molecules are recognized by electron microscopy or by immunohistochemistry? Only incomplete answers are available at present. The nature of the "fibrin" deposited in tumors, or for that matter the "fibrin" deposited in blood vessels or tissues in a variety of disease states, has not been well characterized, a surprising fact in view of the ready availability of biochemical techniques for doing so (37,38). Electron microscopic identification of fibrils with characteristic periodicity certainly distinguishes insoluble fibrin from soluble fibrinogen but the electron microscopic appearance of partially hydrolyzed fibrin or of factor XIII$_a$ polymerized fibrinogen has not yet been determined. On the other hand, the antibodies used in immunofluorescence react strongly with fibrinogen, with non-crosslinked and crosslinked fibrin and with certain of their degradation products (37,38). Immunofluorescence performed on unfixed frozen sections involves washing steps in aqueous buffers that remove all, or nearly all, unbound soluble molecules and therefore fibrinogen as well as soluble fibrinogen and fibrin degradation products should be washed away leaving behind only insoluble fibrins. Reassurance of at least this degree of specificity comes from practical experience with immunofluorescence methodology where in fact highly specific antifibrinogen antibodies stain fibrillar material that resembles crosslinked fibrin by other methodologies (1 μm Epon sections, electron microscopy, urea insolubility) and not fibrinogen (plasma in the lumens of blood vessels doesn't generally stain). However, it must be admitted that we do not presently know the exact chemical nature of the insoluble fibrins observed in tissue sections with antifibrinogen antibodies and the term "fibrin" used throughout this chapter must be interpreted by the reader in that light.

III. FIBRIN IS A COMPONENT OF THE TUMOR MICROENVIRONMENT

As noted above, there have been several scattered studies over the past few decades illustrating the presence of fibrin in one or another tumor; however, there were no reports providing a detailed anatomic localization of fibrin within individual tumors, documenting an evolution of fibrin deposits with tumor growth or even surveying a large number of tumors, particularly autochthonous human tumors, to determine whether fibrin is a common or uncommon feature of tumor growth. About five years ago, our laboratory decided to investigate these questions, studying in depth several transplantable animal tumors as well as certain common human tumors.

A. Guinea Pig Hepato (bile duct) Carcinomas

Initially we undertook a detailed longitudinal study of two well characterized transplantable guinea pig tumors, the line 1 and line 10 hepato (bile duct) carcinomas originally induced with the water soluble carcinogen diethylnitrosamine and syngeneic in inbred strain 2 guinea pigs (39-41). Among other goals, we sought to determine whether fibrin was deposited in such tumors and, if so, how early in tumor growth such deposits appeared, how long they persisted, where they were located and how they changed in quantity and quality with time. In fact, both tumors were found to become invested in a fibrin gel within hours of transplantation of even small cell numbers (e.g., 500,000), a development accompanied, and apparently preceded, by permeability changes in nearby blood vessels. However, subsequent events were different for the two tumors and therefore they will be considered separately.

1. Line 1 carcinomas. In the case of line 1 tumors, fibrin was abundant and tumors appeared as largely translucent, gelatinous papules enveloping centrally placed, irregularly shaped clumps of tumor cells. The bulk of the mass perceived as tumor by the naked eye, in fact 80-95% of the tumor mass as measured by planimetry, was comprised of fibrin gel, a translucent meshwork composed of more or less regularly separated fibrin strands oriented in three dimensions

and interspersed within edema fluid. Only occasional inflammatory cells penetrated this gel, predominantly neutrophils on day 1 and including more lymphocytes, monocytes and macrophages on subsequent days; however, the infiltration by inflammatory cells was at all times relatively minor. Scattered new fibroblasts first appeared at about 48 hr after transplantion, growing from the periphery into the fibrin gel.

Striking microvascular changes accompanied the development and evolution of the fibrin gel. Small blood vessels were leaky and became intensely labeled when colloidal carbon was administered intravenously. In addition to becoming labeled with carbon, the normally flattened and inconspicuous endothelial cells of venules located about the fibrin gel became activated as early as 24 hr after tumor implantation and displayed mitotic figures and increased ^{3}H-thymidine incorporation by radioautography. Microvascular endothelial cell proliferation was maximal at 48 hr at which time new vessel sprouts began to penetrate the fibrin gel.

The tumor mass, whose stroma was still composed largely of fibrin gel, developed an increasingly rubbery consistency by da 6. Fibroblasts proliferated extensively and invaded the fibrin gel replacing it with granulation tissue, the highly vascularized young connective tissue characteristic of wound healing. Collagen was laid down giving line 1 tumors the appearance of a scirrhous carcinoma; nonetheless, abundant fibrin remained evident between collagen fibers. This pattern of growth persisted until the tumor was rejected by a cellular immunological mechanism.

2. Line 10 carcinomas. In contrast to line 1, the highly malignant line 10 carcinoma grew progressively in strain 2 guinea pigs while maintaining a more or less constant histological pattern at all stages of growth. Tumors were composed of rapidly dividing, pleomorphic tumor cells, including giant cells and glandular elements with only minimal stroma. A fibrin investment, though small compared to line 1 tumors, was invariably present. Detectable as early as 8 hr after transplantion, the fibrin gel persisted as a thin, enveloping rim. In contrast to the more abundant fibrin of line 1 tumors that of line 10 carcinomas accounted for less than 10% of the tumor mass and never became extensively organized by fibrous connective tissue. Activation of the microvasculature and angiogenesis resembled that occurring in line 1 tumors. Line 10 tumors excited little in the way of an inflammatory cell response and the immune response proved ineffective in limiting tumor growth.

B. Mouse Breast Carcinomas

Confirmatory results were obtained with the TA3-St breast carcinoma which acquired an abundant fibrin gel within hours of transplantion into syngeneic strain A mice (H.F. Dvorak, unpublished data). Equally interesting results were obtained in studies of the malignant breast tumors arising from the D2 hyperplastic alveolar nodule (D2 HAN) line many weeks after transplantation of D2 HAN to the dermal breast fat pads of virgin female mice. The malignant tumors that arose from these HAN regularly exhibited fibrin deposits by immunofluorescence whereas the premalignant HAN did not (B. Asch and H.F. Dvorak, unpublished data).

C. Human Tumors

Taken together, the detailed animal tumor studies cited above suggested that fibrin is one of the earliest and most consistent markers of malignant tumor stroma, appearing within hours of implantation and persisting throughout the course of tumor growth. Nonetheless, it would be dangerous to draw sweeping conclusions from the study of a handful of animal tumors and we therefore extended this line of investigation to human tumors, selecting infiltrating ductal carcinomas of the female breast and Hodgkin's disease for detailed study. An obvious limitation of studies of human tumors is that examination usually can be performed at only a single, arbitrarily selected and generally rather late stage in tumor biology – at the time of surgical intervention. As a result, little can be said about fibrin deposition at early stages of carcinogenesis or about changes in the amount and distribution of fibrin at various stages in the evolution of tumor growth.

1. Infiltrating ductal carcinomas of the human female breast (42). In agreement with many previous histologic descriptions, this, the most common form of human breast cancer, consists of variably sized groupings of anaplastic epithelial cells separated by abundant fibrous stroma. By orienting sections with care we were able to distinguish peripheral from more central portions of each tumor and to identify the tumor-host interface. Fibrin deposits were found in all of the 14 carcinomas studied. Immunofluorescence with highly specific antisera provided the simplest and most sensitive approach for reliable identification and rough quantitation of fibrin in breast tumors and was positive in all 10 carcinomas to which it was applied. Fibrin was also identified by electron microscopy by virtue of its fibrillar structure and characteristic periodicity.

Fibrin was most abundant in the loose connective tissue at the tumor-host junction and in the immediately surrounding benign breast tissue. It appeared as a fibrillar meshwork inserted between bundles of collagen and fat, independent of the extent of lymphocyte infiltration. In fact, although sometimes traversed by a few fibrin strands, areas of lymphocyte infiltration were generally free of fibrin deposition. Peripherally situated tumor cell nests were often enveloped by a prominent rim of fibrin that separated them from the surrounding connective tissue. Sometimes fibrin strands also penetrated into tumor nests and surrounded smaller groups of tumor cells; however, individual tumor cells were usually not enveloped by fibrin. Small peripheral tumor clumps that were surrounded by numerous lymphoid cells were often enveloped by particularly prominent bands of fibrin-staining material that separated them from the lymphocytes.

Fibrin staining was less extensive in more central portions of the tumor. Here the fibrin deposits surrounding tumor clumps were less abundant, often discontinuous and not infrequently lacking altogether. However, small patchy fibrin deposits remained in the abundant fibrous stroma even in central portions of the tumor.

For comparison with intraductal carcinomas, benign breast tissue (normal, fibrocystic disease, fibroadenoma) was also examined. Immunofluorescence staining for fibrin was negative in normal breast tissue and also in fibrocystic disease. However, moderate fibrin staining was observed in 4 of the 5 fibroadenomas studied. Patchy fibrin deposits analogous to those described in ductal carcinomas were observed at the tumor-breast junction and to a lesser extent in the mature fibrous connective tissue of the tumor stroma. In the single fibroadenoma that was fibrin-negative, the stroma was almost completely hyalinized and epithelial elements were sparse suggesting that the tumor was dormant.

2. <u>Hodgkin's disease and other malignant lymphomas</u> (43). Fibrin deposition was found in all of a series of 17 Hodgkin's disease specimens (15 cases) examined, representing involved lymph nodes from twelve patients and splenic tumors obtained at staging laparotomy from five patients. Two distinct staining patterns were observed: between cells and along collagen fibers. In addition, fibrin deposits were found in areas of tumor necrosis. In cellular areas, a fine fibrillar staining pattern was regularly observed around and between individual cells, aggregating focally into coarse, amorphous deposits. Similar appearing material, shown to represent fibrin, had previously been described in germinal centers of reactive follicles from hyperplastic lymph nodes (44), a finding we confirmed (43). Fibrin deposits were also associated with both long spaced and normal collagen. Fibrin was particularly abundant in areas of newly formed collagen where active fibroblasts and myofibroblasts were numerous. Fibrin became progressively less abundant as collagen fibrils became denser and more mature. Tumors in the spleen stained similarly to those in lymph nodes. It was possible to recognize involved areas of spleen at low magnification by the bright, coarse, fibrillar deposits of fibrin situated between cells and along collagen bundles.

By transmission electron microscropy fibrin appeared as multiple dense, irregularly oriented strands closely associated with the surfaces of individual small and medium lymphocytes, without evidence of associated cell injury or tissue necrosis. In many instances these deposits encased, constricted or deeply invaginated individual lymphocytes. However, fibrin always remained extracellular; phagocytosis of fibrin was not observed. Fibrin was also not observed in intimate association with classical Reed-Sternberg cells; however, some large mononuclear cells, corresponding to "atypical" or "mononuclear" Reed-Sternberg cells, were enveloped in fibrin deposits.

Antibody to fibronectin, when applied to lymph nodes or spleens involved with Hodgkin's disease, produced a reticulin and vascular basement membrane pattern of staining similar to that seen in reactive lymphoid tissues. Some but not all of the intercellular fibrillar material which stained with antibody to fibrin also stained with antifibronectin antibodies; however, the amorphous, eosinophilic, intercellular deposits generally did not stain or stained much more weakly for fibronectin than for fibrin. In general there was less staining for fibronectin but considerably more staining for fibrin in Hodgkin's disease-involved areas of spleen or lymph nodes than in normal or reactive lymphoid tissues.

Three of six non-Hodgkin's lymphomas we examined contained extracellular material which stained with antisera to fibrinogen. All three were large cell lymphomas: two diffuse and one nodular histiocytic lymphoma. Staining took the form of fine intercellular fibrils and scattered coarse deposits. In one case with extensive sclerosis there was also bright staining along collagen bands. The other three cases had either no definite staining for fibrin or only a few intercellular flecks or fibrils.

D. Conclusions

Certain conclusions follow from the preceding discussion. 1) Many, perhaps most, solid malignant autochthonous and transplanted tumors in both man and experimental animals contain fibrin deposits. 2) The amount of fibrin deposited, as a fraction of the total tumor mass, is highly variable but characteristic and relatively constant for a given tumor. 3) Fibrin deposits are often concentrated about clumps of carcinoma cells and particularly at the tumor-host interface. Fibrin is also associated with newly deposited collagen fibers in desmoplastic tumors. In Hodgkin's disease fibrin is also found between and around individual small and medium lymphocytes, cells thought to represent an inflammatory response to the presumed malignant cell element, Reed-Sternberg cells, which were were not enveloped by fibrin. 4) Fibrin was also observed in at least some benign tumors. 5) It seems unlikely that the fibrin observed about tumors represents artifact. The possibility of coagulation occurring in tissues during the course of transplantation or of surgical removal seems unlikely because: a) as noted, the extent and pattern of fibrin deposition were different and characteristic for each individual tumor type, e.g., line 1 and line 10 tumors, growing in solid form in the subcutaneous space, could be distinguished solely on the basis of their characteristic, and very different, patterns of fibrin deposition, b) transplants of HAN (mouse) to the breast or of normal fibroblasts (guinea pig) to the subcutaneous space did not induce persistent fibrin deposition, c) however, tumors arising spontaneously in the mouse breast weeks to months after HAN implantation did exhibit fibrin and d) finally, fibrin staining is not observed by immunofluorescence in normal tissues taken routinely nor is it found in a wide variety of surgical specimens where the underlying pathology would not have been expected to induce clotting in vivo. 6) Though only a small number of tumor types were compared, a correlation was found between the amount of fibrin deposited about transplanted tumors early and the extent of subsequent desmoplasia, i.e., the scirrhous line 1 tumor was characterized at early intervals of growth by abundant fibrin deposits and later by abundant desmoplasia, the medullary line 10 tumor by little early fibrin or late desmoplasia. 7) No simple relationship was found between the amount of fibrin deposited and tumor malignancy, e.g., both highly malignant human breast carcinomas and the relatively nonmalignant line 1 guinea pig bile duct carcinoma were characterized by abundant fibrin, whereas the highly malignant guinea pig line 10 bile duct carcinoma had relatively little associated fibrin. 8) Inflammatory cells did not effectively penetrate the fibrin gel or fibrous connective tissue enveloping any of the tumors studied. Nonetheless, host immunologic defense mechanisms were able to reject at least some tumors (i.e., guinea pig line 1) by causing profound damage to the blood vessels supplying the tumor and leading to massive ischemic tumor necrosis in a manner similar to that involved in the rejection of vascularized skin allografts (45).

IV. TUMOR SECRETED MEDIATORS CAN GENERATE TUMOR ASSOCIATED FIBRIN DEPOSITS

Granting the likelihood that fibrin deposition is a feature of the growth of many malignant tumors, the question arises as to how such fibrin deposits develop. In theory, tumor cells could themselves synthesize fibrinogen but this possibility seems unlikely as a general principle. Indeed, fibrinogen synthesis has only been reported in the case of well differentiated hepatic cells and would be most unexpected for a wide variety of tumor cells arising in multiple body organs and tissues (46). Far more plausible, in our view, is the possibility that tumor fibrin is derived from plasma fibrinogen. Fibrinogen normally circulates in the plasma at a concentration of about 3 mg/ml and enters normal tissue at a very low rate, one that is significantly lower than that of other plasma proteins such as albumin (37). Therefore, deposition of fibrin in solid tumors requires at minimum an increase in normal vascular permeability to plasma proteins and a mechanism for clotting extravasated fibrinogen. The pathogenesis of tumor associated fibrin deposition thus revolves itself into an understanding of the mechanisms by which these two events are accomplished and regulated. Although other possibilities exist (3,38,47) it seems likely that tumors frequently effect fibrin deposition by secreting mediators that enhance vascular permeability and that serve as tissue procoagulants (41,46,47). Recent work has identified and characterized mediators that can account for the fibrin deposits found about tumors:

A. Tumor Secreted Vascular Permeability Factor (PF)

Several years ago we reported that line 10 guinea pig tumor cells cultured for several hours or longer in serum free medium released a factor that enhanced the permeability of normal blood vessels (41,46). Activity was measured using the Miles assay, a sensitive test of vascular permeability in which a dye (such as Evans' blue) is introduced into the circulation of a normal guinea pig and putative permeability factors and various control substances are injected intradermally in the depilated flank skin. Prominent blue spots appear within a few minutes at sites of injection of active substances and activity may be quantitated by dilution until bluing activity is lost. Alternatively, or in addition, iodinated albumin may be administered intravenously along with dye and skin test sites removed and counted for radioactivity as a measure of permeability.

Production of tumor permeability factor (PF) activity was found to be progressive with time of culture and was inhibited when cells were cultured at 4°C or in the presence of puromycin. PF activity apparently did not involve histamine in that it was not inhibited by antihistamines nor did PF provoke histamine release from guinea pig basophils nor degranulation of skin mast cells.

Recently Senger et al. (48,49) greatly extended these initial findings. First, they showed that many tumor cells or cell lines derived from animal species secreted permeability factors in culture. Second, they purified the PF from serum free culture medium of one tumor, guinea pig line 10, some 1,200 fold to virtual homogeneity by a series of column chromatography steps and by SDS polyacrylamide gel electrophoresis. Purified line 10 PF accounts for all of the permeability increasing activity found in line 10 culture supernatants, has an apparent MW of 34-42 K (exhibiting some microheterogeneity) and is active in the picomolar range, about 800 times as active as histamine on a molar basis.

In addition, Senger et al. (48,49) considered the possibility that tumor-secreted permeability factors might have a role in tumor ascites formation. Initial experiments were conducted to determine whether in fact ascites tumor bearing animals exhibited increased permeability of peritoneal lining vessels. Two lines of evidence indicated that such was the case. First, guinea pigs, Syrian hamsters and mice bearing syngeneic ascites tumors (line 10, HSV-NIL8 and TA3-St, respectively) were injected intravenously with colloidal carbon as a probe of leaky blood vessels. Many venules of the peritoneal wall, diaphragm, mesentery and gastrointestinal serosal surfaces were heavily labeled with colloidal carbon whereas comparable vessels in control animals were not. More quantitative evidence was obtained using ^{125}I-labeled serum albumin (^{125}I-HSA) as a probe to measure influx or efflux into or out of the peritoneal cavity. A markedly increased influx of ^{125}I-HSA was evident in the peritoneal cavity as early as one hour after intraperitoneal injection of guinea pig line 10 tumor cells and this influx progressed with tumor growth; in contrast, efflux of ^{125}I-HSA from the peritoneal cavities of line 10 bearing guinea pigs was not significantly altered, even with progressive tumor growth.

Taken together, these observations suggested that tumor ascites is attributable to permeability alterations in peritoneal lining vessels. To determine whether a soluble factor such as the PF purified from line 10 tissue culture might be responsible, Senger et al. (48,49) tested various tumor ascites fluids for permeability enhancing activity using the Miles assay. Cell-free tumor ascites fluids from line 10 and line 1 guinea pig and TA3-St mouse carcinomas and the HSV-NIL8 hamster sarcoma all dramatically and rapidly increased local subcutaneous vascular permeability. By contrast, platelet poor plasmas from the same species or oil induced guinea pig peritoneal exudate fluids expressed little or no such activity. The permeability factor found in line 10 ascites fluid was then purified using the same columns and electrophoretic conditions used to purify the line 10 PF produced in tissue culture. The line 10 ascites PF behaved identically in all of these steps suggesting that the molecules produced in vitro and in vivo were identical. Further evidence for identity was obtained by raising an antibody in rabbits to the PF produced by line 10 cells in vitro. This antibody bound and neutralized virtually all of the vessel permeability increasing activity in line 10, line 1 and 104C 1 guinea pig fibrosarcoma conditioned medium but not the low levels of activity released by guinea pig fibroblasts or smooth muscle cells. The antibody also neutralized the PF activity found in line 10 and line 1 tumor ascites. Initially it was thought that the antibody directed against line 10 PF was species specific, i.e., that it reacted only with guinea pig tumor permeability factors. More recent evidence suggests that this antibody also neutralizes tumor PFs of rat origin, raising the possibility that tumors of several species secrete an antigenically related molecule.

Attempts were next made to characterize the line 10 PF. As noted earlier, line 10 PF was apparently not histamine nor did it act by releasing histamine from basophils and mast cells. Light and electron microscopic studies indicated that line 10 PF did not damage local blood vessels nor did it provoke an inflammatory cell infiltration. Vessels responded equally well to multiple challenges with equivalent doses of line 10 PF administered 30 min apart. The effect of a single intradermal injection was rapid (within 5 min) and transient (little residual increased permeability detectable 20 min after injection) providing further evidence that line 10 PF is not toxic to blood vessels. Line 10 PF does not resemble bradykinin (MW 1,200), plasma kallikrein (MW 108,000) or leukokinins (MW 2,500). It is unlikely that the effects of line 10 PF are mediated through prostaglandin synthesis since neither systemic nor local indomethacin treatment affected the response of vessels to the permeability factor. However, this lack of an indomethacin effect does not rule out the involvement of lipoxygenation products of arachidonic acid metabolism (see Chapter 13).

B. Tumor Associated Procoagulants

An extensive literature describes procoagulant activities (PCA) of various types that have been identified in disrupted tumor cells (3,9,10,50-52). In our view, the biological significance of such findings is open to serious question: it is unclear how much of the PCA expressed by broken cells in vitro would be expressed by living tumor cells in vivo; also extracts of normal as well as malignant cells may exhibit PCA (53-55). More relevant to the clinical situation, and considerably fewer in number, are studies demonstrating expression of procoagulant activity by viable tumor cells (41,56-58) and/or in cell free conditioned medium in which tumor cells have been cultured (41,46,51,59-62). Tumor associated PCA have been described which act at several different stages in the clotting cascade.

1.   __Tissue factor-like activity.__   Tissue   factor   (TF)   is   a
phospholipoprotein that activates by a factor of some 3,000 fold
clotting factor VIIa in its catalysis of factor X to factor Xa. Not
itself a proteinase, tissue factor acts as a cofactor and is thought
to be responsible for initiating the extrinsic pathway of the
coagulation system (63,64). However, tissue factor has also been
found to activate factor IX of the intrinsic pathway (63).

A vast literature dating back to O'Meara (3) reports that tissue
factor is present in tumor cell homogenates but, as noted above, we
question the usefulness of such studies. Several authors (53,65,66)
have reported that small amounts of PCA, presumably TF, are expressed
by living cultured tumor cell lines. In these studies, the PCA of
intact cells was largely dormant and could be greatly enhanced by mild
trypsinization that did not lead to cell death (65).

2.   __Factor X cleaving activities.__ Mucin has been reported to initiate
the conversion of clotting factor X to Xa by a nonenzymatic mechanism
and thereby initiate clotting (67). Such an activity might be of
interest in the case of mucin secreting adenocarcinomas but the
findings have not been confirmed or extended.

More recently Gordon and coworkers described a cysteine
proteinase present in certain tumor cells that directly activates
factor X to Xa (68). This molecule is described in greater detail in
Chapter 6. A cathepsin B-like cysteine proteinase which may be
involved in platelet aggregation is discussed in Chapter 12.

3.   __Shed plasma membrane vesicles that are active at more than a
single step in the clotting cascade.__   Several groups working
independently have reported that tumor cells in culture shed membrane
bounded vesicles. Several different activities (60,61,69-75) have
been attributed to these vesicles, including source of tumor antigens,
virus production, platelet aggregation and procoagulant. Viruses have
been looked for but not found in at least some of the cell lines that
shed vesicles (60,69,75-77). Therefore, shedding cannot be related
only to virus replication. The platelet aggregating properties of
shed vesicles are reviewed in Chapters 10 and 12. The possible role
of vesicle shedding in the dissemination of tumor antigens is beyond
the scope of this review which will concentrate on the procoagulant
function of shed vesicles.

Studies of 14 separate tumor cells of guinea pig, mouse and human
origin revealed that all but one released PCA in short term (4-22 hr)
tissue culture (60,61,75,75). In all 13 instances where PCA was found
in conditioned medium the vast majority could be pelleted by
ultracentrifugation (90 min; 100,000 x g); little or no activity
remained in the supernatant. Examination of ultracentrifuge pellets
from 9 of these tumors in the electron microscope revealed numerous
membrane bounded vesicles with diameters in the low nanometer range.
By analyzing marker enzymes characteristic of different cell
compartments it was found that these vesicles were enriched in enzymes
characteristic of the plasma membrane (e.g., 5'-nucleotidase,

phosphodiesterase I, ouabain sensitive-Na^+-K^+-ATPase) but not in enzymes found in other cellular organelles (e.g., lysosomes, mitochondria, endoplasmic reticulum). Moreover, shedding was apparently a physiological event and did not result from cell death. Viability of cultured cells remained in excess of 95% throughout culture and release of vesicles was inhibited by cold although not by several metabolic inhibitors tested. Finally, the amount of PCA associated with vesicles was substantial when compared with that expressed by the living cells that were the source of vesicles. Thus, in multiple experiments, one milliliter of cell free conditioned medium in which 5,000,000 line 10 or line 1 tumor cells had been cultured for 4 hours contained PCA equivalent to that expressed by 2,500,000 ± 500,000 living line 10 tumor cells or 3,480,000 ± 800,000 living line 1 tumor cells.

The procoagulant activity associated with vesicles was stable to dialysis, to prolonged storage at 4°C, to freezing, to sonication, to temperatures up to 70°C, to a pH range of 1.0 – 11.0 and to proteolysis and was unaffected by diisopropylfluorophosphate. When tested in one stage plasma recalcification assays, vesicles in every instance were most potent in clotting platelet poor plasmas of the species of origin (guinea pig, mouse or human).

A number of tests were performed to identify the site of vesicle PCA within the clotting scheme. In brief, the results indicated that vesicles behaved as tissue factor and in addition acted at other sites in the coagulation cascade requiring phospholipid. Evidence for a tissue factor-like activity was obtained in several different types of experiments. Vesicles of both guinea pig and human tumor origin effectively shortened two stage Pitlick-Nemerson assays. Moreover, human tumor vesicles like tissue factor standards were much more effective in coagulating normal human platelet poor plasma than its factor VII deficient counterpart. More specific assays were also employed. All of 6 human tumor vesicle preparations tested were able to cleave purified ^3H bovine factor X and this activity was entirely dependent on the presence of added factor VIIa. Finally, the PCA expressed by human tumor vesicle preparations was strikingly inhibited by a rabbit antibody (64) prepared against bovine tissue factor in one and two stage assays as well as in the ^3H bovine factor X cleaving assay.

However, not all of the PCA expressed by shed tumor vesicles could be attributed to its action as tissue factor (60,61,75,76). For example, guinea pig sources of tissue factor were found unable to interact with heterologous bovine or human factors VII and X. Thus, neither guinea pig brain tissue factor nor guinea pig tumor vesicles were able to cleave ^3H bovine factor X, react with anti-bovine tissue factor antibody or react in a two-stage Pitlick-Nemerson assay with human factor VII/X concentrates. Nonetheless, tumor vesicles were able to accelerate clotting of factor VII deficient human plasma as well as that of normal human platelet poor plasma. Thus, guinea pig tumor vesicles clearly possessed procoagulant activity(ies) apart from tissue factor. To identify the additional site(s) of such activity detailed clotting studies were performed employing vesicles from line 10 guinea pig carcinomas and singly deficient human plasmas. In brief, though slightly less active than in normal human platelet poor plasma, line 10 vesicles were effective procoagulants in plasmas singly deficient in any one of the intrinsic clotting factors, i.e., factors XII, XI, IX and VIII. However, all factors within the common pathway (factors X, V, II and Ca^{++}) were required for activity. Line 10 vesicles possessed no significant activity as any of the intrinsic or extrinsic clotting factors. Finally, line 10 vesicles neither possessed factor Xa activity nor were they able to generate such activity from factor X; similarly, no evidence of factor Xa or factor Xa generating activity was obtained in studies of several human tumor vesicles, using the highly specific ^{3}H factor X cleaving assay. Taken together, these data suggest that line 10 guinea pig tumor vesicles, in addition to possessing tissue factor-like activity, also act late in the clotting sequence at the level of prothrombinase generation. Prothrombinase, the activity that generates thrombin from prothrombin, is thought to consist of a complex of factors Xa, V, prothrombin and Ca^{++}, all associated with phospholipid. It is very likely that line 10 tumor vesicles provide a phospholipid surface to which these soluble clotting factors bind. The nature and specificity of this binding is currently being investigated.

Shedding of plasma membrane vesicles with procoagulant activity is not a property unique to tumor cells. Oil induced guinea pig macrophages and normal rat fibroblasts, for example, shed similar vesicles in culture (61; L. Van De Water and H.F. Dvorak, unpublished data). Membrane shedding is also not a phenomenon confined to tissue culture. Similar vesicles with procoagulant activity have been identified in ascites fluid from a number of tumors in several species (60). Though in some instances shedding has been associated with virus production, it is clear that in other instances shedding occurs in the absence of detectable viruses.

4.   Thrombin-like and factor XIII-like activities. Both such activities have been described (78) in a single mouse tumor, the YPC-1 plasmacytoma but the findings have not been independently confirmed nor extended to other tumors.

V. SUMMARY AND CONCLUSIONS

Does fibrin deposition have a role in tumor growth and metastasis? Despite several decades of interest in this problem no definitive statement is warranted at this time. However, considerable progress has been made in addressing more preliminary questions. For example, with the application of immunofluorescence and careful transmission electron microscopy it has been possible to determine with certainty that fibrin is deposited in and about a wide variety of human and animal tumors, even though we do not yet know with precision the biochemical nature of the fibrin we visualize. We have, moreover, made considerable progress toward an understanding of the mechanisms by which fibrin may be deposited in and about tumors, mechanisms that most probably involve tumor secreted mediators that increase vascular permeability and trigger clotting. Inflammatory cells of the host may also contribute to tumor fibrin deposition by secreting or shedding

110

analogous mediators (38,47). The progress made to date is exciting in that if fibrin proves to have an important role in tumor growth or metastasis obvious strategic intervention points will be available for therapeutic manipulation. Even if our hopes for fibrin and its role in tumor biology are not realized, the neutralizing antibody raised against the line 10 tumor permeability factor offers promise of blocking what may be the earliest event in tumor parasitization of the host, the capacity of tumors to obtain locally increased nutrients from the plasma by enhancing local microvascular permeability.

At present, the evidence linking fibrin to tumor biology is largely circumstantial: cancer patients have an increased incidence of clotting abnormalities, fibrin is in fact deposited about many tumors, tumors by virtue of the mediators they secrete have the means to deposit fibrin locally. None of this evidence can be taken to indicate conclusively that fibrin has an important role in tumor growth or metastasis. Clearly, attempts to establish such a role are an important goal of future research. In the interim, unhindered by the restraints so often imposed by hard data, it may be useful to examine briefly certain of the possibilities that future investigations need to consider. In our view, fibrin could exert an effect on tumor biology in several different ways:

1. The fibrin deposited about tumors might serve a barrier function. As such it could interfere with tumor invasion while at the same time protecting tumors from the host's immune response. Tumor cells migrating through a fibrin gel would probably require enzymes capable of digesting fibrin at neutral pH; a tumor cell's capacity to express or secrete neutral proteinases might therefore determine its metastatic capacity. Plasminogen activator(s) come to mind as likely candidates in this regard in view of the extensive evidence linking secretion of this proteinase to malignancy.

A fibrin gel might also interfere with the efferent or afferent limbs of the host's immune response. For example, fibrin could inhibit dissemination of tumor associated antigens. Alternatively, fibrin deposits could impede the influx of both antibodies and cells of the host's immune response, limiting their ability to reach tumor cell targets. Suggestive evidence supporting this view comes from morphological studies of both lines 1 and 10 guinea pig bile duct and human breast carcinomas. In all these instances large numbers of lymphocytes accumulated about the tumor mass, but outside the fibrin gel deposits, and relatively few cells penetrated this fibrin to make contact with tumor cells. Moreover, this barrier function was accentuated by desmoplasia and the apparent inability of host inflammatory cells to diapedese from intra-tumor (as compared with extra-tumor) blood vessels such that relatively few inflammatory cells ever penetrated more than a millimeter or two into such tumors (40,42). On the other hand, when breast tumors underwent focal infarction, a not uncommon event, macrophages were able to enter the tumor in great numbers (42). It may be that macrophages are able to migrate through both fibrin and fibrous connective tissues, perhaps by virtue of the proteinases (e.g., plaminogen activator) that they secrete.

2. Tumor associated fibirn might serve as a stimulus to angiogenesis. Evidence favoring a role for fibrin in tumor angiogenesis comes from studies in which fibrin was found to induce new blood vessel formation within 24-48 hr of implantation in the subcutaneous space of normal guinea pigs independent of tumor cells (40). If, therefore, it can be assumed that fibrin is deposited about malignant tumors, angiogenesis would be expected to follow as an automatic consequence and the tumor secreted mediators responsible for enhancing vascular permeability and clotting extravasated fibrinogen may be regarded as de facto "tumor angiogenesis factors." Moreover, when fibrin deposits were abundant, angiogenesis was accompanied by fibrous organization with collagen deposition just as occurs in tumor desmoplasia and in wound healing (40).

Of course the fibrin implantation experiment just described does not prove that fibrin itself is the proximate cause of angiogenesis or of desmoplasia. Indeed, it is unlikely that an insoluble polymer such as fibrin would itself be able to send signals that would attract blood vessels and fibroblasts, cause endothelial cells or fibroblasts to proliferate and induce fibroblast collagen synthesis. However, it must be remembered that fibrin arises from fibrinogen by the splitting off of soluble A and B fibrinopeptides, molecules with a variety of pharmacologic activities (26,28,79,80). Thrombin, the enzyme catalyzing this conversion, is itself a mitogen (81) and could have other roles. Moreover, fibrin deposition is not a static process. Whether deposited in tumors or about healing wounds, fibrin may be expected to undergo continuous remodeling, a process involving fibrinolysis. Indeed, it has been known for many years that tumors are more able than most cells to initiate this process by secreting plasminogen activators that convert plasminogen to plasmin, the major effector proteinase of the fibrinolytic system. A wide variety of relevant biological activities have been proposed for various soluble fibrinogen or fibrin degradation products (27,29-35), but their possible role in angiogenesis or desmoplasia has not been investigated. Finally, it must also be remembered that fibrin deposits in tissue form associations with other molecules. One of these, plasma fibronectin, has a binding site for fibrin and has been described in association with fibrin about tumors. Products of fibronectin degradation (82,83), like those of fibrin, may exhibit biological activities. Indeed, one such product particularly relevant to the present discussion is reported to exhibit chemotactic activity for fibroblasts and could therefore be involved in initiating the desmoplastic response. If this general line of thinking proves correct, the "tumor angiogenesis factor" proposed by Folkman (59) may turn out to be not a single product unique to tumors but rather a series of mediators, closely linked to the physiological process of wound healing that leads to the deposition and modulation of tumor fibrin or fibronectin. As a result, tumor angiogenesis and tumor desmoplasia may come to be regarded not as processes peculiar to malignancy but rather as specialized examples of wound healing, a process whose cardinal features also include fibrin and fibronectin (84) deposition, angiogenesis and fibrous connective tissue (scar) formation.

112

REFERENCES

1. Trousseau A. Clinique Medicale de l'Hotel-dieu de Paris. J.B. Bailliere et Fils, Paris, 5th Edition. 3:94, 1865.
2. O'Meara RAQ and Jackson RD. Ir. J. Med. Sci. 6:327-328, 1958.
3. O'Meara RAQ. Ir. J. Med. Sci. 6:474-479, 1958.
4. Gitlin D and Craig JM. Am. J. Pathol. 33:267-283, 1957.
5. Day ED, Planinsek JA and Pressman D. J. Natl. Cancer Inst. 22:413-426, 1959.
6. Marrack D, Kubala M, Corry P, Leavens M, Howze J, Dewey W, Bale WF and Spar IL. Cancer (Philadelphia) 20:751-755, 1967.
7. Hiramoto R, Yagi Y and Pressman D. Cancer Res. 19:874-879, 1959.
8. Hiramoto R, Bernecky J, Jurandowski J and Pressman D. Cancer Res. 20:592-593, 1960.
9. Zacharski LR, Henderson WG, Rickles FR, Forman WB, Cornell CJ, Forcier RJ, Harrower HW and Johnson RO. Cancer (Philadelphia) 44:732-741, 1979.
10. Donati MB, Davidson JF and Garattini S, eds. Malignancy and the Hemostatic System. Raven Press, New York, 1981.
11. Zacharski LR, Henderson WG, Rickles FR, Forman WB, Cornell CJ, Forcier RJ, Edwards R, Headley E, Kim S-H, O'Donnell JR, O'Dell R, Tornyos K and Kwaan HC. J. Am. Med. Assoc. 245:831-835, 1981.
12. Chan S-Y and Pollard M. J. Natl. Cancer Inst. 64:1121-1125, 1980.
13. Chew EC and Wallace AC. Cancer Res. 36:1904-1909, 1976.
14. Wood S, Holyoke ED and Yardley JH. Proc. Can. Cancer Res. Conf. 4:167-221, 1961.
15. Kinjo M. Br. J. Cancer 38:293-300, 1978.
16. Maat B. Br. J. Cancer 37:369-376, 1978.
17. Vaheri A and Mosher DF. Biochim. Biophys. Acta. 516:1-25, 1978.
18. Nossel HL. N. Engl. J. Med. 295:428-432, 1981.
19. Davie EW, Fujikawa K, Kurachi K and Kisiel W. Adv. Enzymol. 48:277-318, 1979.
20. Folk JE and Finlayson JS. Adv. Protein Chem. 31:1-133, 1977.
21. Hermans J and McDonagh J. Semin. Thromb. Hemostasis 8:11-24, 1982.
22. Robbins KC, Wohl RC and Summaria L. Ann. N.Y. Acad. Sci. 37:588-591, 1981.
23. Reich E. In: Proteases and Biological Control. (Eds. Reich E, Rifkin DB and Shaw E), Cold Spring Harbor, New York, pp. 333-341, 1975.
24. Wiman B and Collen D. Nature (London) 272:549-550, 1978.
25. Marder VJ and Budzynski AZ. Thromb. Diath. Haemorrh. 33:199-207, 1975.
26. Osbahr AJ, Gladner JA and Laki K. Biochim. Biophys. Acta 86:535-542, 1964.
27. Stecher VJ and Sorkin E. Int. Arch. Allergy Appl. Immunol. 43:879-886, 1972.
28. Kay AB, Pepper DS and Ewart MR. Nature (London) New Biol. 243:56-57, 1973.
29. Girmann G, Pees H, Schwarze G and Scheurlen PG. Nature (London) 259:399-401, 1976.
30. Richardson DL, Pepper DS and Kay AB. Br. J. Haematol. 32:507-513, 1976.
31. Belew M, Gerdin B, Porath J and Saldeen T. Thromb. Res. 13:983-994, 1978.
32. Gerdin B and Saldeen T. Thromb. Res. 13:995-1006, 1978.
33. Krzystyniak K, Stachurska J, Ryzewski J, Bykowska K and Kopec M. Thromb. Res. 12:523-530, 1978.
34. Belew M, Gerdin B, Lindeberg G, Porath J, Saldeen T and Wallin R. Biochim. Biophys. Acta 621:169-178, 1980.
35. Plow EF, Freaney D and Edgington TS. J. Immunol. 128:1595-1599, 1982.
36. Francis CW, Marder VJ and Barlow GH. J. Clin. Invest. 66:1033-1043, 1980.
37. Colvin RB and Dvorak HF. J. Immunol. 114:377-387, 1975.
38. Dvorak HF, Galli SJ and Dvorak AM. Int. Rev. Exp. Pathol. 21:119-194, 1980.
39. Churchill WH Jr., Rapp HJ, Kronman BS and Borsos T. J. Natl. Cancer Inst. 41:13-29, 1968.

40. Dvorak HF, Dvorak AM, Manseau EJ, Wiberg L and Churchill WH. J. Natl. Cancer Inst. 62:1459–1472, 1979.
41. Dvorak HF, Orenstein NS, Carvalho AC, Churchill WH, Dvorak AM, Galli SJ, Feder J, Bitzer AM, Rypysc J and Giovinco P. J. Immunol. 122:166–174, 1979.
42. Dvorak HF, Dickersin GR, Dvorak AM, Manseau EJ and Pyne K. J. Natl. Cancer Inst. 67:335–345, 1981.
43. Harris NL, Dvorak AM, Smith J and Dvorak HF. Am. J. Pathol. 108:119–129, 1982.
44. Cooper JH, Haq BM and Bagnell H. J. Pathol. 98:193–199, 1969.
45. Dvorak HF, Mihm MC Jr., Dvorak AM, Barnes BA, Manseau EJ and Galli SJ. J. Exp. Med. 150:322–337, 1979.
46. Dvorak HF, Orenstein NS and Dvorak AM. Lymphokines 2:203–233, 1981.
47. Dvorak HF, Senger DR and Dvorak AM. Cancer Metastasis Rev., in press, 1983.
48. Senger DR, Galli SJ, Dvorak AM, Perruzzi CA, Harvey VS and Dvorak HF. Fed. Proc. Fed. Am. Soc. Exp. Biol. 41:964, 1982.
49. Senger DR, Galli SJ, Dvorak AM, Perruzzi CA, Harvey VS and Dvorak HF. Science 219:983–985, 1983.
50. Gordon SG and Cross BA J. Clin. Invest. 67:1665–1671, 1981.
51. Kinjo M, Oka K, Naito S, Kohga S, Tanaka K, Oboshi S, Yahata Y and Yasumoto K. Br. J. Cancer 39:15–23, 1979.
52. Laki K, Tyler HM and Yancey ST. Biochem. Biophys. Res. Commun. 24:776–781, 1966.
53. Zacharski LR and McIntyre OR. J. Med. 4:118–131, 1973.
54. Green D, Ryan C, Malandruccolo N and Nadler HL. Blood 37:47–51, 1971.
55. Maynard JR, Fintel DJ, Pitlick FA and Nemerson Y. Lab. Invest. 35:542–549, 1976.
56. Khato J, Suzuki M and Sato H. Gann 65:289–294, 1974.
57. Cattan A and Bresson ML. Biomedicine 25:252–254, 1976.
58. Curatolo L, Colucci M, Cambini AL, Poggi A, Morasca L, Donati MB and Semeraro N. Br. J. Cancer 40:228–233, 1979.
59. Folkman J. Adv. Cancer Res. 19:331–358, 1974.
60. Dvorak HF, Quay SC, Orenstein NS, Dvorak AM, Hahn P, Bitzer AM and Carvalho AC. Science 212:923–924, 1981.
61. Dvorak HF, Van De Water L, Dvorak AM, Harvey VS, Anderson D, DeWolf W and Bach R. Fed. Proc. Fed. Am. Soc. Exp. Biol. 41:8, 1982.
62. Gordon SG and Lewis B.J. Cancer Res. 38:2467–2472, 1978.
63. Nemerson Y, Zur M, Bach R and Gentry R. In: The Regulation of Coagulation. (Eds. Mann KG and Taylor FB), Elsevier/North Holland, New York, pp. 193–202, 1980.
64. Bach R, Nemerson Y and Konigsberg W. J. Biol. Chem. 256:8324–8331, 1981.
65. Maynard JR, Heckman CA, Pitlick FA and Nemerson Y. J. Clin. Invest. 55:814–824, 1975.
66. Maynard JR, Dreyer BE, Stemerman MB and Pitlick FA. Blood 50:387–396, 1977.
67. Pineo GF, Brain MC, Gallus AS, Hirsh J, Hatton MWC and Regoeczi E. Ann. N.Y. Acad. Sci. 230:262–270, 1974.
68. Gordon SG. J. Histochem. Cytochem. 29:457–463, 1981.
69. Black PH. Adv. Cancer Res. 32:75–199, 1980.
70. Doljanski F and Kapeller M. J. Theor. Biol. 62:253–270, 1976.
71. Calafat J, Hilgers J, Van Blitterswijk WJ, Verbeet M and Hageman PC. J. Natl. Cancer Inst. 56:1019–1029, 1976.
72. Koch GLE and Smith MJ. Nature (London) 273:274–277, 1978.
73. Raz A, Goldman R, Yuli I and Inbar M. Cancer Immunol. Immunother. 4:5. 4:53–59, 1978.
74. Gasic GJ, Boettiger D, Catalfamo JL, Gasic TB and Stewart GJ. Cancer Res. 38:2950–2955, 1978.

75. Bitzer AM, Carvalho ACA, Davis GL and Dvorak HF. Fed. Proc. Fed. Am. Soc. Exp. Biol. 41:7880, 1981.
76. Dvorak HF, Van De Water L, Bitzer AM, Dvorak AM, Anderson D, Harvey VS, Bach R, DeWolf W and Carvalho ACA. Submitted.
77. Dunkel VC, Bast RC, Gerwin BI, Heine V, Cotter-Fox M and Borsos T. J. Natl. Cancer Inst. 53:591-593, 1974.
78. Laki K, Tyler HM and Yancey ST. Biochem. Biophy. Res. Commun. 24:776-781, 1966.
79. Ratnoff OD. Adv. Immunol. 10:145-227, 1969.
80. Colman RW, Osbahr AJ and Morris RE. Nature (London) 215:292-293, 1967.
81. Glenn KC, Carney DH, Fenton JW II and Cunningham DD. J. Biol. Chem. 255:6609-6616, 1980.
82. Postlethwaite AE, Keski-Oja J, Balian G and Kang AH. J. Exp. Med. 153:494-499, 1981.
83. Tsukamoto Y, Helsel WE and Wahl SM. J. Immunol. 127:673-678, 1981.
84. Clark RAF, Lanigan JM, DellaPelle P, Manseau E, Dvorak HF and Colvin RB. J. Invest. Dermatol. 79:264-269, 1982.

CHAPTER 9. PERSPECTIVES ON THE ROLE OF PLATELETS IN HEMOSTASIS AND THROMBOSIS

FREDERICK OFOSU, MICHAEL R. BUCHANAN AND JACK HIRSH

I. INTRODUCTION

The interaction of platelets with vascular wall structures, plasma proteins and other circulating cells is of fundamental importance in the regulation of hemostasis and in the pathogenesis of thrombosis. When platelets are stimulated, they release biologically active constituents which interact with vessel wall cells, plasma coagulation factors and circulating blood cells to modulate hemostasis. In this review we will discuss platelet adhesion, the platelet release reaction, platelet aggregation, the effects of these phenomena on the coagulation system and their importance in hemostasis and thrombosis.

A. Platelet Adhesion

Platelets do not adhere to the endothelial cell surface of blood vessels under normal circumstances but do adhere to detached endothelial cells and to the underlying basement membrane (1-4). Endothelial cell injury is a primary event in the initiation of thrombosis. The platelet response to injury is influenced by the extent and depth of a vessel wall injury. With minor degrees of injury which cause only endothelial cell desquamation, platelets are exposed to the underlying basement membrane to which they adhere and on which they spread. However, they do not release their constituents and do not aggregate (5). With more marked injury and exposure of deeper structures in the vessel wall, platelets not only adhere to the surface but also undergo the release reaction, aggregate and activate blood coagulation on their surface (6,7). The difference in platelet responses to these two types of injury is likely to be due to the differences in the vessel wall components to which the platelets are exposed (8). Endothelial and smooth muscle cells synthesize different types of collagen which are therefore located at different depths within the vessel wall. Types IV and V collagens are located in the basement membrane and are synthesized by the endothelial cells (9,10). These collagens promote platelet adhesion (4) but do not cause platelet aggregation unless they are in a fibrillar or aggregated form (6,7). The reason why platelet aggregation and release do not occur following exposure of platelets to basement membrane is not entirely clear. A possible explanation is that fibronectin which is synthesized and/or released by both endothelial cells and platelets, and which blocks the ability of collagen to induce the release of serotonin from washed platelets (11), interferes with the platelet-basement membrane interaction. In contrast, types I and III collagen, which are synthesized by smooth muscle cells (12,13) and located in the media of the vessel wall, promote platelet adhesion, aggregation and the release reaction (6,7,14).

At physiological shear rates, platelet adhesion to collagen requires von Willebrand's factor (15), a large multimeric plasma protein, which acts as a link between specific glycoprotein receptors on the platelet surface and subendothelial connective tissue. These platelet glycoprotein receptors are absent in the rare inherited platelet abnormality known as Bernard-Soulier syndrome (16) and the von Willebrand's glycoprotein is absent or defective in patients with von Willebrand's disease (17). Platelet adhesion is defective in both of these conditions.

Other plasma proteins also influence the interaction of platelets with artificial surfaces. The adhesion of platelets to these surfaces is an important limiting factor in their use as vascular prostheses (18-24). The biocompatibility of surfaces with blood has been correlated with the surface charge, contact angle and specific surface groups of a prosthetic material (25). When these materials are implanted in the body and come in contact with blood, their surfaces become rapidly coated with plasma proteins which influence platelet adhesion (18-24). Thus the biocompatibility of these surfaces may not only reflect their inherent inertness to blood but also the inhibitory effect of plasma proteins which coat the surface.

B. Platelet Release Reaction

Platelets contain two morphologically distinct granules, the contents of which are expelled into the ambient fluid upon stimulation (26,27). The dense granules contain serotonin, calcium and adenosine diphosphate (ADP). The alpha granules contain platelet-specific proteins (beta-thromboglobulin and platelet factor 4), proteoglycan, coagulation factors (factor V, fibrinogen), fibronectin and cationic proteins such as the platelet-derived growth factor (mitogenic factor) and permeability and chemotactic factors (28-31). In addition, platelets contain lysosomes which upon stimulation release a number of acid hydrolases (30), but their precise role in platelet function has not been well elucidated.

A number of biological agents including collagen, thrombin, epinephrine, thromboxane A_2 (TXA_2) and other arachidonic acid metabolites cause platelets to release their granular contents (32-35). With relatively weak stimuli, only the contents of alpha granules are released, but with stronger stimuli the contents of the dense granules are also released (36). Physiologically, ADP is the most important substance released from the dense granules. It induces platelet shape change and promotes platelet aggregation. However, ADP is rapidly hydrolyzed to AMP by ADP plasma phosphohydrolase and is subsequently dephosphorylated to adenosine. Components released from the alpha granules also contribute to platelet aggregation and activate the coagulation system by as yet unknown mechanisms. Gerrard et al. (37) reported abnormal platelet function in two patients with gray platelet syndrome. In the syndrome, dense granules and lysosomes are normal, but there is a deficiency of alpha granules.

C. Platelet Aggregation

Platelet aggregation is induced by a number of stimuli including ADP, thrombin, TXA_2, collagen and epinephrine. The aggregation reaction is preceded by a change in platelet shape which is mediated by a contractile microtubular system within the platelet. This response is characterized morphologically by platelet pseudopod formation. At least three independent mediators of platelet aggregation have been identified. These are ADP, TXA_2 and thrombin. ADP is released from platelet dense granules in response to collagen, thrombin, epinephrine and TXA_2 (29-31). The mechanism of ADP-induced aggregation has not been clearly elucidated but appears to be dependent upon the presence of a specific platelet glycoprotein receptor which is absent in the rare congenital platelet disorder, thrombasthenia. Thrombasthenic platelets do not aggregate with ADP, but when thrombin or collagen are used thrombasthenic platelets undergo the release reaction, however, they do not aggregate (38).

Thrombin induces platelet aggregation by a number of mechanisms. It stimulates platelets to release ADP (30). It activates platelet membrane phospholipases and thus initiates the formation of TXA_2 (39). It also can induce platelet aggregation independently of the former two mechanisms by a third mechanism which is as yet poorly understood (40).

Activation of the platelet arachidonic acid pathway results in the formation of products which promote further platelet aggregation. Platelet arachidonic acid is oxidized to the endoperoxides, PGG_2 and PGH_2, by a reaction which utilizes molecular oxygen and which is catalyzed by the enzyme cyclooxygenase. The endoperoxides are subsequently converted to TXA_2 (the principal product) and to a number of other prostaglandins (PGD_2, PGE_2 and $PGF_{2\alpha}$). TXA_2 promotes platelet aggregation directly and also acts synergistically with ADP and other stimuli (thrombin and collagen) to augment the platelet release reaction (41, see also Chapter 13). The endoperoxide, PGH_2, is also thought to induce platelet aggregation (42).

At least one lipoxygenase derivative (12-hydroxy-eicosatetraenoic acid, 12-HETE) produced by the platelets appears to be important in regulating platelet function. Dutilh and co-workers (43) have suggested that lipoxygenase products are necessary for irreversible platelet aggregation. Schaffer (44) has suggested that deficiency in platelet lipoxygenase activity seen in patients with myeloproliferative disease may be responsible for hemorrhagic complications seen in those patients. We have recently reported that products of the lipoxygenase pathway may be necessary for platelet adhesion (45). In addition, platelet-derived lipoxygenase products are chemotactic for leukocytes and may be important for the recruitment of leukocytes to the site of thrombosis. Leukocytes have procoagulant activity (46-48) and leukocyte-derived thromboplastin activity is markedly enhanced in granulocytes which have ahdered to vessel wall segments (49).

D. Coagulant Activities of Platelets

Conceptually, the principal role of platelets in blood coagulation could be associated with any or all of the initiation, propagation and inhibition of thrombin generation in plasma (50). Platelets appear to be the site for the activation of factor X and prothrombin. Platelets provide a membrane surface on which several of the clotting factors for the intrinsic activation of factor X and prothrombin bind, interact and subsequently generate coagulant activities (51). Stimulated platelets secrete a number of clotting factors including fibrinogen, factor V, factor VIII (as factor VIII:RAg), factor XI (60,61) and factor XIII (52-63). Under certain conditions, erythrocytes, leukocytes and endothelial cells can provide an activity equivalent to platelets in supporting the formation of a fibrin clot (64).

E. Role of Platelets in Contact Activation

It is well known that, on recalcification, the clotting times of platelet poor plasmas are considerably longer than the clotting time of platelet rich plasmas from which they were derived. Recalcification times of plasma and both rate and amount of plasma thrombin generation are a function of platelet count (65). The recalcification times of platelet rich plasma are shortened by the addition of ADP in concentrations that do not promote platelet aggregation. This effect of ADP has been termed contact-product forming activity of platelets meaning the ability of platelets to trigger intrinsic coagulation in the presence of ADP by activating factor XII adsorbed onto the platelet surface (66). When platelets are activated with collagen under conditions which do not lead to aggregation of platelets, they shorten the recalcification time of plasma by an additional mechanism that bypasses requirements for factor XII (66). This precept is based on the observation that no differences in the clotting times are observed between factor XII-deficient and normal plasma under the same conditions (67). The mechanism for the factor XII-independent coagulant activity of platelets apparently involves a kallikrein-dependent proteolytic activation of factor XI in the absence of factor XII (68). Thus, there are two independent but related mechanisms by which platelets seem to participate in contact activation of blood.

Platelets also participate in several non-contact factor dependent reactions of blood coagulation. For example, platelets shorten the clotting times of plasma treated with calcium and the factor X activator isolated from Russell's viper venom (69). Like recalcification times of plasma, the Russell viper venom clotting times are a function of platelet concentration. Biggs (70) has suggested that platelets provide the phospholipid surface for several reactions of coagulation. Miletich et al. (71) have shown that in a purified system consisting of factor Xa, calcium and prothrombin, the rate of thrombin formation is linearly related to platelet count. These non-contact-coagulant activities of platelets will be discussed below in the section on the formation of factor X activator and prothombinase complexes.

II. INTERACTION OF PLATELETS WITH COAGULATION FACTORS

   A. Interactions of Platelets with Factor VIII

      Human factor VIII/von Willebrand's factor protein has two distinct biological activities: (1) the correction of the prolonged clotting time associated with factor VIII:C deficiency or hemophilia A and (2) the correction of the prolonged bleeding times associated with von Willebrand's disease (vWD). It is now generally accepted that the clotting entity and vWD factor are two separate moieties which are closely associated (74). The vWD factor is measured by its ability to cause platelets to aggregate in the presence of the antibiotic ristocetin (73,74). von Willebrand's disease factor is usually present in normal amounts in hemophilia A plasma. It is a large molecular weight glycoprotein which elutes in the void volume of Sepharose 4B and is generally associated with the factor VIII:C when isolated from plasma. von Willebrand's disease factor and factor VIII:C activity can be dissociated with 0.25 M $CaCl_2$ (75,76). Heterologous antisera to vWD factor are used in the measurement of this glycoprotien in normal, hemophilia A and vWD patients. The plasma levels of vWD factor are generally reduced in vWD patients. Electrophoretic mobilities of this protein are abnormal in some vWD patients (74,77-79). von Willebrand's disease factor is released from platelets (74,75). Binding of vWD factor to platelets via a specific protein receptor is a prerequisite for platelet aggregation induced by ristocetin (80,81). This interaction is also involved in the adherence of platelets to subendothelium. It is not known whether when bound to platelets the vWD factor serves as the platelet receptor for factor VIII:C, the factor required for the efficient conversion of factor X to factor Xa by factor IXa (see below). It is likely that factor VII:C and vWD factor circulate as a complex in plasma as the two activities co-elute on Sepaharose 4B columns. It is not known whether factor VIII:C binds to platelets directly, but it has been demonstrated that factor VIII:C binds firmly to phospholipid vesicles (82). In the presence of phospholipid, vWD factor and VIII:C dissociate and the VIII:C is preferentially bound to phospholipid (83). The contribution of vWD factor to platelet adhesion to subendothelium is discussed in the section on platelet adhesion.

   B. The Interaction of Platelets with Factor V

      Factor V is one of several platelet constituents secreted upon the activation of platelets (56-58). Tracy et al. (84) have demonstrated that platelet factor V and plasma factor V are immunologically identical. Factor V has been shown to bind to platelets with a high affinity. Like factor V, factor Va binds to platelets with a Kd of 3 nM. In addition to these sites however, factor Va has 900 additional high affinity sites (Kd = 0.3 nM) per platelet (84). Binding of factor V and factor Va does not require platelet activation (84). This contrasts sharply with factor X and factor Xa. Only factor Xa is capable of binding to the platelet receptor with high affinity. The platelet receptor for factor Xa is available only on activated platelets (71). Recent data by Pusey et al. (85) demonstrate that factors V and Va bind to phospholipid. These observations raise the possibility that the binding of factor V or factor Va to platelets may essentially be due to binding of the glycoproteins to platelet phospholipids.

Kane et al. (86) have demonstrated that platelet lysate (obtained by freeze-thawing) contains a proteinase that is not thrombin which is capable of activating purified factor V. The physiological significance of the platelet factor V activator is unknown at this time.

C. Interactions of Platelets with Vitamin K-Dependent Clotting Factors

While there is good evidence that prothrombin, factor IX and factor X can bind to negatively charged phospholipids (87), the ability of any of these procoagulants to bind with high affinity to platelets in the absence of factor V has not been demonstrated (71). To date, thrombin and factor Xa are the only vitamin K-dependent clotting factors that have been shown to bind specifically to platelets (71,87,88). Specific receptors for thrombin have been identified on platelets. Platelet bound factor Va is the receptor for factor Xa on platelets (71,87,88). It is noteworthy that the receptors for factor Xa (approximately 200-300 per platelet) are best expressed when the platelets are activated. The specificity of the interaction of factors Xa-Va on platelets is evident from observations that only factor Xa is capable of displacing platelet bound factor Xa (65). Factor X, factor IX, factor IXa and prothrombin do not displace factor Xa from its binding site on the platelet (71). Interestingly, prothrombin appears to enhance factor Xa binding to platelets (71). The calcium-dependent binding of factor Xa to activated platelets results in the formation of prothrombinase complex (89). An undetermined number of non-specific binding sites on the platelet for factor Xa (or X) have also been described (71). Even though no specific binding sites on platelets for prothrombin, factor X or factor IX have been described, it is evident that the calcium- and phospholipid-dependent interactions of prothrombin with platelets are required for thrombin generation, since thrombin generation by the prothrombinase complex proceeds efficiently only with prothrombin as substrate and not when either prethrombin I or prethrombin II is the substrate (88). Binding between platelets and factor X, factor IX and prothrombin may not be readily demonstrated by the methods that are currently in use. In order to demonstrate complex formation filtration through oil is necessary (71). Dissociation constants greater than 10 nM may not be demonstrable under such conditions. It is doubtful whether such tight binding is necessary for the expression of functional binding as the functional binding of calcium to prothrombin has a dissociation constant of approximately 10 μM (89).

D. The Role of Platelets in the Intrinsic Activation of Factor X
    and Prothrombin

    Platelets have been shown to provide procoagulant phospholipid
for blood coagulation (91,92). This is readily apparent with the
effect of RVV-X (factor X activator purified from Russell's viper
venom) on recalcified platelet poor plasma and platelet rich plasma
are compared (69). There are several reasons why few definitive
studies that assess the role of platelets in the intrinsic activation
of factor X have been undertaken for a system consisting of purified
clotting factors. Human factor VIII:C has not been purified to
homogeneity. However, because factor VIII:C and factor V are
functionally similar, one may speculate that factor VIII:C, like
factor V, binds tightly to platelets (or activated platelets),
particularly since factor VIII:C has been shown to bind to
phospholipid vesicles (83). Upon binding to platelets, factor VIII:C
may serve as the platelet receptor for factor IXa. To date, no
binding of factor IXa or factor IX to platelets has been described.
The unavailability of homogeneous preparations of factor VIII:C has
prevented the description of the kinetic parameters that characterize
the interaction of factor VIII:C with factor IX or with factor X. The
role of phospholipid and activated factor VIII:C in the activation of
bovine factor X by factor IXa has been investigated by van Dieijen et
al. (93). The phospholipid serves primarily to reduce the Km to below
the plasma concentration of factor X. Activated factor VIII serves to
increase the Vmax by 5 orders of magnitude. Platelets may play a
similar role to phospholipid in the activation of factor X. Vehar and
Davie (94) have purified bovine factor VIII:C and have demonstrated
that in the bovine system, prior activation of the factor VIII:C by
either thrombin or factor Xa (in the presence of calcium and
phospholipid) is a prerequisite for the expression of the cofactor
activity of factor VIII:C.

The role of platelets in the intrinsic activation of factor X has been
explored by Walsh and Biggs (95). In a reconstituted plasma system,
it was evident that the activation of factor X by factor IXa and
factor VIIIa generated in situ was dependent upon the availability of
platelets or coagulant phospholipids (95). In this experimental
system, platelets from normal and factor V deficient plasma were
equally effective in supporting the activation of factor X by factor
IXa and factor VIIIa. Interestingly, platelets appeared to protect
factor Xa from inactivation by its inhibitors present in the
reconstituted plasma. Recent work by van Dieijen et al. (93) suggests
that the role of platelets is primarily the provision of an efficient
catalytic surface for the activation of factor X by factor IXa as
evidenced by the decrease in the Km from 2,000 μ M to 58 nM.

    The role of platelets in the activation of prothrombin by the
prothrombinase complex has been to a large extent defined. The
prothrombinase complex consists of factor Xa bound to its receptor
(factor Va) on the platelet surface (65,87,91). Calcium is required
for the interaction of factor Xa with platelet bound factor Va (96).
Calcium is also required for the expression of cofactor activity of
factor Va and is required to stabilize the interactions of the heavy
and light chains of factor Va as both subunits are necessary for the

expression of the cofactor activity (96,97). Factor Va on the platelet surface forms a 1:1 stoichiometric complex with factor Xa (87). Assembly of the prothrombinase complex does not require the presence of prothrombin (91). Binding of the substrate to prothrombinase for its activation to thrombin is probably calcium-dependent, as efficient conversion of prothrombin and thrombin has been demonstrated only for prothrombin with its gamma-glutamyl-carboxyl residues intact (88,89). The relative rate of conversion of prothrombin to thrombin by the full prothrombinase complex is 300,000-fold greater than the rate achieved with the enzyme (factor Xa) alone (87).

E. Platelet Activation as it Relates to the Conversion of Prothrombin to Thrombin

Zwaal and collaborators have compared apparent efficiencies of the prothrombinase complex formed under a variety of conditions where the principal conditions used for platelet activation are varied (64). Either collagen-treated platelets or thrombin-treated platelets were more effective than gel-filtered platelets as surfaces for the activation of prothrombin by factor Xa. The concentrations of collagen and thrombin used to activate the platelets were suboptimal for platelet aggregation. No exogenous factor V or Va was added and thus factor V/factor Va was also rate limiting (64). The activation of the platelets with a constant suboptimal concentration of collagen and thrombin led to a synergistic increase in the rate and amount of thrombin generation. One of the consequences of the interactions of platelets with either collagen or thrombin was the appearance of phosphatidyl serine on the platelet surface (64). Platelet activation as measured by prothrombin activation thus results in the appearance of a coagulant phospholipid and hence to increased interactions of factor V/Va, factor Xa and prothrombin with platelets (64,96,97). It is significant that during the course of platelet activation the changes that occur at the platelet surface initially appear to favor the activation of factor X. The surface, better suited for the activation of prothrombin, develops subsequent to the formation of the "factor-tenase" surface (62). It is unlikely that the appearance of this phospholipid on the surface of activated platelets accounts alone for the ability of activated platelets to enhance activation of prothrombin by factor Xa. van Zutphen et al. (100) have compared the ability of synthetic coagulant phospholipid vesicles with that of platelet phospholipid fractions (obtained by freeze-thawing bovine platelet suspensions) to shorten the clotting time of the plasma as a function of phospholipid concentration. The platelet phospholipid fraction was obtained from sonicated freeze-thawed platelet suspensions. At low phospholipid concentrations, the two phospholipid sources had equivalent ability to shorten the clotting time of bovine plasma. At higher phospholipid concentrations, however, the sonicated platelets provided the better surface for activation by the addition of factor V or factor Va. However, added factor V/factor Va was not as efficient as factor V/factor Va bound to the platelet membrane in catalyzing prothrombin activation. This raises the possibility that, in addition to providing the coagulant phospholipid, the intact activated platelet membrane probably has additional components that serve to make it a more efficient receptor for factor Va than phospholipids alone (99).

III. OTHER POTENTIAL CONSEQUENCES OF PLATELET ACTIVATION

The release of other granular contents of platelets likely accompanies release of factor V/factor Va from platelets upon activation. One particular constituent that may influence thrombin generation is platelet factor four (PF4). The antiheparin activity of this basic protein is well known (100,101). Glycosaminoglycans such as heparin sulphate and dermatan sulphate can inhibit thrombin generation in plasma (101,102). If, as is likely, PF4 is able to neutralize the potential anticoagulant activity of vessel wall glycosaminoglycans PF4 could play an important role in the propagation of thrombin generation.

REFERENCES

1. Tschopp TB, Baumgartner HR, Silberbauer K and Sinzinger H. Haemostasis 8:19-29, 1979.
2. Cazenave JP, Blondowska D, Richardson M, Kinlough-Rathbone RL, Packham MA and Mustard JF. J. Lab. Clin. Med. 93:60-70, 1979.
3. Stemmerman MB, Spaet TH. Bull. N.Y. Acad. Med. 48:289-301, 1972.
4. Cazenave JP, Packham MA, Kinlough-Rathbone RL and Mustard JF. Adv. Exp. Med. Biol. 102:31-47, 1978.
5. Madri JA, Dreyer B, Pitlick FA and Furthmayr. Lab. Invest. 43:303-315, 1980.
6. Barnes MJ, Bialey AJ, Gordon JL and MacIntyre DE. Thromb. Res. 18:375-388, 1978.
7. Wang CL, Miyata T, Weksler B, Ruben AL and Stenzell KH. Biochim. Biophys. Acta 544:568-577, 1978.
8. Trelstad RL. In: Collagen-Platelet Interactions (Ed. Gastpar H), Schattauer Verlag, Stuttgart, p. 153, 1978.
9. Howard BV, Macarak EJ, Gunson D and Kefalides NA. Proc. Natl. Acad. Sci. USA 73:2361-2364, 1976.
10. Sage H, Crouch E and Bornstein P. Biochemistry 18:5433-5442, 1979.
11. Bensusan HB, Koh TL, Henry KG, Murray BA and Culp LA. Proc. Natl. Acad. Sci. USA 75:5864-5868, 1978.
12. Trelstad RL. Biochem. Biophys. Res. Commun. 57:717-725, 1974.
13. Scott DM, Horwood R, Grant ME and Jackson DS. Connect. Tissue Res. 5:7-13, 1977.
14. Balleisen L, Gay S, Marx R and Kuhn K. Klin. Wochenschr. 53:903-905, 1975.
15. Turritto VT and Baumgartner HR. Microvasc. Res. 17:38-54, 1979.
16. Degos L, Tobelem G, Lethielluex P, Levy-Toledano S, Caen J and Colombani J. Blood 50:899-903, 1977.
17. Caen JP, Michel H, Tobelem G, Bodevin E and Levy-Toledano S. Experientia 33:91-93, 1976.
18. Mason RG. Prog. Hemostasis Thromb. 1:141-164, 1972.
19. Mason RG, Mohammad SF, Chuang HY and Richardson PD. Semin. Thromb. Hematol. 3:98-116, 1976.
20. Friedman LI, Liem H, Grabowski EF, Leonard EF and McCord CW. Trans. Am. Soc. Artif. Intern. Organs 16:63-76, 1970.

21. Turitto VT and Leonard EF. Trans. Am. Soc. Artif. Intern. Organs 18:348-353, 1972.
22. Grabowski EF, Herther KK and Didesheim P. J. Lab. Clin. Med. 88:368-374, 1976.
23. Feuerstein IA, Brophy JM and Brash JL. Trans. Am. Soc. Artif. Intern. Organs 21:427-435, 1975.
24. Turitto VT, Muggli R, Baumgartner HR. Trans. Am. Soc. Artif. Intern. Organs 24:568-578, 1978.
25. Salzman EW and Merrill EW. In: Hemostasis and Thrombosis. Basic Principles and Clinical Practice (Eds. Colman RW, Hirsh J, Marder VJ and Salzman EW), J.B. Lippincott, Philadelphia, pp. 931-943, 1982.
26. Hovig T. Thromb. Diath. Haemorrh. 8:455-471, 1962.
27. White, JG. In: Platelets: Production, Function, Transfusion and Storage (Eds. Baldini MG and Ebbe S), Grune & Stratton, New York, pp. 235-252, 1974.
28. Buckingham S and Maynert EW. J. Pharmacol. Exp. Ther. 143:332-339, 1964.
29. Holmsen H, Day HJ and Storm E. Biochim. Biophys. Acta 186:254-266, 1969.
30. Holmsen H and Day JH. J. Lab. Clin. Med. 75:840-855, 1970.
31. Kaplan KL, Broekman MJ, Chernoff A, Lesznik GR and Drillings M. Blood 53:604-618, 1979.
32. Mustard JF, Perry DW, Kinlough-Rathbone RL and Packham MA. Am. J. Physiol. 228:1757-1765, 1975.
33. Packham MA, Kinlough-Rathbone RL, Reimers H-J, Scott S and Mustard JF. In: Prostaglandins in Hematology (Eds. Silver MJ, Smith JB and Kocsis JJ), Spectrum, New York, pp. 247-276, 1977.
34. Kinlough-Rathbone RL, Reimers JJ and Mustard JF. Science 192:1011-1012, 1976.
35. Packham MA. Thromb. Haemostasis 36:269-272, 1976.
36. Holmsen H. Thromb. Haemostasis 38:1030-1040, 1977.
37. Gerrard JM, Philips DR, Rao GHR, Plow EF, Walz DA, Ross R, Harker LA and White JG. J. Clin. Invest. 66:102-109, 1980.
38. Nurden AT and Caen JP. Nature (London) 255:720-722, 1975.
39. Lewis N and Majerus PW. J. Clin. Invest. 48:2114-2123, 1969.
40. Packham MA, Kinlough-Rathbone RL, Reimers HJ, Scott S and Mustard JF. In: Prostaglandins and Hematology (Eds. Silver MJ et al.), Spectrum, New York, pp. 247-276, 1977.
41. Kinlough-Rathbone RL, Packham MA and Mustard JF. Thromb. Res. 11:567-580, 1977.
42. Needleman P, Whitaker MO, Whyche A, Watters K, Sprecher H and Raz A. Prostaglandins 19:165-181, 1980.
43. Dutilh CE, Haddeman E, Don JA and Ten Hoor F. Prostaglandins Med. 6:111-126, 1981.
44. Schaffer AI. N. Engl. J. Med. 306:381-384, 1982.
45. Buchanan MR, Butt RW, Markham B and Hirsh J. Thromb. Haemostasis 50 (Suppl. 1):101, 1983.
46. Lerner R, Goldstein R and Cummings G. Proc. Soc. Exp. Biol. Med. 138:145-148, 1971.
47. Niemetz J. J. Clin. Invest. 51:307-313, 1972.
48. Kociba GJ, Loeb WF and Wall RL. J. Lab. Clin. Med. 79:778-787, 1972.
49. Rivers RP, Hathaway WE and Westen WL. Br. J. Haematol. 30:311-316, 1975.
50. Tobb-Smith AHT. Br. J. Haematol. 13:618-636, 1967.
51. Sizma JJ. Thromb. Haemostasis 40:163-167, 1978.
52. Lopaciuk S, Lovette KM, McDonagh J, Chaung HTK and McDonagh RP. Thromb. Res. 8:453-465, 1976.
53. Kaplan KL, Broekman J, Chernoff A, Lesznik GR and Drillings M. Blood 53:604-618 , 1979.
54. Keenan JP and Solum NO. Br. J. Haematol. 23:461-488, 1972.

55. Breederveld K, Giddings JC, tenCate JW and Bloom AL. Br. J. Haematol. 29:405-412, 1975.
56. Osterud B, Rapaport SI and Lavine KK. Blood 49:819-834, 1977.
57. Giddings JC, Shearn SAM and Bloom AL. Br. J. Haematol. 39:569-577, 1978.
58. Slot JW, Bouma BN, Montgomery R and Zimmerman TS. Thromb. Res. 13:871-881, 1978.
59. Zucker MB, Broekman MJ and Kaplan KL. J. Lab. Clin. Med. 94:675-682, 1979.
60. Lipscomb MS and Walsh PN. J. Clin. Invest. 63:1006-1011, 1979.
61. Tuszynski GP, Bevacona SJ, Schmaier AH, Cloman RW and Walsh PN. Blood 59:1148-1156, 1982.
62. Luscher EF. Schweiz Med. Wochenschr. 87:1220-1221, 1957.
63. McDonagh J, Kiesselbach TH and Wagner RH. Am. J. Physiol. 216:508-513, 1969.
64. Zwaal RFA and Coenraad Hemnker H. Haemostasis 11:12-39, 1982.
65. Miale JB. Laboratory Medicine. Hematology. Chapter 15. Fourth edition. C.V. Mosby Co., St. Louis, MO, pp. 1054-1193, 1972.
66. Walsh, PN. Br. J. Haematol. 22:237-254, 1972.
67. Walsh PN. Br. J. Haematol. 22:393-405, 1972.
68. Walsh PN and Griffin JH. Blood 57:106-118, 1981.
69. Fantl P and Ward HA. Aust. J. Exp. Biol. Med. Sci. 36:497-504, 1958.
70. Biggs R. In: Human Blood Coagulation, Hemostasis and Thrombosis (Ed. Biggs R), Blackwell, Oxford, pp. 66-80, 1976.
71. Miletich JP, Jackson CM and Majerus PW. J. Biol. Chem. 253:6908-6916, 1978.
72. Hoyer LW. Blood 58:1-13, 1981.
73. Bouma BN, Wiegerink Y and Sixma JJ. Nature (London) New Biol. 136:104-106, 1972.
74. Zimmerman TS, Ratnoff OD and Powell AE. J. Clin. Invest. 50:244-254, 1971.
75. Weiss HJ and Hoyer LW. Science 182:1149-1151, 1973.
76. Sussman II and Weiss HJ. Thromb. Haemostasis 40:316-325, 1978.
77. Bloom AL. Semin. Hematol. 17:215-227, 1980.
78. Zimmerman TS, Abilgaard CF and Meyer D. N. Engl. J. Med. 301:1307-1310, 1979.
79. Meyer D, Obert B, Pietu G, Lavergue JM and Zimmerman TS. J. Lab. Clin. Med. 95:590-602, 1980.
80. Kao KJ, Pizzo SV and McKee PA. J. Clin. Invest. 63:656-664, 1979.
81. Kao KJ, Pizzo SV and McKee PA. Proc. Natl. Acad. Sci. USA 76:5317-5320, 1979.
82. Andersson L-P and Brown JE. Biochem. J. 200:161-167, 1981.
83. Lajmanovich A, Hudry-Clergeon G, Freyssinet J-M and Marguerie G. Biochim. Biophys. Acta 678:132-136, 1981.
84. Tracy PB, Paterson JM, Nesheim ME, McDuffie FC and Mann KG. J. Biol. Chem. 254:10354-10361, 1979.
85. Pusey ML, Mayer LD, Jason Wei G, Bloomfield VA and Nelsestven GI. Biochemistry 21:2562-2579, 1982.
86. Kane WH, Mruk JS and Majerus PW. J. Clin. Invest. 70:1092, 1982.
87. Nesheim ME, Taswell JB and Mann KG. J. Biol. Chem. 254:10952-10962, 1979.
88. Stenflo J and Dahlback B. In: The Regulation of Coagulation (Eds. Mann KG and Taylor FB), Elsevier/North Holland, New York, 1980.
89. Mann KG, Predergast FG and Bloom JW. In: The Regulation of Coagulation (Eds. Mann KG and Taylor FB), Elsevier/North Holland, New York, pp. 3-9, 1980.
90. Milstone JH. Fed. Proc. Fed. Am. Soc. Exp. Biol. 23:742-778, 1964.
91. Nesheim ME, Eid S and Mann KG. J. Biol. Chem. 256:9874-9882, 1981.
92. Marcus AJ, Zucker-Franklin D, Safier LB and Ullman HL. J. Clin. Invest. 45:14-27, 1966.
93. Van Dieijen G, Tans G, Rosing J and Hemker HC. Biochemistry 256:3433-3442, 1981.
94. Vehar GA and Davie EW. Biochemistry 19:401-410, 1980.
95. Walsh PN and Biggs R. Br. J. Haematol. 22:743-760, 1972.

96. Guinto ER and Esmon CT. J. Biol. Chem. 257:10038-10043, 1982.
97. Esmon, CT. J. Biol. Chem. 254:964-973, 1979.
98. Bevers EM, Comforius P and Zwaal FRA. Eur. J. Biochem. 122:81-85, 1982.
99. Bevers EM, Comforius P, van Rijn JLM, Hemker HC and Zwaal RFA. Eur. J. Biochem. 122:429-436, 1982.
100. van Zutphen H, Bevers EM, Hemker HC and Zwaal RFA. Br. J. Haematol. 45:121-131, 1980.
101. Rucinski B, Niewiarowski S, James P, Walz DA and Budzynski A. Blood 53:47-62, 1979.
102. Handin RI and Cohen HJ. J. Biol. Chem. 251:4273-4278, 1976.

CHAPTER 10. MECHANISMS OF PLATELET AGGREGATION BY MURINE TUMOR CELL SHEDDINGS

GABRIEL J. GASIC, TATIANA B. GASIC AND GWENDOLYN J. STEWART

I. INTRODUCTION

Cells from a variety of animal and human neoplasms can induce the aggregation of platelets in plasma (1-3). While the mechanism of this effect has not been fully elucidated preliminary evidence suggests that several mechanisms may exist. With human tumor cells platelet aggregation may be induced via mechanisms involving the leakage of tumor cell ADP (2,4,5; see also Chapters 11 and 12). In rodents aggregation may occur with both whole cells and cell sheddings. This suggests that the aggregating activity of intact cells is mediated by the spontaneous release of some subcellular component. We found that a mixture of membrane vesicles and cytoplasmic dense granules were shed (6). Normal cells are also capable of shedding a small amount of material which is much less active in platelet aggregation (6,7).

In this chapter we will limit our consideration to the platelet aggregating activity of material shed from murine tumors and possible mechanisms by which shed material aggregates platelets.

II. EXPERIMENTAL SYSTEMS

Three different murine tumor cell lines and one murine virally transformed fibroblastic cell line will be considered: 1. a spontaneous mouse mammary tumor (15091A) studied extensively by Gasic and associates (1,2,8-10), 2. a murine renal adenocarcinoma studied by Hara et al. (11), 3. a fibroblastic cell line transformed by SV40 virus studied by Karpatkin and associates (3,4,7,12) and 4. MCA6. The 15091A and MCA6 cells were grown intraperitoneally as ascites tumors. In addition, 15091A cells were also grown on biocarrier beads in tissue culture. The murine renal adenocarcinoma and the transformed fibroblastic cell line were grown as monolayers in tissue culture.

All of these cells spontaneously shed membrane vesicles, however, the amount of shed material can be greatly increased by treatment with urea (7), isotonic low ionic strength medium (11) or mild trypsinization (13). The shed vesicles were collected by differential centrifugation. Karpatkin and associates (7) and Hara et al. (11) used these vesicles without further purification. On the other hand Gasic and associates purified the shed vesicles by sucrose density gradient centrifugation (9,13). Vesicles with or without further purification were capable of inducing aggregation of rat, rabbit or human platelets in heparinized plasma. Aggregation of washed or gel filtered platelets from rats, rabbits or humans required a minimal amount of platelet poor plasma (PPP).

III. PLATELET-VESICLE INTERACTIONS

A. Platelet Aggregating Activity Shed Spontaneously by Cells

1. Spontaneous shedding of vesicles by 15091A. In Figure 1A (x 8,250) the surfaces of ascitic 15091A cells can be seen to be covered by cytoplasm filled membrane protrusions that take the form of microvilli or rounded blebs with a broad base. In Figure 1B (x 17,000) are shown tumor cell sheddings composed of membrane vesicles with cytoplasm and dense granules which appeared to be ribosomes. Two fractions could be further purified by sucrose density centrifugation. One fraction was composed of membrane vesicles (Figure 1C, x 32,000) and the other fraction composed of dense granules (Figure 1D, x 31,800).

2. Activity of vesicles isolated by sucrose density gradient centrifugation. Addition of these vesicles to rat platelet rich plasma (PRP) caused irreversible aggregation with as little as one μg of protein. The aggregation was preceded by a lag period of one or more minutes depending upon the protein concentration of the fraction added. The higher the concentration of vesicle protein, the shorter was the lag period. This aggregation coincided with platelet secretion as shown by lumiaggregometry studies (Figure 2). Possible mechanisms for this aggregation might include physical adhesion or binding of vesicles to platelets, the release of platelet activating agents such as ADP or a cathepsin B-like proteinase (see also Chapter 12) and activation of the clotting cascade leading to the generation of thrombin, even in the presence of heparin.

A typical aggregometry tracing of purified vesicle-induced platelet aggregation (rat PRP) is shown in Figure 2A. The lag period is indicated by I, the rapid aggregation period by II and the plateau of maximal aggregation by III. In Figure 2B is shown a typical tracing from the lumiaggregometer. The binding of vesicles was complete for almost a minute before platelet ADP release. Platelet ADP release then continued during the period of rapid aggregation.

Vesicles labeled with ^{125}I were used to establish that binding of vesicles preceded platelet aggregation and occurred even in the presence of levels of prostacyclin or dibutyryl cAMP which blocked subsequent platelet aggregation. Vesicle binding was proportional to the concentration of vesicles added. Prior addition of unlabeled vesicles decreased the binding of ^{125}I-labeled vesicles. Once vesicles had bound, they could not be displaced by addition of unlabeled vesicles, indicating irreversible binding.

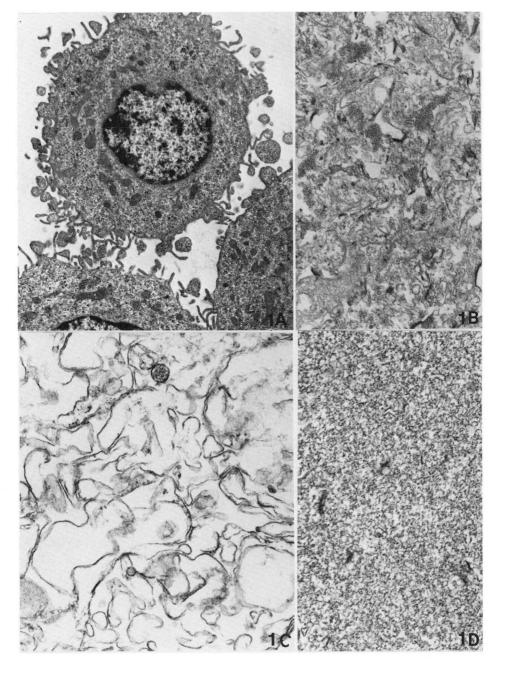

130

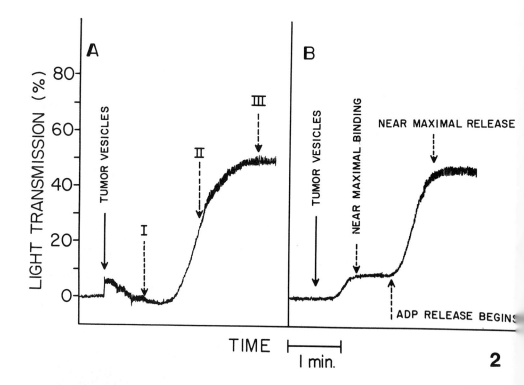

Ultrastructural support for the binding of vesicles to platelets is evident in Figure 3: Figure 3A (x 25,000), rat platelets to which no vesicles were added and Figure 3B (x 25,000), rat platelets (treated with PGI_2 before the addition of vesicles) with numerous membrane vesicles in close proximity to the platelets. The frequency of vesicles in close proximity to platelets increased with increasing vesicle concentration.

Gel filtered rat platelets no longer bound vesicles nor aggregated. However, if a small aliquot of heparinized plasma was added back into the system, binding took place and aggregation proceeded in the usual manner. Thus, we concluded that plasma cofactors were essential for both events.

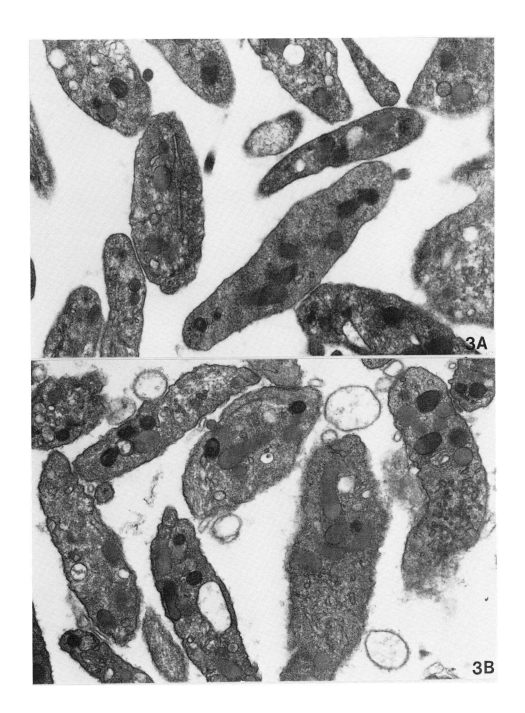

A subsequent series of experiments indicated that divalent cations and complement were necessary cofactors for vesicle binding to platelets. Rat plasma that was depleted of C3 by treatment with zymosan or cobra venom or C4 deficient guinea pig plasma or serum no longer supported vesicle binding. While complement and divalent cations were required for vesicle binding they were not sufficient for platelet aggregation. Aggregation required the presence of the vitamin K-dependent plasma proteins of the clotting cascade (14) as shown by the failure of rat plasma from coumadin treated rats to support aggregation after vesicle binding (8,10). The role of thrombin in platelet aggregation was further investigated by the use of specific synthetic inhibitors of thrombin such as DAPA (4) and compound 805 (10). Final concentrations of inhibitors in the range of 1 to 5 μM completely inhibited aggregation of platelets by tumor vesicles in rat PRP. Hirudin, a natural, specific and irreversible inhibitor of thrombin (11-15), also prevented platelet aggregation at a level of 80 units/ml.

Ultrastructural evidence for the role of thrombin generation in platelet aggregation induced by tumor vesicles is shown in Figure 5. In platelet aggregation induced by ADP (Figure 4A, x 11,250) and by collagen (Figure 4B, x 11,250), the platelets demonstrated gross shape change and degranulation and were tightly aggregated. However, no fibrin was evident. A low magnification survey of a tumor vesicle-induced platelet aggregate using the same heparinized rat PRP as that used in Figure 4 is shown in Figure 5A (x 14,000). In this case dark strands resembling fibrin are dispersed throughout the aggregate. In a higher magnification (Figure 5B, x 31,8000) some of the strands demonstrate the typical periodicity of fibrin. This observation may be explained by the presence in platelets, probably in the lysosomes, of an enzyme that can degrade heparin (16,17).

Vesicles of 15091A cells isolated by Cavanaugh et al. (9 and Chapter 12) induced a typical two phase aggregation of washed human platelets in the presence of Ca^{++} and a small amount of human plasma. The aggregation was prevented by inhibitors of cysteine proteinases such as leupeptin and antipain but not by inhibitors of serine proteinases such as aprotinin or soybean trypsin inhibitor (9). The same authors also found that homogenates of the vesicles contain cathepsin B-like activity and that activity could be inhibited by the same inhibitors that blocked platelet aggregation. The cathepsin B-like proteinase was apparently a proenzyme which required proteolytic cleavage for full activity (see Chapter 12).

Although a cathepsin B-like enzyme appears to be involved in induction of platelet aggregation it is not yet clear whether the proteinase is acting directly on the platelet membrane, presumably when vesicles bind to platelets or whether it is capable of activating clotting factor X (18 and Chapter 6), thereby leading to thrombin generation.

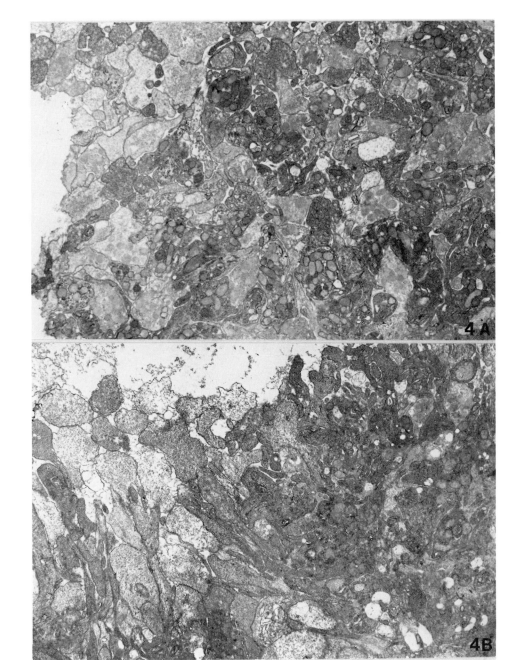

4A

4B

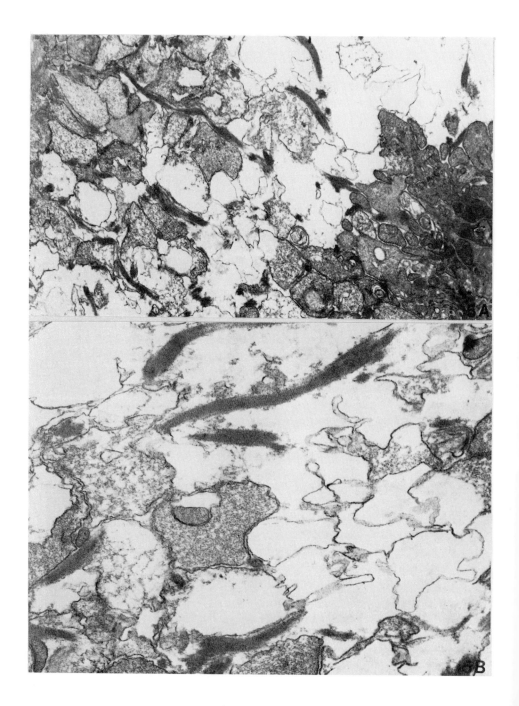

B. Platelet Aggregating Activity Released by Augmented Shedding

1. **Isotonic low ionic strength medium.** Confluent monolayers of a
mouse renal adenocarcinoma cell line were incubated at 37°C for 24 hr
in the presence of an isotonic low ionic strength solution. After
incubation the medium was collected and the shed material isolated and
concentrated by vacuum filtration. This preparation induced platelet
aggregation in the same manner as did whole cells with a typically
prolonged lag period preceding aggregation. The platelet aggregating
material was completely sedimentable (2600 x g, 10 min). Platelet
aggregation required Mg^{++} and plasma (5%). One important component of
plasma was fibrinogen which could itself partially restore the maximal
aggregation of washed rabbit platelets. The investigators attributed
platelet aggregation to the release of ADP from platelets directly
activated by contact with vesicles; vesicles were shown in close
contact with platelets. The addition of ADP-degrading enzymes to the
system or treatment of platelets with aspirin suppressed the
aggregation. In contrast, they felt that thrombin was not involved
since platelets aggregated in the presence of heparin and hirudin.
However, this remains to be resolved since rat platelets were induced
to aggregate by vesicles from 15091A cells in heparinized PRP and in
the presence of low levels of hirudin. The activity of membrane
fragments could not be extracted as a soluble material and apparently
depended on an intact membranous structure.

2. **Urea.** The amount of platelet aggregating activity shed from
cultured tumor cells was substantially augmented by urea treatment.
Originally this was done by Pearlstein et al. (7) using an SV40
virally transformed mouse fibroblastic cell line. In this study
confluent monolayers of transformed cells in a shaker incubator were
treated with 1 M urea. After one hour of incubation at 30°C the
medium was collected, centrifuged to remove floating cells and the
cell-free supernatant dialyzed and concentrated to 1/100 of their
original volume.

This concentrate induced typical platelet aggregation of
heparinized rabbit or human platelet rich plasma and of gel filtered
rabbit platelets in the presence of Ca^{++} and a small amount of PRP
following the typical lag period of 1-2 min. The material was
particulate and sedimentable at 100,000 x g for 60 min. Karpatkin et
al. (12) identified two plasma cofactors that were necessary for
platelet aggregating activity, one sensitive and one resistant to
heating at 56°C for 30 min. The heat-labile factor appeared to be one
or more components of the complement system as indicated by tests for
C3. Plasma decomplemented by cobra venom factor or zymosan did not
support platelet aggregation. However, guinea-pig plasma genetically
deficient in C4 supported platelet aggregation indicating that the
classical pathway of complement activation was not involved.

These investigators demonstrated the binding of platelet
aggregating material to platelets by covalently binding the shed
material to Sepharose beads and adding the beads to PRP or gel
filtered platelets free of plasma. Following platelet aggregation the
association of the aggregating material and platelets was evident from

the adherence of platelets and platelet clumps to the surface of the coated beads.

The process of urea-induced shedding of vesicles was investigated by the present authors. Ascitic 15091A cells were extracted with urea according to the method of Pearlstein et al. (7). Urea treatment considerably increased the amount of material that was shed by the cells. A vesicle component and a dense granule component were isolated by sucrose density gradient centrifugation. This material induced aggregation of platelets and very likely constitutes the physical basis of the platelet aggregating material described by Pearlstein et al. (7).

The ultrastructural basis for the urea-enhanced release of platelet aggregating material from ascitic 15091A cells is illustrated in Figure 6. In Figure 6A (x 8,250) is a control cell with typical microvilli and round blebs on the surface. In Figure 6B (x 8,250) are shown the deep clefts in the membrane of urea treated cells. Figure 6C (x 20,500) shows a mixture of membrane vesicles and dense granules shed from the cells. Figure 6D (x 17,000) shows a purified fraction of membrane vesicles and Figure 6E (x 32,000) shows a purified fraction of dense granules. The appearances of the crude shed material and of the purified fractions were indistinguishable from that of spontaneously shed material.

3. Trypsin. Agents other than urea were capable of inducing vesiculation of the plasma membrane (18) and also increased the shedding of platelet aggregating material. In our experience tryspin is such an agent. Ascitic 15091A and MCA6 that were treated by mild trypsinization released material that aggregated platelets while the cells themselves retained the ability to aggregate platelets. However, prolonged (18 hr) treatment with trypsin destroyed the ability of the cells to aggregate platelets, presumably because the ability of the cells to produce vesicles was exhausted. Interestingly the capacity of the cells to aggregate platelets was restored when the cells were incubated in trypsin-free culture medium under conditions permitting the synthesis of membrane proteins, i.e., in the absence of inhibitors of protein synthesis such as cycloheximide and puromycin (13).

IV. CONCLUSIONS

The ability of murine tumor cells to shed material with platelet aggregating activity was a basic characteristic of these cells as indicated by the diversity of systems that were used for its demonstration. Furthermore, the shed material was able to induce aggregation of a variety of platelets ranging from rat to human. The shed material induced platelet aggregation by at least three mechanisms: the release of ADP, the release of a cathepsin B-like proteinase and the activation of the clotting cascade. Different mechanisms were demonstrated in different systems but this may be a consequence of experimental design rather than differences between tumors. Careful investigation may demonstrate that all three

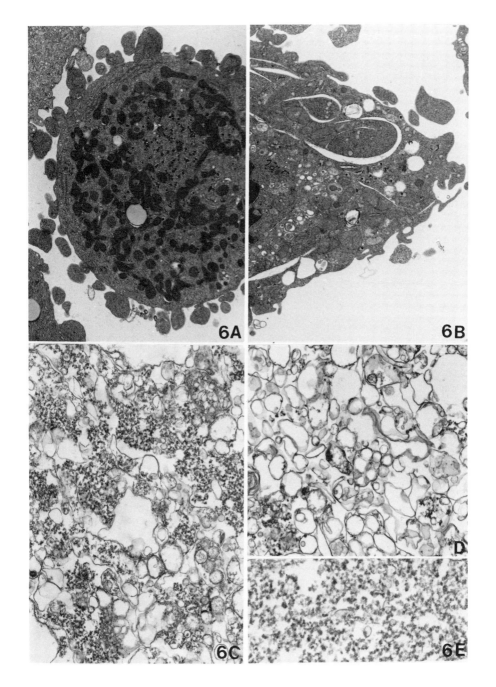

activities are present in material shed from all tumors. The third component of complement appeared to be required for the binding of vesicles to platelets while the clotting cascade was required for platelet aggregation. The role of direct platelet activation through vesicle binding and the role of a cathepsin B-like cysteine proteinase remain to be established (see also Chapter 12).

REFERENCES

1. Gasic GJ, Gasic TB, Galanti N, Johnson T and Murphy S. Int. J. Cancer 11:704-718, 1981.
2. Gasic GJ, Koch PAG, Hsu B, Gasic TB and Niewiarowski S. Z. Krebsforch. 86:263-277, 1976.
3. Karpatkin S and Pearlstein E. Ann. Intern. Med. 95:636-641, 1981.
4. Pearlstein E, Ambrogio C, Gasic G and Karpatkin S. Cancer Res. 41:4535-4539, 1981.
5. Bastida E, Ordinas A, Giardina SL and Jamieson GA. Cancer Res. 42:4348-4352, 1982.
6. Gasic GJ, Boettiger D, Catalfamo JL, Gasic TB and Stewart GJ. Cancer Res. 38:2950-2955, 1978.
7. Pearlstein E, Cooper L and Karpatkin S. J. Lab. Clin. Med. 93:332-344, 1979.
8. Gasic GJ, Catalfamo JL, Gasic TB and Avdalovic N. In: Malignancy and the Hemostatic System (Eds. Donati MB, Davidson JF and Garattini S), Raven Press, New York, pp. 27-35, 1981.
9. Cavanaugh PG, Sloane BF, Bajkowski A, Gasic GJ, Gasic TB and Honn KV. Clin. Exp. Metastasis (in press).
10. Gasic GJ, Gasic TB. In: Interaction of Platelets and Tumor Cells (Ed. Jamieson GA), Alan R. Liss, New York, pp. 429-443, 1982.
11. Hara Y, Steiner M and Baldini MG. Cancer Res. 40:1217-1223, 1980.
12. Karpatkin S, Smerling A and Pearlstein E. J. Lab. Clin. Med. 95:994-1001, 1980.
13. Gasic GJ, Gasic TB and Jimenez SA. Lab. Invest. 36:413-419, 1977.
14. Stenflo, J. Adv. Enzymol. Relat. Areas Mol. Biol. 46:1-36, 1978.
15. Markwardt F. Methods Enzymol. 19:924-932, 1970.
16. Wasteson A, Glimelius B, Busch C, Westermark B, Hedlin C-H and Norling B. Thromb. Res. 1:309-321, 1977.
17. Oosta GM, Faverau LV, Beeler DL and Rosenberg RD. J. Biol. Chem. 257:11249-11255, 1982.
18. Gordon SG and Cross BA. J. Clin. Invest. 67:1665-1671, 1981.

CHAPTER 11. HETEROGENOUS MECHANISMS OF TUMOR CELL-INDUCED PLATELET AGGREGATION WITH POSSIBLE PHARMACOLOGIC STRATEGY TOWARD PREVENTION OF METASTASES

SIMON KARPATKIN AND EDWARD PEARLSTEIN

I. INTRODUCTION

Recent reports from several laboratories have emphasized the role of platelets in the development of certain tumor metastases (for review see 1). Platelets interact with certain tumor emboli, and in so doing, appear to enhance their survival in vivo. Both platelets as well as tumor cells adhere to subendothelial basement membrane. Platelets secrete permeability factors (2,3) as well as tumor cell growth factors (4-7), which theoretically should assist in tumor cell penetration of the vessel wall and development of extravascular secondary tumor colonies.

Our laboratory has been interested in the ability of certain tumors to aggregate platelets in vitro, in order to better understand the mechanism and significance of tumor cell-platelet interaction in vivo. We have grouped tumors into three groups based on different mechanisms of tumor-induced platelet aggregation from studies (8-12) of ten different tumor cell lines (Table 1). The first group consists of virally-transformed SV40 murine fibroblasts (SV3T3 cells) (8,9) and polyoma (PW20) transformed rat renal sarcoma cells (10). Both require cell surface sialic acid for platelet aggregating activity. SV3T3 cells (studied more extensively) require surface phospholipid and trypsin-sensitive protein, divalent cation, serum complement and a stable plasma factor for activity (8,9). The cell surface sialic acid content of ten different PW20 rat renal sarcoma lines, selected on their varying ability to metastasize in vivo, correlates positively with their ability to aggregate platelets as well as their ability to metastasize ($r = 0.85$) (10).

The second group of tumor conssits of four spontaneous human adenocarcinomas of the colon (11): HCT-8, LoVo, SW-403 and SW-620, and an undifferentiated murine tumor, HUT-20. In contrast to the virally-transformed lines, these tumors aggregate platelets via their procoagulant activity (generation of thrombin). They are inhibited by specific thrombin inhibitors [dansylarginine N-(3-ethyl-1,5-pentanediyl) amide; DAPA and 805) and do not require cell surface sialic acid, trypsin-sensitive protein or serum complement for activity. They do require cell surface phospholipid and divalent cation.

The third group of tumors (12) consists of spontaneous human HM29 melanoma, a spontaneous murine B16F10 melanoma and a carcinogen-induced CT26 murine adenocarcinoma of the colon. These tumors do not require cell surface sialic acid or phospholipid, and do not require serum complement. They do not aggregate platelets via the generation of thrombin. Tumor-induced platelet aggregation is not inhibited by specific thrombin inhibitors. They do require a trypsin-sensitive surface protein for activity.

Table 1. Heterogenous Mechanisms of Tumor-Induced Platelet Aggregation.

	Sialic Acid and Complement Requiring	Thrombin Generating	Phospholipase A_2 Insensitive and Trypsin Sensitive
Tumors	SV3T3 PW20 Rsa[a]	LoVo HCT-8 Hut-20 SW-403[a] SW-620[a]	HM29 B16F10 CT26
Enzymes			
Neuraminidase	+[b]	–	–
Trypsin	+	–	+
Phospholipase A_2	+	–	–
Cobra Venom	+	–	–

[a]Refers to tumors which have been partially studied, and appear to fit into these groups: (i.e., PW20-Rsa is sensitive to neuraminidase, SW-403 and SW-620 are sensitive to inhibition by DAPA).

[b]+ or – refer to tumors which are inhibited (+) or not inhibited (–) from aggregating platelets by this treatment.

Various anti-platelet agents (those which enhance cyclic AMP levels; those which specifically inhibit thrombin; and those which inhibit prostaglandin synthesis) were found to be heterogenous in their ability to interfere with tumor-induced platelet aggregation. This correlated with the mechanism by which the tumor cells aggregated platelets.

II. MATERIALS AND METHODS

A. Tumor Cell Lines and Tissue Culture Media

All cell lines were grown in tissue culture media supplemented with 2 mM glutamine, 100 units/ml penicillin and 100 μg/ml streptomycin, and harvested at confluence. Tissue culture supplies were obtained from Grand Island Biological Co., Grand Island, NY.

SV3T3 mouse fibroblast cells were obtained from the Imperial Cancer Research Fund, London, and grown in Dulbecco's Modified Eagle's Medium (E4) containing 10% calf serum, as previously described (8). HCT-8 spontaneous human colon adenocarcinoma cells were obtained through the courtesy of Dr. E. Cadman of Yale University Medical School, New Haven, CT and grown in RPMI 1640 containing 10% fetal bovine serum, as described previously (11). LoVo spontaneous human colon adenocarcinoma cells were obtained through the courtesy of Dr. B. Drewinko of M.D. Anderson Hospital, Houston, TX, and grown in McCoy's medium 5A containing 15% fetal bovine serum, as described previously (11). HUT-20 cells, an anaplastic murine tumor cell line, was obtained through the courtesy of Dr. Addi Gazdar of the Veterans Administration Hospital, Washington, DC. The line was grown in RPMI 1640 containing 10% Bobby calf serum. B16F10 (high lung colonizing ability) and HM29 spontaneous human melanoma cells were obtained through the courtesy of Dr. J-C Bystryn at our institution, and CT26, N-nitroso-N-methylurethane-induced mouse undifferentiated carcinoma cells (13-16) were obtained through the courtesy of Dr. M.H. Goldrosen at Roswell Park Memorial Institute, Buffalo, NY and grown in the same media as the B16F10 cells.

The PW20 family of tumor cell lines was derived from a culture of the polyoma virus-induced PW20 Wistar-Furth rat renal sarcoma (obtained from H.O. Sjogren, Univ. of Lund, Sweden) by varying conditions of passage in tissue culture and passage through syngeneic animals by Salk and Yogeeswaran (10,17). The spontaneous metastatic behavior of the tumor cell lines was evaluated in syngeneic Wistar-Furth rats by Salk and Yogeeswaran (10,17). The percent sialylation of the exposed cell surface glycoconjugates was determined by using the galactose oxidase/sodium boro[^{3}H]hydride-labeling technique as described (10,18).

Unless otherwise noted, tumor cells were harvested from tissue culture dishes with brief trypsin-EDTA treatment as described previously (11). They were washed three times and suspended in Veronal buffer (0.03 M sodium barbital - 0.12 M NaCl buffer, pH 7.4) and quantitated in a hemocytometer. Trypan blue exclusion, for viability, was greater than 90%.

PAM. A platelet aggregating material (PAM) could be extracted from some of the tumor cell lines with 1 M urea, followed by dialysis, as described previously (8). This PAM is enriched with membrane vesicles.

B. Platelet Aggregation

Platelet-rich plasma (PRP) and platelet-poor plasma were prepared as described previously (8,9), employing heparin, 5 units/ml final concentration (Liquamin, Organon, Inc., West Orange, NJ) or trisodium citrate, 0.38% (w/v) final concentration. Platelets were obtained from New Zealand white rabbits in order to facilitate comparisons because some of the murine cell lines did not aggregate human platelets. Gel-filtered platelets were prepared (19) employing Sepharose 6B (Pharmacia Fine Chemicals, Piscataway, NJ).

Aggregation was performed turbidometrically, employing a Bio-Data aggregometer (Bio-Data, Willow Grove, PA) (8-12). ADP (grade 1, Sigma Chemical Co., St. Louis, MO) was employed as a positive control agonist at 10 μM final concentration. Apyrase [grade 1, from potato with 1.9 units ADPase/mg protein (Sigma Chemical Co.)] was employed to eliminate potential ADP leakage from tumor cells. (This is noted when tumor cells aggregate platelets in the absence of a lag period, and can be eliminated by preincubation of tumor cells with 2-3 units/ml ADPase at 37°C for 2 min prior to addition of tumor cells to PRP, or by extensively washing the tumor cells.)

C. Variables Affecting Platelet Aggregation

Aggregation inhibition was defined as 50% reduction of the maximal slope of the velocity of platelet aggregation noted after an initial lag period of usually 1-3 min.

1. Enzyme treatment. All enzymes and reagents were obtained from Sigma Chemical Co. Washed tumor cells were incubated with either neuraminidase (1 unit/ml, type V) plus 2 mM PMSF or boiled (10 min) phospholipase A_2 (25 μg/ml, bee venom). They were then washed in sodium barbital buffer (as above) and utilized for aggregation studies as described previously (8-12). Trypsin treatment was performed directly on tissue cell monolayers and the cells removed and prepared for aggregation as described previously (11).

2. Treatment of platelet-rich plasma with complement activators. Purified cobra venom factor (20 units/ml final concentration) from Naja naja Kaouthia (Cordis Laboratories, Miami, FL) was incubated with 0.4 ml of platelet-rich plasma for 30 min at 37°C, follwed by addition of tumor cell suspension and apyrase. Control aggregation with 1   M ADP was not affected by a similar 30 min incubation with cobra venom factor (9).

D. Pharmacologic Agents Interfering with Tumor-Induced Platelet Aggregation

In a typical experiment, 50 μl of varying concentration of pharmacological agent in buffer, or buffer alone, were preincubated with 0.4 ml of heparinized PRP in an aggregometer cuvette for 3 min at 37°C prior to the addition of 50 μl of tumor cell suspension containing apyrase.

1. Anti-thrombin agents. DAPA was synthesized and kindly supplied by Dr. Kenneth Mann, Mayo Foundation, Rochester, MN. This highly-specific synthetic competitive inhibitor of thrombin has a Ki for fibrinogen of 0.1 μM (20). Another highly specific synthetic competitive inhibitor, No. 805, was kindly supplied by Dr. Y. Amari of Mitsubishi Chemical Industries, Ltd., Tokyo, and Dr. S. Okamura of

Kobe University, Japan. This compound selectively inhibits the interaction of thrombin with fibrinogen with a Ki of 0.019 μM (21,22).

2. Platelet aggregation inhibitors which elevate cyclic AMP Levels. Prostacyclin (PGI_2) and 6-keto-PGE_1 (a more stable analogue of PGI_2) were kindly supplied by Drs. U.F. Axen, G. Neil and J. Pike of the Upjohn Co., Kalamazoo, MI. These reagents were freshly dissolved in 0.05 M Tris-HCl buffer, pH 9.3-9.4, prior to use. Dibutryl cyclic AMP was obtained from Sigma Chemical Co. and dissolved in Veronal buffer prior to use.

3. Platelet aggregation inhibitors which interfere with prostaglandin synthesis by inhibiting platelet cyclooxygenase activity. Sodium ibuprofen solution (50 mg/ml) was obtained through the courtesy of the Upjohn Co. and diluted in 0.9% (w/v) NaCl prior to use. Indomethacin was obtained from Sigma Chemical Co. and dissolved in 1% (v/v) DMSO (Sigma) diluted in veronal buffer.

III. RESULTS

A. Tumors which Require Complement, a Vesicular Cell Surface, Sialo-Lipoprotein Component, Divalent Cation and a Stable Plasma Factor for Platelet Aggregation Activity

SV3T3 cells can aggregate PRP anticoagulated with sodium citrate (0.3% w/v) as well as heparin (5 units/ml).

1. Whole cells. Intact SV3T3 transformed cells were capable of inducing platelet aggregation after a lag period of 1 to 2 min (Figure 1). When 50 μl of transformed cells at an initial concentration of 10 cells/ml were added to 0.4 ml of PRP, the final maximal level of aggregation (optical density change) reached was 80% of that achieved by the addition of 20 μM ADP. The normal 3T3 line was also capable of inducing moderate aggregation following a slightly longer lag period than that observed with the transformed cell. However, the final percentage of aggregation induced by the normal cell line was approximately 40% of the ADP control (Figure 1). Treatment of monolayers of intact SV3T3 cells with 2.5 mg/ml trypsin completely abolished its ability to aggregate platelets (Figure 2).

2. Urea extract. A urea extract of SV3%3 cells induced platelet aggregation at a final concentration of 40 μg/ml protein (Figure 3). In contrast, medium contditioned by the same cell type for an identical length of time required approximately five-fold to ten-fold higher concentration of protein to induce a similar degree of aggregation (data not shown). Dilution of the extracted SV3T3 cell line PAM by a factor of 20 (from 40 to 2 μg/ml) resulted in a loss of activity (Figure 3), demonstrating the sensitivity of the system to dilution. Normal 3T3 cell extracts, at 40 μg/ml, were capable of inducing only slight aggregation after a prolonged lag period (Figure 3).

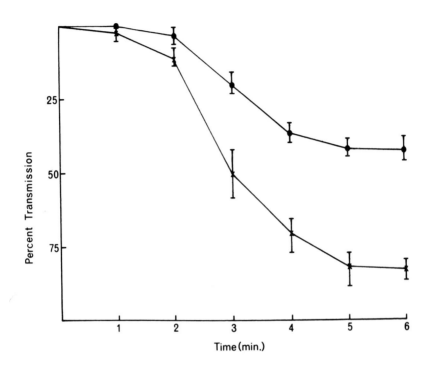

FIGURE 1. Induction of Rabbit Platelet Aggregation in Heparinized PRP by 10,000,000 Intact 3T3 (o) or SV3T3 (x) Cells. Each point (±SEM) represents the average of four experiments. [From Pearlstein et al. (8) with permission.]

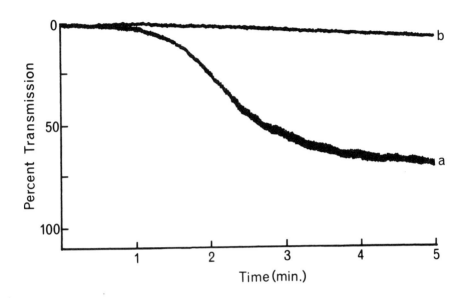

FIGURE 2. Induction of Rabbit Platelet Aggregation in Heparinized PRP by 1,000,000 Intact SV3T3 Cells before (a) and following (b) Treatment of Monolayer Cells with 0.25 ml of 0.25% Trypsin for 5 min at 37°C. Trypsin was neutralized with 0.5 ml of 0.25% soybean trypsin inhibitor prior to the preparation of the cell suspension for the aggregation assay. Subsequently, 0.05 ml of cells was added to 0.4 ml of PRP. Data taken from one of five experiments with similar results. [From Pearlstein et al. (8) with permission.]

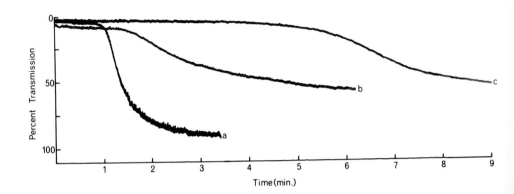

FIGURE 3. Induction of Rabbit Platelet Aggregation in Heparininzed PRP by 1 M Urea Extracts from SV3T3 and 3T3 Cells. Final protein concentration of (a) 40 μg/ml or (b) 2 μg/ml and (c) 40 μg/ml. Data taken from one of 20 experiments with similar results. [From Pearlstein et al. (8) with permission.]

The transfomred cell extract was more effective in heparin-PRP than in citrate-PRP, as were the intact cells, in agreement with the results of others (23).

3. Inhibitors of PAM. As shown in Table 2, several compounds which inhibit the secondary wave of platelet aggregation (24) also prevented PAM induction of platelet aggregation. Thus 5 mM EDTA, 0.05 mM indomethacin, 0.1 mM adenosine, and 0.1 mM N6,0^{2}-dibutyrl cyclic AMP all inhibited PAM activity.

Table 2. Inhibition of PAM-Induced Aggregation with Inhibitors of the Platelet Release Reaction[a]

Inhibitor	Aggregating Agent	Percent Aggregation
Veronal buffer	PAM	100
Veronal buffer	20 μM ADP	100
5 mM EDTA	PAM	0
0.1 mM dBcAMP[b]	PAM	1-30
0.1 mM dBcAMP	20 μM ADP	0
0.1 mM adenosine	PAM	0
0.1 mM adenosine	20 μM ADP	0
0.05 mM indomethacin	PAM	10

[a]All inhibitors were incubated with heparinized rabbit PRP for 6-9 min at 37° C prior to the addition of PAM, 10 μg/ml. Inhibitor concentration is that achieved following dilution of inhibitor in PRP. Each experiment was performed 3 or more times. [From Pearlstein et al. (8) with permission.]

[b]dBcAMP = N^6, $O^{2'}$-dibutyrl cyclic AMP.

4. Release of ^{14}C-serotonin. Direct measurement of the release reaction was performed by quantitating ^{14}C-serotonin release from aggregated platelets. The results, shown in Table 3, indicate that PAM accomplishes irreversible aggregation by inducing platelet release.

Table 3. Release of ^{14}C-Serotonin Following Addition of PAM to Heparinized Rabbit PRP[a]

Addition	CPM in Supernatant	% Release
Veronal buffer	399	2
20 μM ADP	387	2
PAM	10,255	53
Sonication	19,350	100

[a]Percent release was calculated as radioactivity in PAM-containing supernatant minus background radioactivity (buffer) divided by total radioactivity taken up by the platelet suspension. Results are an average of 2 determinations. [From Pearlstein et al. (8) with permission.]

5. <u>Non-inhibitors of PAM</u>. Certain proteinases induce platelet aggregation (25), and tumor cells frequently synthesize higher levels of proteinases than do their normal counterparts (26,27). Therefore, an attempt was made to inhibit PAM with several selective serine proteinase inhibitors known to interfere with transformed cell plasminogen activation (28). All inhibitors were assayed for activity on appropriate substrates prior to use. For example, 2.5 mM DFP inhibited thrombin-induced platelet aggregation at a concentration of 0.1 g/ml. The results given in Table 4 clearly indicate that PAM activity is not related to any increase in serine proteinase activity associated with transformed cell plasma membranes. Thus EACA (0.8 mM), soybean trypsin inhibitor (50-500 μ g/ml), trasylol (50 units/ml), PMSF (2 mM), and DFP (2.5 mM) had no significant effect on platelet aggregation (see also Chapter 12).

Table 4. Effect of Proteinase Inhibitors on PAM-Mediated Platelet Aggregation[a]

Inhibitor	Final Concentration	Percent Aggregation
Veronal buffer	—	100
EACA	0.8 mM	95
Soybean trypsin inhibitor	50-500 μg/ml	98
Trasylol	50 U/ml	95
PMSF	2.0 mM	90
DFP	2.5 mM	82

[a]Inhibitors were incubated with PAM for 4-5 min at 20°C prior to addition to PRP. Each experiment was performed 2 or more times. [From Pearlstein <u>et al</u>. (8) with permission.]

6. <u>Centrifugation of PAM</u>. The urea-extracted PAM from SV3T3 cells can be pelleted by centrifugation at 100,000 x g for 1 hr at 4°C. The results shown in Figure 4 clearly demonstrate that all the activity was recoverable in the pellet, with no residual PAM remaining in the supernatant. The ability to pellet the material provided a means of removing enzyme from the enzyme-treated PAM in order to discriminate between the effect of enzyme on PAM and on the platelet surface.

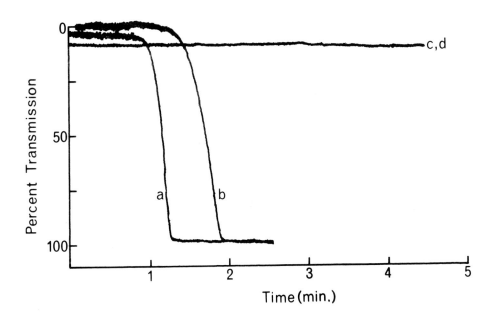

FIGURE 4. Platelet Aggregation following Sedimentation of PAM by Ultracentrifugation. (a) Original SV3T3 extract; (b) resuspended extract pellet in original volume of Veronal buffer following centrifugation at 100,000 x g for 1 hr; (c) supernatant following centrifugation; and (d) 3T3 extract pellet following centrifugtion and resuspension of pellet in veronal buffer. The difference in lag period between a and b is not significant. [From Pearlstein et al. (8) with permission.]

7. Effect of boiling, enzymes, non-ionic detergents or sonication on PAM and PRP. The following treatments, listed in Table 5, completely destroyed PAM activity: (1) boiling for 15 min (partial activity could be restored, following boiling, by storage for several weeks at 4°C); (2) crystalline trypsin at 1 mg/ml; (3) neuraminidase at 2 mg/ml in the presence of 2 mM PMSF; (4) boiled phospholipase A_2 at 0.1 µg/ml; (5) non-ionic detergents, NP-40 (0.1%) and Tween 80 (0.1%); (6) sonication for 15 sec at 0°C. Beta-Galactosidase at 5 mg/ml had no effect on PAM.

149

150

PAM was washed by centrifugation and resuspended in fresh buffer prior to mixing with platelets in order to ensure that these enzymes or compounds did not affect platelets directly, making them unresponsive to PAM. Furthermore, platelet aggregation could be induced by addition of fresh PAM to PRP containing inactivated PAM. Therefore, the effect was on PAM directly, not on platelet receptors for PAM.

Table 5. Effect of Boiling, Enzymes, Non-Ionic Detergents and Sonication on PAM Activity[a]

Treatment	Final Concentration or Time	Percent Aggregation	N[b]
Boiling	15 min	0	3
Boiling and storage at 0°C for 2 weeks	–	30–40	2
Trypsin-TPCK	1 mg/ml	0	5
Neuraminidase	2 mg/ml	0	5
Phospholipase A_2	0.1 µg/ml	0	5
NP-40	0.1%	0	3
Tween-80	0.1%	0	3
Sonication	15 sec	0	2
β-Galactosidase	0.5 mg/ml	83	2

[a]All enzymes, in 10 µl volume, were incubated with 100 µl of PAM, 100 µg/ml, for 1 hr at 37°C. PAM was then sedimented at 100,000 x g for 1 hr at 4°C, and the pellet was resuspended in 100 µl of veronal buffer. Of this material, 50 µl were used for platelet-aggregation studies with heparinized rabbit platelet rich plasma. [From Pearlstein et al. (8) with permission.]

[b]N = number of experiments.

8. Requirement of a labile plasma factor. In the absence of plasma (gel-filtered platelets), PAM-induced aggregation did not occur (Figure 5a and b). However, the addition of plasma to a final concentration of 10% completely restored PAM-mediated aggregation, which followed a typical lag period of 1 to 2 min. This restoration by plasma was concentration-dependent.

9. Studies on the lag period and activation of PAM. The lag period
routinely observed preceding the aggregation could be shortened or
eliminated by preincubating PAM with plasma prior to its addition to
GFP (Figure 5c) or platelet-rich plasma (data not shown). This
preincubation served to activate PAM. When PAM was incubated with
plasma for 10 min at 37°C and the mixture was added to platelets, the
lag period was reduced from 1 to 2 min to less than 0.5 min. The
reduction in lag period was dependent on the duration of
preincubation, with maximal reduction occurring after 10 to 15 min.

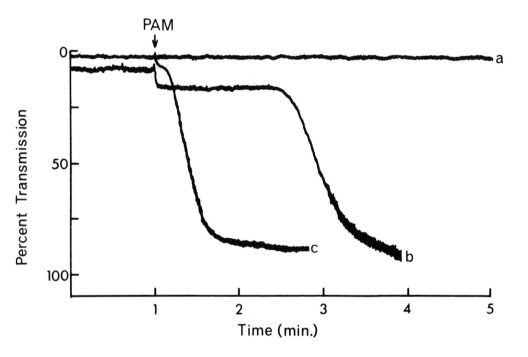

FIGURE 5. Aggregation of 0.4 ml of Gel-Filtered Platelets (GFP) by 50
µl of PAM (20 µg) in the Absence (a) or the Presence (b) of 10%
Plasma. Plasma was added at time zero. Preincubation of PAM with an
equal volume of plasma for 10 min at 37°C prior to its addition (50
µl) to GFP abolished the lag period (c). [From Karpatkin et al. (9)
with permission.]

PAM did not lose its aggregating activity after heating at 56°C for 30 min. In contrast, heating of plasma to 56°C for 30 min resulted in the complete loss of its ability to support PAM-induced aggregation of GFP (Figure 6a and b). However, when PAM and plasma were incubated for 10 min at 37°C and then heated for 30 min at 56°C, the mixture was capable of supporting platelet aggregation with a shortened lag period (Figure 6c and d).

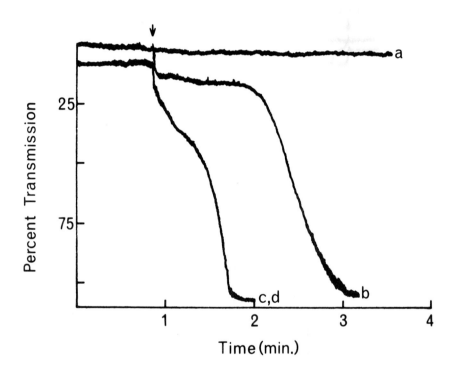

FIGURE 6. Aggregation of 0.4 ml of GFP with 50 μl of PAM (20 μg). Reconstitution at time zero with 50 μl of (a) plasma heated to 56°C for 30 min or (b) plasma plus PAM added at arrow. Plasma was incubated 1:1 with PAM for 10 min at 37°C with (c) or without (d) subsequent heating to 56°C for 30 min. Fifty microliters of this mixture was then added to the GFP. [From Karpatkin et al. (9) with permission.]

10. <u>Nature of the heat-labile factor</u>. The heat-labile factor(s) appears to be a protein(s) of the complement system since treatment of PRP with cobra venom (Figure 7) diminished the plasma factor activity in a time-dependent fashion. The ability of the plasma factor to support PAM aggregation of GFP was reduced to > 20% of control levels by 45 min of incubation and essentially abolished by 75 min of incubation. Plasma from inbred strains of guinea pigs genetically

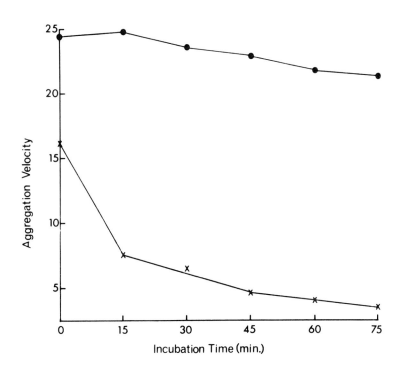

FIGURE 7. Inactivation of the Aggregation-Promoting Activity of Plasma by Cobra Venom. PRP was incubated with cobra venom as described in Methods for the indicated times. PAM was added immediately, and platelet aggregation was measured turbidometrically. Aggregation velocity was measured as the slope of a tangent drawn parallel to the steepest part of the aggregation curve and is plotted in arbitrary units of optical density change per unit time. Control PRP was incubated under identical conditions with an equivalent volume of buffer. X, cobra venom; o, control. [From Karpatkin <u>et al</u>. (9) with permission.]

154

deficient in the fourth component of complement was as capable of supporting PAM-induced aggregation of guinea pig platelets as normal guinea pig plasma. This implies that the classical pathway of complement activation is not involved in PAM activity. Zymosan-treated plasma was incapable of supporting PAM-induced aggregation of GFP, strongly suggesting the requirement for an intact complement system to allow activation of the alternative pathway in the presence of platelets (Figure 8).

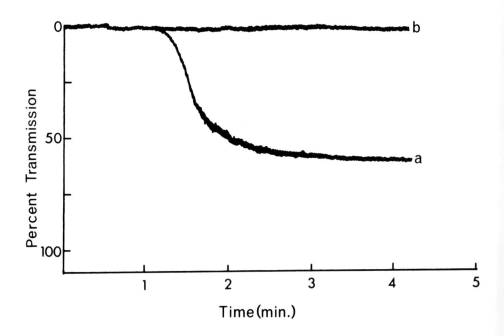

FIGURE 8. Aggregation of 0.4 ml of GFP with 50 µl of PAM (20 µg) in the Presence of 50 µl of (a) Normal Plasma Incubated at 37°C for 1 hr or (b) Plasma Treated with Zymosan at 37°C for 1 hr. [From Karpatkin et al. (9) with permission.]

155

11. **Binding of PAM to platelets by employing PAM coupled to Sepharose beads.** PAM-Sepharose beads can aggregate platelets in PRP as well as GFP in the presence of plasma. A 50 µl volume of a suspension of derivatized beads was added to 0.4 ml of PRP or 0.4 ml of GFP contianing 50 µl of plasma. Data are presented in Figure 9 for PRP. After platelet aggregation, binding of PAM to platelets can be visualized by the adherence of platelets and platelet clumps to the surface of PAM-coated beads (Figure 9A) but not to beads coated with bovine serum albumin (Figure 9B) or fibronectin or to underivatized beads which have been added to PRP and aggregated by exogenous PAM (Figure 9C).

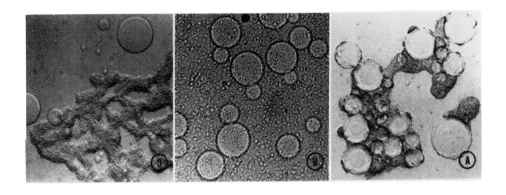

FIGURE 9. Aggregation of 0.4 ml of PRP with 50 µl of Sepharose 4-B Beads. Beads coated with (A) PAM or (B) bovine serum albumin or (C) 50 µl of underivatized beads were added to PRP followed by 50 µl (20 µg) of PAM. [From Karpatkin et al. (9) with permission.]

12. **Requirement of a stable plasma factor.** We have demonstrated that PAM activity is sedimentable at 100,000 x g for 1 hr. This physical property has enabled us to demonstrate that a multistep process occurs during PAM-plasma interaction. When PAM was activated by incubating it with plasma for 10 min at 37°C and subsequently subjected to centrifugation, platelet aggregating activity was recoverable in the pellet. However, the expression of this activity still required a plasma factor (Figure 10). Plasma previously heated to 56°C will also restore PAM aggregation ability as long as the initial activation of PAM was induced with unheated plasma (Figure 10d). Rabbit fibrinogen (2 mg/ml) did not restore PAM aggregation ability (Figure 10e). The heat-stable factor was precipitable with 50% saturated ammonium sulfate and was stable to dialysis (data not shown).

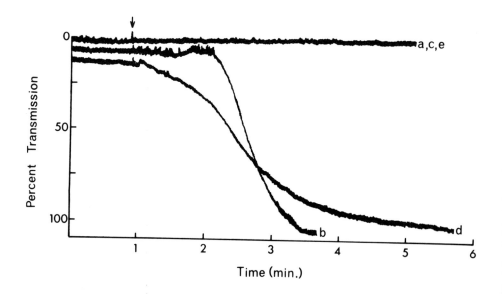

FIGURE 10. Requirement of a Heat-Stable Plasma Factor for PAM-Induced Platelet Aggregation. PAM was activated by preincubation with plasma for 10 min at 37°C and then sedimented by centrifugation at 100,000 x g. The sediment was resuspended in veronal buffer and compared to "unactivated" fresh PAM. Aggregation of 0.4 ml of GFP with (a) 50 μl fresh PAM (20 μg); (b) 50 μl of fresh PAM in the presence of 50 μl of fresh plasma, (c) 50 μl of fresh PAM in the presence of 50 μl of 56°C-heated plasma; (d) 50 μl of activated PAM in the presence of 50 μl of 56°C-heated plasma; and (e) 50 μl of activated PAM in the presence of rabbit fibrinogen (2 mg/ml). Plasma was added at zero time and PAM added at the arrow. [From Karpatkin et al. (9) with permission.]

It therefore appears that at least two plasma factors support PAM aggregation: one that was labile to heating at 56°C (and is probably a complement component) and the other which was stable to heating at 56°C (Figure 11).

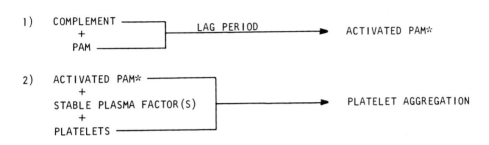

FIGURE 11. Proposed Sequence of Events during PAM-Induced Platelet Aggregation. [From Karpatkin et al. (9) with permission.]

13. Correlation between in vivo metastatic potential, platelet aggregating activity and cell surface sialylation of 10 metastatic-variant derivatives of a rat renal sarcoma cell line. The PW20 virally-transformed SV40 3T3 mouse fibroblasts. However, their requirement for cell surface sialic acid for platelet aggregation (see below) and the ability to extract PAM from these cells, suggests a platelet aggregating mechanism similar to the SV40 3T3 cell lines.

14. Metastatic properties. The percentage of animals developing one or more spontaneous metastatic lesions after primary tumor excision ranged from 0% to 100%, with lesions appearing in the lung, mediastinal lymph nodes, abdominal viscera and external lymph nodes.

15. Platelet aggregation. The maximum average velocity of platelet aggregation induced by the PAM ranged from 1.5 to 100 units of light transmission per min. A significant correlation was observed between the platelet-aggregating activity of the PAM and the metastatic potential of the tumor cell lines from which the PAM was derived (correlation coeficient, r = 0.68, probability, P < 0.03) (10).

16. Sialic acid content of PAM. The sialic acid content of the PAM ranged from 1.5 to 24.7 mg per 100 mg of protein. PAM preparations from the three least metastatic cell lines, which were the least active with respect to platelet-aggregating ability, contained the lowest levels of sialic acid. A good correlation was observed between the platelet-aggregating activity of the PAM and its sialic acid content ($r = 0.60$, $P < 0.06$), and between the metastatic potential of the cell lines and the sialic content of the PAM ($r = 0.69$, $P < 0.03$) (10).

17. Sialylation of cell surface glycoconjugates. The percent sialylation of the exposed cell surface Gal and GalNAc residues ranged from 13% to 77%, with the three lowest values observed in the three least metastatic cell lines. A significant correlation was observed between cell surface sialylation and metastatic potential ($r = 0.83$, $P < 0.003$), cell surface sialylation and the platelet-aggregating activity of the PAM ($r = 0.85$, $P < 0.002$), and cell surface sialylation and the sialic acid content of the PAM ($r = 0.74$, $P < 0.02$) (10).

B. Tumors which Aggregate Platelets via the Generation of Thrombin

PAM could not be extracted from this group of tumors. This group of tumors will not aggregate PRP anticoagulated with 0.32% sodium citrate but will aggregate PRP anticoagulated with heparin (5 units/ml).

1. Platelet aggregation by LoVo, HCT-8 or Hut-20 Cells is independent of complement. To facilitate comparisons between human lines and SV3T3-induced aggregation, rabbit PRP was often used since SV3T3 cells do not aggregate human PRP and rabbit PRP responded similarly to responder human PRP.

SV3T3 PAM-induced aggregation is impaired and the lag period prolonged when rabbit complement is inactivated with cobra venom factor or zymosan. No such effect was noted when LoVo, HCT-8 or HUT-20 cells (100,000) were used as the aggregating agent, using either rabbit PRP (Figure 12) or human PRP (data not shown).

2. Treatment of LoVo, HCT-8, Hut-20 and SV3T3 tumor cells with enzymes. The PAM extract of the animal tumor cell line SV3T3 is sensitive to treatment with trypsin, neuraminidase or phospholipase A_2. These experiments were repeated with intact SV3T3 cells and compared to LoVo, HCT-8, and Hut-20 cells (Figure 13), since PAM cannot be prepared from the three nonvirally transformed cell lines. Although SV3T3 cells lost their platelet aggregability following treatment with trypsin, neuraminidase, or phospholipase A_2, the LoVo, HCT-8, and Hut-20 cells were only affected by phospholipase A_2 treatment (data not shown for LoVo cells).

3. Recalcification time. Because clot formation was noted 10 to 15 min after platelet aggregation with three spontaneous tumor cells, but not with SV3T3 cells, thrombin generation was measured, using recalcification time of citrated rabbit platelet poor plasma (PPP). LoVo was more potent than HCT-8 or Hut-20 cells. Similar results were obtained with human plasma. This was dependent on cell concentration (Table 6). Similar results were obtained with PRP (data not shown). SV3T3 cells had a negligible effect on the recalcification time. For example, 100,000 cells had no effect; 1,000,000 cells shortened the recalcification time from 10.0 to 7.8 min.

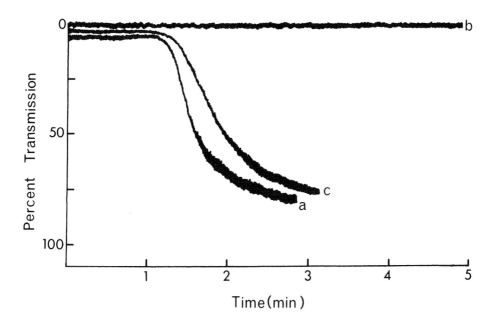

FIGURE 12. Aggregation of Rabbit PRP with SV3T3, LoVo, HCT-8, and Hut-20 Cells with or without Treatment with Cobra Venom. Aggregation induced by SV3T3 in (a) control or (b) cobra venom-treated PRP. Aggregation by LoVo, HCT-8, or Hut-20 cells in control or cobra venom-treated PRP (c); these curves were superimposable. [From Pearlstein et al. (11) with permission.]

160

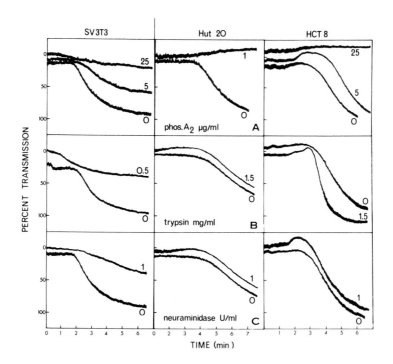

FIGURE 13. Comparison of Platelet Aggregation Induced by Enzyme-Treated Tumor Cells. One tumor cell line representing each mechanism was exposed to either phospholipase A_2, trypsin or neuraminidase for 1 hr at 37°C and washed with veronal buffer. 50 μl of a tumor cell suspension containing 500,000 cells in buffer was preincubated for 2 min at 37°C with 5-10 μl apyrase (2-3 units) and then added to 0.4 ml of heparinized rabbit PRP. The percentage of light transmission was recorded with a Bio-Data platelet aggregometer. Controls of untreated cells (enzyme concentration, 0) were similarly incubated in buffer for 10 hr at 37°C. [From Lerner et al. (12) with permission.]

Table 6 also demonstrates the effect of trypsin, neuraminidase, or phospholipase A_2 on the ability of tumor cells to shorten the recalcification time of rabbit PPP. As with platelet aggregation results, trypsin and neuraminidase had no effect on the recalcification time, whereas phospholipase A_2 did have an effect.

Table 6. Effect of Cell Concentration and Enzyme Treatment on Recalcification Time of Rabbit Platelet Poor Plasma by LoVo, HCT-8 and Hut-20 cells[a].

	Recalcification time (min)		
	Buffer		
No. of Cells	LoVo	HCT-8	Hut-20
0	18.0	18.0	18.0
1,000	3.0	11.5	7.5
10,000	1.5	4.5	5.0
100,000		1.4	3.5
500,000			2.4
1,000,000			1.5
1,000,000		0.4	
	Recalcification time (min)		
	Neuraminidase		
No. of Cells	LoVo	HCT-8	Hut-20
0	18.5	18.5	18.5
1,000			
10,000	1.5		
100,000			
500,000			2.3
1,000,000			
1,000,000		0.4	
	Recalcification time (min)		
	Phospholipase A_2		
No. of Cells	LoVo	HCT-8	Hut-20
0	20.0	20.0	20.0
1,000			
10,000	3.5		
100,000			
500,000			> 25.0
1,000,000			
1,000,000		10.0	
	Recalcification time (min)		
	Trypsin		
No. of Cells	LoVo	HCT-8	Hut-20
0	19.0	19.0	19.0
1,000			
10,000	1.0		
100,000			
500,000			2.8
1,000,000			
1,000,000		0.5	

[a]Cells (0.1 ml) treated previously with buffer or the indicated enzymes for 1 hr at 37°C were washed and then incubated with 0.1 ml of 50 mM $CaCl_2$ for 2 min at 37°C in a plastic tube. PPP (0.1 ml) was added, and the clotting time was recorded. [From Pearlstein et al. (11) with permission.]

Table 7 demonstrates the effect of tumor cells on the recalcification times of coagulation factor-deficient human plasmas. LoVo, HCT-8 and Hut-20 cell-induced shortening of the recalcification time was noted with Factor XII-deficient plasma, but not with Factor II-, V-, X- or VII-deficient plasmas. The data suggest that these cell lines were activating the coagulation system via activation of Factor VII by the extrinsic tissue pathway.

Table 7. Effect of LoVo, HCT-8 and Hut-20 Cells on the Recalcification Time of Coagulation Factor-Deficient Plasmas[a].

Test Plasma	Clotting Time (min)			
	Buffer	LoVo	HCT-8	Hut-20
Normal	36.3	1.3	3.2	3.5
XII-deficient	>60.0	1.3	3.3	4.5
IX-deficient	>60.0	1.2	4.0	7.0
V-deficient	>60.0	ND[b]	ND	40.0
VII-deficient	26.0	7.0	23.0	31.0
X-deficient	>60.0	3.8	19.0	19.0
II-deficient	>60.0	>60.0	>60.0	>60.0

[a]Cell suspension (0.1 ml; 100,000 cells) in Veronal buffer was incubated with 0.1 ml of $CaCl_2$ for 2 min at 37°C in a plastic tube. The reaction was started by addition of 0.1 ml test plasma and the clotting time was recorded. Representations of 2 to 5 experiments. [From Pearlstein et al. (11) with permission.]

[b]ND, not determined

4. Effect of DAPA, a specific thrombin inhibitor. The ability of human tumor cells to aggregate platelets via the generation of thrombin was examined by the use of a highly specific thrombin inhibitor, DAPA. Figure 14 demonstrates complete inhibition of tumor-induced rabbit platelet aggregation by DAPA at 4 to 15 μM, using 500,000 LoVo, HCT-8 and Hut-20 cells. Similar results were obtained with human PRP. At higher concentrations, DAPA had an effect on SV3T3 cells. However, 20-fold fewer cells and a 30-fold greater DAPA concentration were required to demonstrate this effect.

C. Tumors Which Require a Trypsin Sensitive Protein for Platelet Aggregating Activity

A third group of tumors was found not to be sialic acid-dependent, complement requiring, phospholipase A_2 sensitive, or thrombin generating. This group of tumors was found to be uniquely trypsin sensitive with respect to its ability to aggregate platelets. PAM can be extracted from this group of tumors, which can aggregate citrated PRP more completely than heparinized PRP.

1. __Effect of enzyme treatment of tumor cell lines on platelet aggregation.__ Figure 13 represents a comparison of the effects of enzyme treatment on three tumor cell lines. Displayed are platelet aggregation curves induced by a representative tumor for each mechanism: sialic acid-dependent, complement-requiring, SV3T3 cells; thrombin-generating, HCT-8 cells; and trypsin-sensitive, uniquely phospholipase A_2 insensitive, CT26 cells. The tumor-induced platelet aggregation of SV3T3 cells is inhibited by pretreatment of these cells with phospholipase A_2, trypsin or neuramindase. CT-26-induced platelet aggregation is inhibited solely by pretreatment of the tumor cells with trypsin. Similar results were obtained for B16F10 and HM29 cell lines (data not shown).

2. __Effect of complement inhibition on tumor-induced platelet aggregation.__ When complement is inactivated in PRP with cobra venom, only SV3T3 cells lose their ability to induce platelet aggregation. HCT-8 and CT26 cells, representatives from the other two groups, are not affected (Figure 15). No inhibition was obtained with LoVo, Hut-20, B16F10 and HM29 cells (data not shown).

D. Effect of Pharmacologic Agents on the Three Mechanisms of Tumor-Induced Platelet Aggregation

1. __Effect of specific thrombin inhibitors on tumor-induced platelet aggregation.__ Preincubation of PRP with varying concentrations of DAPA, a specific thrombin inhibitor, resulted in complete inhibition of thrombin-induced platelet aggregation by HCT-8 cells at 4 μM (similar results were obtained using LoVo cells). In contrast, platelet aggregation induced by SV3T3 and CT26 cells was insensitive to the effects of DAPA, revealing no inhibition at 40 μM and 92 μM respectively (Table 8). The results using B16F10 and HM29 cells similarly revealed an insensitivity to DAPA (data not shown). The specificity of these results was confirmed by employing another highly-specific thrombin inhibitor, No. 805 (Table 8). LoVo and HCT-8-induced platelet aggregation was inhibited at 2 μM while the other tumor cell lines were insensitive at approximately ten-fold higher concentration (19 μM). Similar differences were noted with the different tumor groups with respect to their ability to generate procoagulant activity in a plasma recalcification time (see below).

2. __Effect of tumor cell lines on recalcification time.__ Table 9 demonstrates comparative recalcification times of citrated rabbit platelet-poor plasma employing six different tumor cell lines. The spontaneous human adenocarcinoma cells of the colon, LoVo and HCT-8, markedly shortened the recalcification time compared to the virally-transformed SV3T3 murine fibroblast cells. The melanomas, murine B16F10 and human HM29, and the murine undifferentiated colon carcinoma CT26 were significantly less active than LoVo and HCT-8 cells.

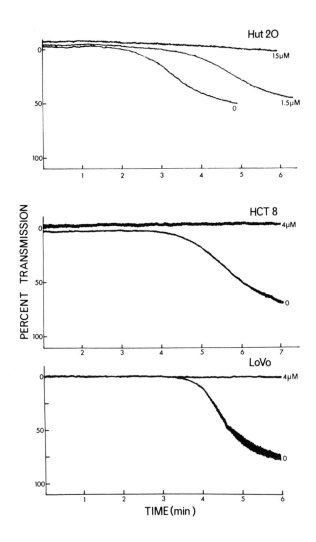

FIGURE 14. Effect of DAPA on Platelet Aggregation Induced by Hut-20, HCT-8 or LoVo Cells. Heparinized rabbit PRP (0.35 ml) was preincubated with 50 µl of DAPA in veronal buffer at 37°C for 3 min prior to the addition of 50 µl of 500,000 tumor cells. Concentration of DAPA is given in µM. [From Pearlstein et al. (11) with permission.]

COBRA VENOM U/ml

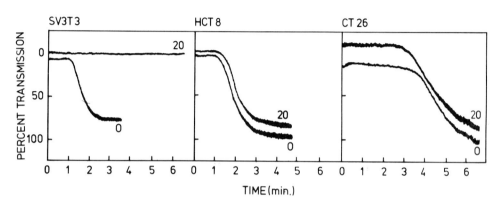

FIGURE 15. Effect of Cobra Venom Treatment of Platelet Rich Plasma (PRP) on Platelet Aggregation Induced by Tumor Cells. Tumor cells were preincubated with apyrase (as above) and then added to PRP that had been treated with purified cobra venom factor (20 units/ml) for 30 min at 37°C. Comparisons were made with control PRP that had been treated with buffer only.

3. Effect of pharmacologic agents which elevate cyclic AMP levels. A ten-fold higher concentration of prostacyclin is required to inhibit HCT-8 (and LoVo; not shown)-induced platelet aggregation as compared to that required to inhibit SV3T3 or CT26 (as well as B16F10 and HM29; not shown)-induced aggregation. Compared to prostacyclin, a ten-fold higher concentration of 6-keto-PGE$_1$ was required to inhibit tumor-induced platelet aggregation by SV3T3 or CT26 cells (Table 8). This is consistent with data reporting that prostacyclin is approximately ten-fold more potent than 6-keto-PGE$_1$ as a platelet aggregation inhibitor (see Chapter 14). Compared to prostacyclin, a ten-fold greater concentration of 6-keto-PGE$_1$ was also required to inhibit platelet aggregation induced by the thrombin generating cells, LoVo and HCT-8, confirming the specificity and relative sensitivity of inhibition of tumor cell induced-platelet aggregation. This was further substantiated by employing dBcAMP as a platelet inhibitory substance. Again aggregation of the thrombin generating tumors was ten-fold less sensitive compared to the two other groups (Table 8).

Table 8. Effect of Pharmacologic Agents on Tumor Cell-Induced
Platelet Aggregation[a]

		Mechanisms of Tumor-Induced Platelet Aggregation		
		Complement-Requiring	Thrombin-Generating	Trypsin-Sensitive Phospholipase A_2 Insensitive
			50% Inhibition At	
Pharmacologic Agent				
DAPA	(μM)	> 40.0[b]	4.0	> 92.0
No. 805	(μM)	> 19.0	2.0	> 19.0
Prostacyclin	(μM)	0.01	0.1	0.01
6-keto-PGE$_1$	(μM)	N.D.[c]	1.0	1.0
dBc AMP	(mM)	0.1	> 1.0	0.1
Ibuprofen	(mM)	N.D.	10.0	0.1
Indomethacin	(mM)	0.1	1.0	0.1

[a]Heparinized PRP (0.4 ml) was preindubated with 50 μl of
pharmacologic agent diluted in appropriate buffer at 37°C for 3 min.
50 μl of tumor cells (500,000) treated with 2-3 units of apyrase were
then added and platelet aggregation recorded. Inhibition of
aggregation was defined as a 50% decrease in the maximal slope of the
velocity of platelet aggregation in the absence of pharmacologic
agent. The tumor cell lines employed were SV3T3, LoVo, HCT-8, CT26,
B16F10 and HM29 cell lines. [From Lerner et al. (12) with
permission.]

[b]> signifies not inhibited at this concentration.

[c]N.D., not determined

4. Effect of pharmacologic agents which inhibit prostaglandin
synthesis. The cyclooxygenase inhibitors ibuprofen and indomethacin
were employed to determine their effect on tumor-induced platelet
aggregation induced by the three different tumor groups. Again, the
thrombin generating tumors, LoVo and HCT-8, were at least ten-fold
less sensitive when compared to the other two groups (Table 8).

IV. DISCUSSION

These data indicate the presence of at least three different
mechanisms of tumor-induced platelet aggregation in the seven
different tumor cell lines which have been carefully surveyed (Table
1): a mechanism found in virally-transformed SV3T3 cells which
requires serum complement, a stable plasma factor, divalent cation,
and a sialo-lipoprotein vesicular (PAM) component of the tumor
membrane; a second mechanism found in two spontaneously metastatic
human adenocarcinomas of the colon, LoVo and HCT-8, which operates by

the activation of the coagulation system, via the tissue factor pathway and appears to require a phospholipid component of the tumor membrane. The ability of these tumors to aggregate platelets is not sensitive to neuraminidase or trypsin but is sensitive to phospholipase A_2. The third mechanism is found in a spontaneously metastatic human melanoma (HM29) and murine melanoma (B16F10) as well as a carcinogen-induced metastatic murine colon carcinoma (CT26), in which the ability of the tumors to aggregate platelets is dependent upon the presence of a vesicular (PAM) trypsin-sensitive protein. The platelet aggregating ability of these tumors is not sensitive to neuraminidase or phospholipase A_2.

Table 9. Effect of Various Tumor Cell Lines on the Recalcification Time of Citrated-Rabbit Platelet-Poor Plasma[a]

Cell Line	Recalcification Time (min)
Veronal Buffer	17.1
SV3T3	13.8
HCT-8	1.5
LoVo	0.7
B16F10	7.1
HM29	14.3
CT26	6.8

[a]0.1 ml of tumor cell suspension (100,000 cells) in veronal buffer was incubated with 0.1 ml of 50 mM $CaCl_2$ for 2 min at 37°C in a plastic tube. The reaction was started by addition of 0.1 ml of the same citrate-rabbit plasma, and the clotting time recorded. Test tubes were inverted every 30 sec. Data are representative of 3 experiments. [From Lerner et al. (12) with permission.]

It is now apparent that: (1) heterogenous mechanisms do exist for the aggregation of platelets by tumor cells; (2) all human tumor cell lines do not aggregate platelets via their procoagulant activity (i.e., HM29); (3) all spontaneously metastatic lines do not aggregate platelets via their procoagulant activity (i.e., HM29, B16F10) and (4) various antiplatelet pharmacologic agents interfere with tumor-induced platelet aggregation in a manner which is related to the mechanism of tumor-induced platelet aggregation. Thus the thrombin generating tumors are uniquely sensitive to highly specific thrombin inhibitors, whereas the other two groups of tumors are at least ten-fold more sensitive to drugs which elevate cyclic AMP or inhibit prostaglandin synthesis.

Since the initial report of Gasic et al. (29) on the inhibition of tumor metastasis by the induction of thrombocytopenia in the host, there have been several conflicting reports on the ability of anti-platelet agents to inhibit metastases. Thus although Gasic and

168

co-workers (30) reported beneficial effects from the use of aspirin in mice injected with MCA2 and T241 fibrosarcoma cells, and Kolenich and associates (31) made similar observations on a BW10232 adenocarcinoma of rabbits, Wood and Hilgard (32) obtained negative results with a V2 carcinoma of rabbits and Hilgard and colleagues (33) obtained negative results in a careful study with Lewis lung carcinoma in mice employing various antiplatelet agents: aspirin, bencyclane, RA233 (a dipyridamole derivative). Furthermore, although Gordon et al. (34) obtained positive results with a Wilm's tumor of Wistar-Furth rats, equivocal results were obtained with a neuroblastoma (C1300) of mice, and negative results with an NIH renal adenocarcinoma of mice, employing pentoxifylline (a phosphodiesterase inhibitor) as an antiplatelet agent. However, in a recent report, Honn et al. (35) have obtained positive results on the inhibition of metastases from a B16 amelanotic melanoma in mice employing a combination of prostacyclin and theophylline.

In another series of studies, Stringfellow and Fitzpatrick (36,37) provided data indicating that prostaglandin modulation could affect in vivo metastases. They examined the production of prostaglandin D_2 (an inhibitor of platelet aggregation) by B16F1 and B16F10 malignant melanoma cells. The moderately metastatic F1 line produced five-fold more prostaglandin D_2 than the highly metastatic F10 (36). Of particular interest was the observation that pretreatment of F1 and F10 cells with indomethacin increased the number of metastases for F1 cells 5.8 fold compared to 1.5 fold for F10 cells (37).

These in vivo observations support the probability of heterogenous mechanisms for the interaction of tumor cells with platelets in the host. OUr data are relevant in this regard and could possibly explain the apparent contradictory results reported by different workers employing different tumors and different antiplatelet agents.

There has been recent interest in the initiation of clinical trials on the effect of antiplatelet agents on tumor metastases. We would like to suggest that knowledge of the in vitro mechanisms of tumor-platelet interaction may be helpful in understanding the pathophysiology of tumor metastases. Selection of appropriate antiplatelet pharmacologic agents, derived from these in vitro studies, may be helpful in the treatment of metastases.

REFERENCES

1. Karpatkin S and Pearlstein E. Ann. Intern. Med. 95:636-641, 1981.
2. Nachman RL, Weksler B and Ferris B. J. Clin. Invest. 51:549-556, 1972.
3. Packham MA, Nishizawa EE and Mustard JF. Biochem. Pharmacol. 17 (Suppl):171-184, 1968.
4. Cowan DH and Graham J. In: Interaction of Platelets and Tumor Cells (Ed. Jamieson GA), Alan R. Liss, New York, pp. 249-268, 1982.
5. Eastment CT and Sirbasku DA. J. Cell. Physiol. 97:17-28, 1978.
6. Hara Y, Steiner M and Baldini MG. Cancer Res. 40:1212-1216, 1980.
7. Kepner N and Lipton A. Cancer Res. 41:430-432, 1981.

8. Pearlstein E, Cooper LB and Karpatkin S. J. Lab. Clin. Med. 93:332–344, 1979.
9. Karpatkin S, Smerling A and Pearlstein E. J. Lab. Clin. Med. 96:994–1001, 1980.
10. Pearlstein E, Salk PL, Yogeeswaran G and Karpatkin S. Proc. Natl. Acad. Sci. USA 77:4336–4339, 1980.
11. Pearlstein E, Ambrogio C, Gasic G and Karpatkin S. Cancer Res. 41:4535–4539, 1981.
12. Lerner WA, Pearlstein E, Ambrogio C and Karpatkin S. Int. J. Cancer 31:463–469, 1983.
13. Brattain MG, Strobel-Stevens J, Fine D, Webb M and Sarrif AM. Cancer Res. 40:2142–2146, 1980.
14. Griswold DP and Corbett TH. Cancer (Philadelphia) 36:2441–2444, 1975.
15. Sato N, Michaelides MC and Wallack MK. Cancer Res. 41:2267–2272, 1981.
16. Tan MH, Holyoke ED and Goldrosen MH. J. Natl. Cancer Inst. 56:871–874, 1976.
17. Salk P and Yogeeswaran G. Fed. Proc. Fed. Am. Soc. Exp. Biol. (Abstract) 37:1760.
18. Yogeeswaran G, Sebastian H and Stein BS. Int. J. Cancer 24:193–202, 1979.
19. Tangen D and Berman HJ. Adv. Exp. Med. Biol. 34:235–243, 1972.
20. Nesheim ME, Prendergast FG and Mann KG. Biochem. 18:996–1003, 1979.
21. Nagano W, Okamoto S, Ikezawa K, Minura K, Matruoka A, Hujikata A and Tamao Y. Thromb. Haemostasis 46:0128A, 1981.
22. Tamao Y, Hara H, Kikumota R and Okamoto S. Thromb. Haemostasis 46:0130A, 1981.
23. Gasic G, Koch PAG, Hsu B, Gasic TB and Niewiarowski S. Z. Krebsforsch 86:263–277, 1976.
24. Weiss HJ. N. Engl. J. Med. 293:531–541, 1975.
25. Davey MG and Luscher EF. Thromb. Diath. Haemorrh. 20(Suppl.):283, 1966.
26. Ossowski L, Unkeless JC, Tobia A, Quigley JP, Rifkin DB and Reich E. J. Exp. Med. 137:112–126, 1973.
27. Goldberg AR. Cell 2:95–102, 1974.
28. Hynes RO and Pearlstein E. J. Supramol. Struct. 4:1–14, 1976.
29. Gasic GJ and Gasic TB. Proc. Natl. Acad. Sci. USA 48:1172–1177, 1962.
30. Gasic GJ, Gasic TB, Galanti N, Johnson T and Murphy S. Int. J. Cancer 11:704–718, 1973.
31. Kolenich JJ, Mansour EG and Flynn A. Lancet (Letter) 2:714, 1972.
32. Wood S Jr. and Hilgard P. Lancet (Letter) 2:1416–1417, 1972.
33. Hilgard P, Heller H and Schmidt CG. Z. Krebsforsch 86:243–250, 1976.
34. Gordon S, Witul M, Cohen H, Sciandra J, Williams P, Gastpar H, Murphy GP and Ambrus JL. J. Med. 10:435–441, 1979.
35. Honn KV, Cicone B and Skoff A. Science 212:1270–1272, 1981.
36. Fitzpatrick FA and Stringfellow DA. Proc. Natl. Acad. Sci. USA 76:1765–1769, 1979.
37. Stringfellow DA and Fitzpatrick FA. Nature (London) 282:76–78, 1979.

CHAPTER 12. TUMOR CYSTEINE PROTEINASES, PLATELET AGGREGATION AND METASTASIS

BONNIE F. SLOANE, PHILIP G. CAVANAUGH AND KENNETH V. HONN

I. CYSTEINE PROTEINASES

Cysteine proteinases are a subclass of endopeptidases which require activation by thiol reagents (1). This group of enzymes includes the plant proteinase papain, the lysosomal cysteine proteinases (cathepsins B, H and L) and the cytosolic calcium-activated neutral proteinases (CANP). Sequence homologies among the cysteine proteinases suggest that they may have a common evolutionary origin. Takio et al. (2) compared the amino acid sequences of papain and of rat liver cathepsins B and H and found substantial sequence homologies among the three. Surrounding the active site cysteine, cathepsin B has 10 of 11 and cathepsin H 9 of 11 amino acids found in papain. Overall, however, cathepsin H is more closely homologous to papain than to cathepsin B. A peptide containing the active site cysteine residue of chicken skeletal muscle CANP was isolated and found to consist of 7 residues of which 3 are common to the active sites of papain and cathepsin B (3) and cathepsin H (2). Bajkowski and Frankfater (4,5) have provided evidence that there are functional homologies as well as structural homologies between the active sites of cathepsin B and papain.

The lysosomal cysteine proteinases, cathepsins B, H and L, have pH optima from 6.2 to 6.8 (6), suggesting that these proteinases might have some activity if released from the acid environment of the lysosome into the cytoplasm or into the extracellular matrix. However, these enzymes are unstable above pH 7.0 (7). The one exception is the cathepsin B-like enzyme released from tumors which has increased stability at pH's above 7.0 (8 and see below). Cathepsin B has been the most thoroughly studied of the lysosomal cysteine proteinases. Cathepsin B has dipeptidylpeptidase activity against glucagon (9) and aldolase (10) as well as broad specificity as an endopeptidase against protein substrates such as hemoglobin (11), myosin (12,13), actin (12), troponin (13), tropomyosin (13) and insulin (14). Cathepsin B has also been shown to have activity against several components of the extracellular matrix, degrading proteoglycans (15), fibronectin (16) and the nonhelical portion of collagen (17), types I, II, III and IV (18). In addition to degrading collagen, cathepsin B can act as a regulatory enzyme in collagen degradation by activating latent collagenase (19). Sylven (20) reported that cathepsin B can degrade cellular attachment proteins at pH 7.1 as evidenced by cell detachment from glass.

There have been fewer studies of the proteolytic activities of cathepsins H and L, but they may well overlap with those of cathepsin B. Against synthetic substrates cathepsin H has aminopeptidase activity as well as endopeptidase activity (21). Katunuma and Kominami (17) recently reported that cathepsin H degraded troponin-T but not myosin, actin or tropomyosin. In contrast to cathepsins B and H, cathepsin L has more activity against protein substrates than against synthetic substrates (22). For example, the specific activity of cathepsin L for degradation of insoluble tendon collagen at pH 3.5 is 5-10 fold greater than that of cathepsin B (23). The susceptibility of myofibrillar proteins to degradation by cathepsin L is greater than to degradation by cathepsins B or H (7). Tropomyosin can, however, be degraded by cathepsin B but not by cathepsin L (7).

Calcium activated proteolytic enzymes have been referred to in the literature as calcium-activated proteases (CAP or CAF), calcium-dependent cysteine proteinases (calpain) and calcium-activated neutral proteinases (CaANP or CANP). Two forms of CANP have been purified from a number of tissues, one requiring millimolar levels of calcium for activation and the other micromolar levels of calcium (24-27). CANP has been shown to have broad activity (for review see 28). These activities include the ability to activate regulatory enzymes such as phosphorylase b kinase in skeletal muscle, adenylate cyclase in platelets (29) and the epidermal growth factor receptor (a protein kinase; 30), to degrade cytoskeletal proteins (31) including those from skeletal muscle (32) and platelets (33) and to modulate membrane functions in platelets and endothelial cells and thereby inhibit thrombin-induced platelet aggregation as well as thrombin-induced production of prostacyclin by endothelial cells (34).

II. TUMOR PROTEOLYTIC ENZYMES AND METASTASIS

The malignancy of a tumor can be attributed to its ability to metastasize to secondary sites. This process which is termed the "metastatic cascade" involves an intricate series of sequential events which are diagrammed schematically in Figure 1 and listed below:

1. Invasion of the primary tumor into normal tissue.

2. Detachment of tumor cells from the primary tumor.

3. Direct shedding of tumor cells into circulation or intravasation into the microvasculature or lymphatics.

4. Hematogenous dissemination and possible interaction with circulating host platelets.

5. Arrest of a tumor cell-platelet thrombus in the microvasculature or direct adhesion of tumor cells to endothelial or de-endothelianized surfaces with subsequent thrombus formation.

172

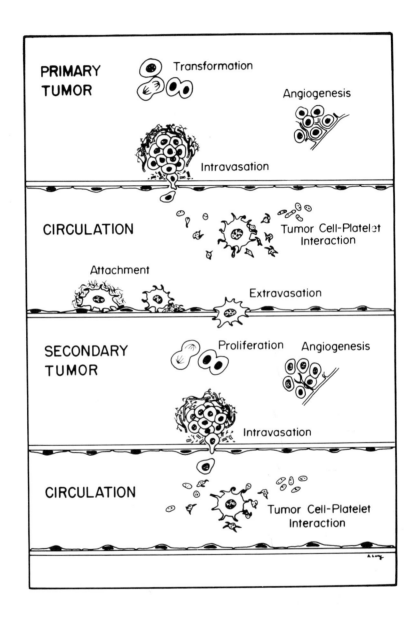

FIGURE 1. Schematic Diagram of the Metastatic Cascade. [From Honn et al. (124) with permission.]

6. Extravasation through the vessel wall into normal tissue or organ of secondary arrest.

7. Immediate growth into a secondary metastatic tumor (or dormancy).

It is intuitive that in order to metastasize a tumor cell must pass through connective tissue barriers during steps 1, 3 and 6 above.

The extracellular matrix or connective tissue consists primarily of proteins such as collagen, proteoglycans and glycoproteins. Thus, proteolytic enzymes released from tumor cells or present on the tumor cell surface should facilitate tumor cell invasion. Liotta et al. (35) and Recklies and Poole (16) have recently reviewed, respectively, the role of collagenases in tumor cell invasion and of proteinases in tissue destruction during tumor growth. The roles of collagenases and of plasminogen activators in basement membrane degradation and in tumor invasion and metastasis are discussed in Chapter 21.

There are other steps in the metastatic cascade (as diagrammed in Figure 1) which may also be mediated by or facilitated by proteolytic enzymes. These include tumor cell proliferation, angiogenesis, tumor cell detachment from the primary tumor and tumor cell interaction with host cells. In many cases the roles of proteinases have not been demonstrated directly but indirectly by use of inhibitors. Radiation- and chemical-induced carcinogenesis in vitro and in vivo can be inhibited by the microbial proteinase inhibitors, antipain and leupeptin (36-39). Proliferation of tumor cells in vitro can also be reduced by proteinase inhibitors (40,41) whereas proliferation of normal cells in vitro can be stimulated by exogenous proteinases (42) including a proteinase released by virally-transformed cells in culture (43). Inhibitors of angiogenesis have been shown to inhibit the activity of several classes of proteinases (44,45). Detachment of cells from substrata as well as preparation of single cell suspensions from solid tissues is readily accomplished by the proteolytic action of several classes of proteinases. Limited proteolysis of the cell surface may also lead to increased cell-cell adhesion such as the induction of platelet aggregation by exogenous proteinases (46).

Activity of any single proteinase or class of proteinases is not likely to be an absolute requirement for tumor cells to metastasize. More conceivably, there is a proteolytic metastatic cascade in which one or more proteinases or one or more classes of proteinases act in concert and in turn may activate others (see also Chapter 21).

III. TUMOR CYSTEINE PROTEINASES AND METASTASIS

A. Cysteine Proteinase Activity in Tumors

A number of in vivo studies (20, 47-50) have provided suggestive evidence that activities of lysosomal enzymes may correlate with tumor malignancy. Elevated lysosomal enzyme activities in tumors have been suggested to be due to the presence of necrotic tumor cells or of invading macrophages or lymphocytes (51,52) but this does not appear to be valid for elevated lysosomal proteinase activities. As early as 1957 Sylven and Malmgren (53) reported that the youngest and most rapidly growing tumors had the highest lysosomal proteinase activity. Shamburger and Rudolph (54) also reported that lysosomal proteinase activity was highest in the youngest skin carcinomas.

In our laboratories we have established that activity based on DNA or protein of a cathepsin B-like cysteine proteinase (CB) is highest in homogenates of solid tumors of B16F1 and F10 melanoma variants of $\leq$ 1 g in wet weight (55). We have also found that CB activity based on DNA or protein is highest in homogenates of solid tumors of the Lewis lung carcinoma (3LL) and an amelanotic variant of the B16 melanoma (B16a) of $\leq$ 1 g in wet weight. Specific activity of CB has been reported to be elevated in the parent line of a murine methylcholanthrene-induced fibrosarcoma (3AM) and 18 of its clones when compared to activity in normal muscle (56). However, in another manuscript (57) from the same laboratory the specific activity of CB was reported to be less in one clone of the fibrosarcoma than in normal liver. We routinely find that the specific activity of CB is greater in murine and human tumors of spontaneous origin than in liver and spleen from non-tumor bearing mice or humans.

We demonstrated that CB activity based on DNA or protein in homogenates of solid B16F1 and B16F10 tumors correlates with their lung colonization potential (55,58) and that CB activity based on DNA in homogenates of solid B16a and 3LL metastatic variants correlates with their potential to spontaneously metastasize to the lungs from a subcutaneous tumor (Figure 2). In contrast, McLaughlin et al. (56) did not find any correlation betweeen the specific activity of CB and the metastatic potential of the chemically-induced 3AM tumor and its 18 clones. McLaughlin et al. (56) suggested that correlates of proteolytic activity and metastatic potential "based on a comparison of only two cell variants [as in our study of B16F1 and F10 tumors; 55,58] may in fact be fortuitous." However, our recent study of CB activity in three additional B16a variants (BL6, O13 and B15b) confirms our earlier work (55,58). Using these three variants plus the B16F1 and F10, Nicolson and co-workers (59) were able to demonstrate a positive correlation between activity of a heparan sulfate endoglycosidase and "the malignant behavior of [the] B16 cells and their ability to colonize the lung" (see also Chapter 20). In our laboratories we have been able to demonstrate positive correlations among CB activity, activity of the heparan sulfate endoglycosidase and the lung colonization potential of the five B16 variants.

Solid tumors contain a multiplicity of cell types (macrophages, lymphocytes and stromal cells as well as tumor cells) any of which could account for CB activity. Therefore, many studies have utilized cultured tumor cells. In vitro studies have demonstrated both correlations between lysosomal proteinase activity or CB activity and metastasis and the lack of such correlations (55,56,58,60-65). In our hands, as subcutaneous tumors, the B16F1 and F10 variants demonstrated a positive correlation between lung colonization potential and CB activity (55,58). However, as cultured cells, these variants exhibited either a positive correlation or no correlation between lung

175

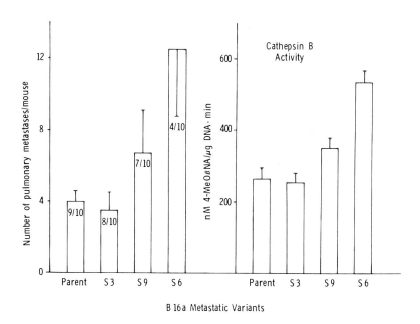

B 16a Metastatic Variants

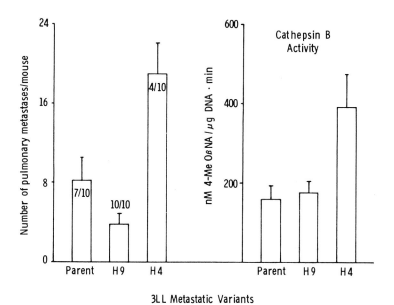

3LL Metastatic Variants

FIGURE 2. Spontaneous Pulmonary Metastasis (left) and Cathepsin B-Like Activity (right) of B16a (upper) and 3LL (lower) Metastatic Variants. Number of surviving mice is indicated within bars on left.

colonization potential and CB activity (55). Other laboratories have recently reported that the phenotype of malignant cells can change in culture in either the direction of increased or decreased malignancy (66,67). In other studies of cells in culture, CB activity exhibited a negative correlation with transformation (62,63) and a positive correlation with differentiation (63). In contrast, we have demonstrated that CB activity in cultures of chemically-transformed 10T½ fibroblasts (clones 15 and 16) was elevated over that in cultures of the parent clone 8 (68). Clones 15 and 16 have been shown to be tumorigenic in vivo (69) and were also tumorigenic in our hands. The malignancy of some cell lines which are transformed in vitro has been questioned by Poste (70) since several of these cell lines including the Nil hamster cells used in one of the studies which demonstrated a negative correlation between CB activity and malignancy (63) are tumorigenic prior to transformation by tumor viruses.

One can also determine whether CB activity is a property of the tumor cells in a solid tumor by isolating the tumor cells. Centrifugal elutriation has been used to separate and synchronize tumor cell subpopulations from solid tumors (71,72) and from multicellular tumor spheroids (73). We employed centrifugal elutriation to separate viable tumor cells from nonviable tumor cells and host cells and demonstrated definitively that CB activity is a property of viable tumor cells in rodent solid subcutaneous tumors. Eighty to ninety percent of the CB activity (based on DNA) in dispersed and elutriated cells of B16F1 and F10 melanoma variants was separated with the viable tumor cells (58). In B16a, 3LL, Walker 256 carcinosarcoma (W256), 15091A mammary adenocarcinoma, M5076 reticulum cell sarcoma and B16BL6, B16B15b and B16013 melanoma variants > 92% of the CB activity separated with the viable tumor cells (Figure 3). Of the cells in this fraction > 95% are tumor cells, < 2% lymphocytes, < 1% monocytes, $\stackrel{<}{-}$ 3% PMNs (Figure 4). The purity of these fractions was determined by having a minimum of 500 cells/fraction identified and enumerated individually by two cytotechnicians. Thus our studies demonstrate in four distinct rodent transplantable tumor types [melanoma, adenocarcinoma, carcinosarcoma and a reticulum cell sarcoma of macrophage origin (74)], including six variants of the melanoma, that CB activity is associated with the tumor cells.

In contrast, Graf et al. (75) have reported that CB activity in frozen sections of a rabbit subcutaneous V2 carcinoma was not associated with the tumor cells. By histochemical staining they localized CB activity in fibroblasts and PMNs at the invasion front of the tumor whereas by immunofluorescent staining, using an antibody to inactivated cathepsin B from rabbit liver, they localized reaction

FIGURE 3. Cathepsin B-Like Cysteine Proteinase Activity in Fractions Isolated from Subcutaneous Tumors by Centrifugal Elutriation. β fraction (striped bar) contains viable tumor cells (see Figure 4) and α fraction (black bar) contains necrotic tumor cells and host cells. Activity expressed as percentage of total (α + β) activity. Values equal x̄ ± SEM where indicated or the average of two experiments.

FIGURE 3

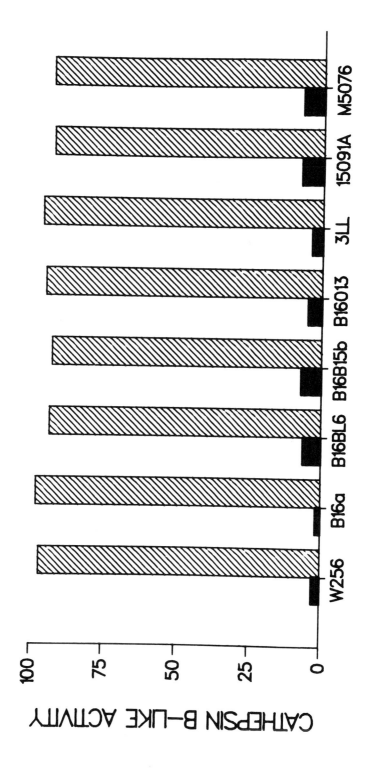

product in the fibroblasts, PMNs and in the extracellular matrix surrounding the tumor cells. We cannot at this time account for the discrepancy between our results and those of Graf et al. (75) although Recklies et al. (76) found that CB released from human breast tumor explants did not cross-react with an antibody to human liver cathepsin B unless the secreted CB had been destabilized by mercurial compounds.

Labrosse and Liener (77) reported that collagenolytic activity with an acid pH optimum (pH 4.2) which is present in homogenates of a methylcholanthrene-induced fibrosarcoma (3AM) is associated with the tumor cells isolated from the tumor and not with the macrophages or lymphocytes which had infiltrated the tumor. Labrosse and Liener (77) did not identify this acid collagenase but suggested that it might be CB or a collagenolytic cathepsin. This tumor acid collagenase activity might also be attributed to cathepsin L (22,23) although Kirschke et al. (78) have reported that negligible activity of cathepsin L is present in the rat Jensen sarcoma or in several human carcinomas.

We have reported that cathepsin H activity in homogenates of B16a solid tumors (79) or of 15091A ascites cells and membrane vesicles shed by these cells in culture (80) is negligible. In more recent studies of 8 rodent tumor lines we have found that cathepsin H activity is substantially less than CB activity in all but the M5076 reticulum cell sarcoma of macrophage origin. In these 8 lines, from 75-98% of the cathepsin H activity was associated with the viable tumor cells separated by centrifugal elutriation.

B. Cysteine Proteinase Activity Released from Tumors

Of particular relevance to tumor invasion and metastasis is the increasing body of literature on release of CB activity from human and animal tumors. Poole and co-workers have shown that up to eleven times more CB activity is released from malignant human breast tumors than from normal breast tissue or nonmalignant tumors (81,82). Other groups have reported elevation of CB activity in pancreatic fluid of patients with pancreatic cancer (83), in serum of women with diverse invasive neoplastic diseases (64,84) including vaginal adenocarcinomas (85) and in urine of women with gynecological cancers (86). Poole and co-workers (81,82) have hypothesized that the CB activity released from human breast carcinoma explants is released from viable tumor cells. They base this hypothesis on two facts: 1. the CB activity released from explants of the invasive and growing edge of the tumor

FIGURE 4. Cellular Composition of β Fraction Isolated from Subcutaneous Tumors by Centrifugal Elutriation. Striped bar = tumor cells; white bar = lymphocytes; black bar = polymorphonuclear leukocytes; cross-hatched bar = monocytes. Composition expressed as a percentage of total cells counted per fraction (minimum of 500). Values equal $\bar{x}$ ± SEM where indicated or the average of two experiments.

FIGURE 4

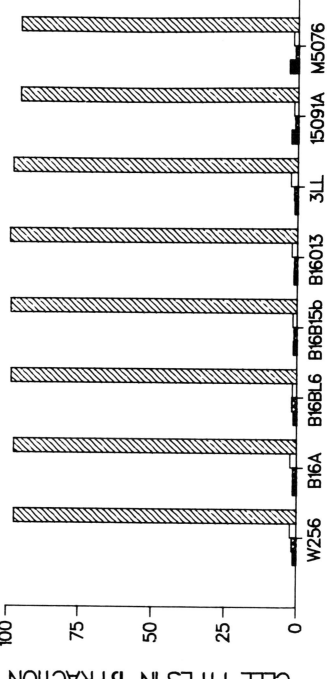

CELL TYPES IN β-FRACTION

W256   B16A   B16BL6   B16B15b   B16O13   3LL   15091A   M5076

was higher than that from explants of the central necrotic core and 2. protein synthesis was required for release of CB activity. Protein synthesis was also required for release of CB activity from murine breast carcinoma explants (87).

Studies with tumor cells in culture have revealed that CB activity is released from tumor cells. Pietras and co-workers (64) have demonstrated that neoplastic cervical cells release CB activity and that the amount of activity released correlated with the rate of cell proliferation. In our laboratories we have demonstrated that B16F1 and F10 (55), B16a (88) and 15091A (80) cells release CB activity into the culture medium. CB activity released from both 15091A cells (80) and B16a cells is both nonsedimentable and sedimentable (associated with membrane vesicles spontaneously shed from these cells in culture). Although we have been able to measure CB activity in the culture medium of several tumor lines of epithelial origin, to date we have not been able to measure CB activity in the culture medium of $10T\frac{1}{2}$ fibroblasts either normal (clone 8) or chemically transformed (clones 15 and 16; 68). The most suggestive evidence that CB is released from tumor cells in vivo is that provided by Mort et al. (89). Ascites fluid from women with ovarian carcinoma was shown to possess CB activity. They concluded that the ascites cells were the source of the CB activity since ascites cells placed in culture released CB activity whereas sera from the same patients had no CB activity. In addition, this group of workers have since demonstrated that resident or stimulated peritoneal macrophages do not release CB activity into the culture medium (87). However, this latter study used murine macrophages.

The presence or absence of CB activity in the medium of cultured tumor cells may reflect the length of time the tumor cells were in culture and the number of passages in vitro. When we established B16F1, F10 variants in culture using tumor cells isolated from a subcutaneous tumor, we found that CB activity could not be measured in the culture medium of the primary cultures (55). Substantial CB activity was present in the medium of 3rd passage cells, but the activity was reduced by the 6th passage. Recklies et al. (87) reported that release of CB activity from explants of murine breast tumors decreased after culture periods of 9-11 days and they presumed that this decrease was due to loss of viability of the explants. We have found that the CB activity released into the culture medium of B16a cells seems to be related to the number of passages in vivo as a subcutaneous tumor before establishment in vitro as well as to the number of passages in vitro. Recklies et al. (87) similarly reported that the secretion rates of CB activity from explants of the first transplant generation of a spontaneous tumor were significantly less than from explants of the spontaneous tumor.

In contrast to cathepsin B from normal tissues, CB released from tumors seems to possess properties which could enable it to possess proteolytic activity extracellularly. Mort et al. (8) and Recklies et al. (87) established that CB released from human and murine breast tumor explants was greater in molecular weight than human liver cathepsin B and more stable to inactivation above neutral pH than human liver cathepsin B. We ourselves have found that CB activity released from tumor cells retains stability at alkaline pH (Table 1). This is also true for CB activity in the membrane vesicles spontaneously shed from 15091A cells in culture (80 and Table 1). This latter CB activity is also more heat stable, retaining 68% of its activity after exposure to 56°C for 30 min whereas the CB activity in the 15091A tumor cells retained only 14% of its activity (80).

Table 1. pH Stability of Tumor Cathepsin B-Like Cysteine Proteinase Activity[a].

Tumor Type	Solid sc Tumor	Cultured Tumor Cells	Culture Medium	Shed Vesicles
B16a	< 5%[b]	< 5%	62 ± 5%	–
15091A	< 5%	16%	67 ± 5%	85%

[a]Aliquots were preincubated at pH 8.0 and 37°C for 30 min without thiol activator (DTT) prior to fluorometric assay at pH 6.2 as previously described (55,58).

[b]Values represent percentage of original activity remaining.

Mort et al. (89) reported that the CB present in human ascites fluid due to ovarian carcinoma was inactive or latent and that it could be proteolytically activated by pepsin. This was also true for the CB released by the ascites cells in culture. Pepsin activation of the released CB resulted in a reduction in molecular weight, as judged by gel filtration, from 41,000 to 33,000 M_r. Mort et al. (89) postulated that the latent CB released from tumor cells was either an enzyme-inhibitor complex or an inactive precursor. In a recent study Mort et al. (90) demonstrated by SDS-PAGE under reducing conditions that pepsin activation of latent ascites CB results in a change in M_r from 40,000 to 32,000, CB running as a single band in both cases. Therefore, they feel that latent CB is an inactive precursor rather than an enzyme-inhibitor complex.

We have confirmed that CB released from B16a cells in culture or CB in membrane vesicles spontaneously shed from 15091A cells in culture (80) can be activated by pepsin. A number of other proteolytic enzymes tested were unable to activate the latent CB released from cultured B16a cells. However, the latent B16a CB underwent autoactivation with time and could be activated by thiol-disulfide interchange reactions. Latent collagenase has been shown to be activated by thiol-disulfide interchange reactions although activation in this case is actually due to inactivation of an inhibitor (91).

Release of CB from tumor cells in culture suggests that CB m.y at some point in time be associated with the plasma membrane. Pietras and Roberts (92) performed subcellular fractionations of control and neoplastic human cervical cells and found CB activity (alkaline and heat stable) associated with a plasma membrane fraction of neoplastic cells, but not of the control cells. Bohmer et al. (93), on the other hand, found that activity of an acid cysteine proteinase was similar in plasma membranes purified from normal bovine lymphoid cells and from bovine lymphosarcoma cells. However, in this latter study a nonspecific substrate (^{125}I-casein) was utilized and the acid cysteine proteolytic activity was not assayed in the presence of a thiol activator. Thus the comparison of acid cysteine proteinase activities in the two plasma membrane fractions was not performed under optimal conditions. Tumor cells grown in tissue culture have been shown to shed plasma membrane derived vesicles by a number of laboratories (94-96). Poste and Nicolson (96) found that the lung colonization potential of the B16F1 melanoma (low potential) could be increased by fusing shed vesicles from B16F10 cells (high potential) with B16F1 cells. Since we had previously established that CB activity is higher in the B16F10 cells (55,58) and that B16F1 and F10 cells release CB (55), we assayed membrane vesicles shed from 15091A cells in culture for CB activity and established that the vesicles possessed CB activity.

Membrane-associated CB could possess proteolytic activity when free CB would not, not only due to increased pH and heat stability, but also to inability of proteinase inhibitors to bind to a membrane-associated enzyme. We found that CB activity in 15091A vesicles seemed to be less susceptible to inhibition by a cysteine proteinase inhibitor than was CB activity in the 15091A tumor. CB activity in 15091A tumor cells was inhibited > 99% by 5 μM Z-Phe-Ala-CHN$_2$ whereas the CB activity released into the culture medium could only be inhibited by 87 ± 2%. Steven et al. (97) have reported that a trypsin- like proteinase present on the surface of Ehrlich ascites cells could be inhibited by low MW proteinase inhibitors but not by high MW inhibitors. This prompted a detailed study by Steven and co-workers (98) in which they showed a significantly reduced ability of proteinase inhibitors to inactivate proteinases which were bound to "artificial membranes" as compared to the same enzyme free in solution. CB released from tumor cells which are in contact with the extracellular matrix such as the basement membrane of the blood vessel wall may also be protected from inhibition by proteinase inhibitors. Campbell et al. (99) have established that proteolysis by elastase released from neutrophils cannot be prevented by proteinase inhibitors when the neutrophils are in contract with their connective tissue substrate (in this case fibronectin).

C. Tumor Cysteine Proteinases and Platelet Aggregation

Aggregation of platelets in vitro can be induced by tumor cells, by membrane vesicles spontaneously shed from tumor cells in culture and by a membrane-derived fraction of the tumor cells (94,100-103). Platelet aggregation can also be induced in vitro by ADP, collagen, platelet activating factor and such proteinases as thrombin, trypsin and papain. There appear to be at least two mechanisms for tumor cell-induced platelet aggregation, one dependent on ADP release from tumor cells and another dependent on the generation of thrombin (104-106). Karpatkin, Pearlstein and co-workers (107,108) have characterized a platelet aggregating material from SV40 transformed murine 3T3 fibroblasts and a polyoma virus-induced rat renal sarcoma cell line (see also Chapter 11). This material required a lipid, a protein and a sialic acid component for activity. Similar results were reported by Hara et al. (102) for murine renal adenocarcinoma and neuroblastoma cell lines. In both cases the aggregating activity appeared to be membrane associated and required the presence of a plasma factor and Ca^{2+} to induce aggregation of washed platelets. The membrane association of tumor cell aggregating activity is further substantiated by the work of Gasic et al. (95,101) which demonstrated that spontaneously shed membrane vesicles (SSMV) from tumor cells induce aggregation of platelets (in the presence of Ca^{2+} and a plasma factor).

Tumor cells are not only able to induce platelet aggregation, but also can induce coagulation of plasma. A tumor cell procoagulant has been identified which appears to directly (109,110) or indirectly (111) activate factor X. Dvorak et al. (111) demonstrated that tumor cell SSMV possess procoagulant activity (see also Chapter 8). Gordon and co-workers (110,112) have purified a tumor cell procoagulant which directly activates factor X and have identified this as a cysteine proteinase based on its irreversible inhibition by iodoacetamide and its dithiothreitol-reversible inhibition by $HgCl_2$, phenylmethyl-sulfonylfluoride and diisopropylfluorophosphate (see also Chapter 6).

The sequence homology at the active site and active site groove between papain and cathepsin B (2) and the fact that papain has been shown to induce platelet aggregation (46) led us to speculate that one tumor cell principle which might be responsible for inducing platelet aggregation could be CB. We demonstrated that inhibition of CB activity in B16a cells correlates inversely with the ability of those cells to induce platelet aggregation in vitro (79). Proteinase inhibitors of varying specificity for cysteine and serine proteinases were tested for their ability to inhibit B16a-induced aggregation of washed human platelets (Figure 5). The most effective inhibitors were cysteine proteinase inhibitors [leupeptin, antipain and iodoacetic acid (IAA)] and the least effective were serine proteinase inhibitors [soybean trypsin inhibitor (SBTI) and aprotinin]. In order to mimic the proaggregatory activity of CB we utilized the commercially available plant cysteine proteinase, papain. Addition of papain ($\geq$ 0.02 U, Sigma) to washed human platelets induced aggregation. As with the B16a tumor cells, the most effective proteinase inhibitors against papain-induced platelet aggregation were cysteine proteinase inhibitors and the least effective were serine proteinase inhibitors. Both B16a-induced and papain-induced platelet aggregation were accompanied by an elevation of thromboxane A_2 levels which could also be blocked by the cysteine proteinase inhibitor, leupeptin. CB activity in the B16a tumor cells (Figure 5) and the proteolytic activity of papain were both effectively inhibited by the same cysteine proteinase inhibitors that blocked B16a-induced and papain-induced platelet aggregation.

184

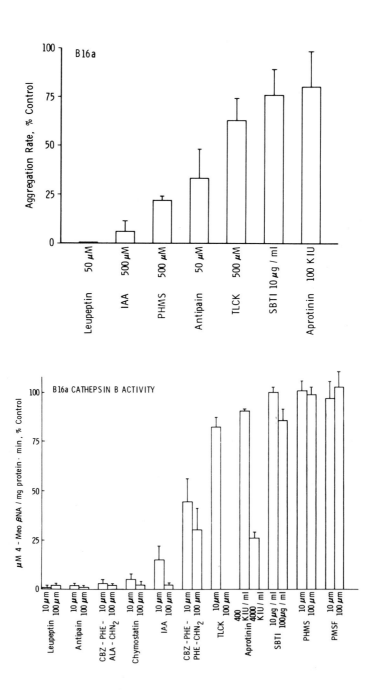

FIGURE 5. Effect of Proteinase Inhibitors on B16a-Induced Platelet Aggregation (upper) and B16a Cathepsin B-Like Cysteine Proteinase Activity (lower; 79).

We also compared the effects of a spectrum of proteinase inhibitors on the induction of platelet aggregation by 15091A cells, and by membrane vesicles spontaneously shed from these cells, with the effects of these inhibitors on CB activity in homogenates of these cells or vesicles (80 and Table 2). Among the proteinase inhibitors tested, leupeptin and antipain (competitive cysteine proteinase inhibitors) inhibited 15091A-induced platelet aggregation to the greatest extent; at a final concentration of 50 μM leupeptin was twice as effective as antipain. The degree of inhibition by these proteinase inhibitors varied with the platelet donor. IAA and iodoacetamide, compounds known to preferentially alkylate sulfhydryl groups and thus irreversible inhibitors of cysteine proteinases, partially inhibited 15091A-induced platelet aggregation. The results with leupeptin, antipain, IAA and iodoacetamide all suggest that a cysteine proteinase is in part responsible for the induction of platelet aggregation by tumor cells. This conclusion is also supported by the observation that two reversible serine proteinase inhibitors, aprotinin and SBTI, had little effect.

We also tested the effects of proteinase inhibitors on platelet aggregation induced by 15091A SSMV (80 and Table 2). The results were similar to the inhibition pattern observed for platelet aggregation induced by 15091A cells. Aprotinin and SBTI had little effect on aggregation whereas leupeptin, IAA and antipain demonstrated approximately the same degree of inhibition of vesicle- as of cell-induced aggregation. The ability of the series of proteinase inhibitors to inhibit CB activity in 15091A cells and SSMV paralleled their inhibition of 15091A cell- and 15091A SSMV-induced platelet aggregation (Table 2).

Our studies indicate that an inverse correlation exists between the inhibition of CB activity in B16a cells, 15091A cells and 15091A vesicles and their ability to induce platelet aggregation (79,80). The cysteine proteinase CANP has also been shown to modulate membrane functions in platelets (34). Since the activity of CANP can be inhibited by leupeptin and antipain (113), there is the possibility that the induction of platelet aggregation by tumor cells might be due to CANP. However, CANP rather than inducing platelet aggregation has been shown to inhibit thrombin-induced platelet aggregation (34). The inhibition of CANP by leupeptin and antipain is dependent upon the presence of Ca^{2+} although the $[Ca^{2+}]$ necessary for inhibition is not clear (113). Recently McGowan et al. (114) demonstrated that 100 μM leupeptin can totally inhibit exogenous platelet CANP but only partially inhibit endogenous CANP.

Although tumor cell CB appears to be involved in induction of platelet aggregation, it is not clear from our studies if CB is acting directly on the platelet membrane or, alternatively, is acting through the generation of thrombin (as B16a and 15091A tumor cells and 15091A SSMV do not induce aggregation of washed platelets in the absence of a small amount of platelet poor plasma). Further suggestive evidence that the latter mechanism may be primary are the reports by Gordon and co-workers (110,112) that a tumor cell cysteine proteinase directly activates factor X, thus leading to the generation of thrombin. It may well be that the active protein component of tumor cell platelet

186

Table 2. Effect of Proteinase Inhibitors on 15091A-Induced Platelet Aggregation and on 15091A Cathepsin B-Like Cysteine Proteinase (CB) Activity (80).

Inhibitor	Concentration	Aggregation Rate[a]		Concentration	CB Activity[b]	
		15091A Cells (200,000 cells)	15091A Vesicles (10 µg protein)		15091A Cells	15091A Vesicles
Leupeptin	50 µM	21.6 ± 9.0	34.5 ± 12.3	5 µM	9.4 ± 2.7	0 ± 0
Iodoacetic Acid	500 µM	55.2 ± 17.1	55.3 ± 19.5	50 µM	3.0 ± 0.6	0 ± 0
Z-Phe-Ala-CHN$_2$	–			1 µM	11.7 ± 2.2	0 ± 0
Antipain	50 µM	57.0 ± 2.5	69.5 ± 16.9	5 µM	13.5 ± 2.7	1.7 ± 1.7
Aprotinin	4000 KIU/ml[c]	73.5 ± 6.9	84.0 ± 4.6	2000 KIU/ml	91.0 ± 9.4	61.8 ± 3.1
Z-Phe-Phe-CHN$_2$	–			1 nM	97.0 ± 8.5	90.3 ± 6.6
Soybean trypsin inhibitor	10 µg/ml	116.8 ± 4.5	95.8 ± 7.9	100 µg/ml	108.5 ± 0.5	80.7 ± 11.8

[a] Aggregation rate is defined as the percentage change in transmission per unit of time and expressed as a percentage of the control; $\bar{x}$ ± SEM of four experiments.

[b] CB activity in nmol of reaction product formed per mg of protein per min and expressed as a percentage of the control; $\bar{x}$ ± SEM of four experiments.

[c] KIU = kallikrein inactivator units.

activating material (102,106,107,115,116) and of tumor cell procoagulant (111,112) is CB. Suggestive evidence that CB may possess both platelet aggregating and procoagulant activities can be derived from the ability of semi-purified leech salivary gland extract to inhibit CB activity of B16a cells and tumor cell-induced platelet aggregation and coagulation (117). Further studies are in progress with CB purified from murine and human tumors to validate our hypothesis that CB is a tumor cell proaggregatory principle and/or a tumor cell procoagulant. We predict that tumor CB will only be able to induce platelet aggregation and/or coagulation as a membrane-associated enzyme and that CB will be one proteinase in a tumor cell proteolytic cascade leading to platelet aggregation and/or coagulation.

IV. SUMMARY

There are potential problems with the hypothesis that tumor cell-derived CB may play a role in tumor invasion and metastasis. One is that cathepsin B purified from a number of normal human and animal tissues, including human liver, is inactivated by exposure to pH's >7.0 (11). This suggests that tumor CB may have little activity when not inside the acid environment of the lysosome, i.e., may not possess activity extracellularly. An additional problem in terms of CB acting extracellularly is the presence of proteinase inhibitors such as α_2-macroglobulin (α_2M) and α_1- and α_2-thiol proteinase inhibitors (α_1, α_2TPIs). Starkey and Barrett (118) have examined the interaction between purified human liver cathepsin B and α_2M. Activity of cathepsin B was reduced 20% against small synthetic substrates and was reduced 50% against protein substrates by α_2M. Human plasma α_1, α_2TPIs have been shown to be much less effective against cathepsin B than against cathepsins H or L, papain or the cytoplasmic CANP (119). Sasaki et al. (119) proposed that the most probably target for α_1, α_2 TPIs in vivo is CANP.

If CB does play a role in tumor invasion and metastasis, one might expect that administration of cysteine proteinase inhibitors in vivo would result in decreased metastasis, yet the results to date have been inconsistent. Yamamoto et al. (120) reported that leupeptin decreased the number and incidence of lung colonies formed after i.v. injection of rat ascites hepatoma cells. In contrast, Giraldi et al. (121) found that leupeptin did not affect spontaneous metastasis of Lewis lung carcinoma. These contrasting results may be due to leupeptin inhibiting a proteinase which acts in the latter half of the metastatic cascade or once the tumor cells have entered the circulatory system. An alternative explanation is that in vivo leupeptin can either inhibit or stimulate the activity of cathepsin B as reported recently by Sutherland and Greenbaum (122). Yet another explanation could be that leupeptin inhibits cysteine proteinases at low concentrations but both cysteine and serine proteinases at high concentrations (123).

There is not yet definitive proof that tumor CB plays a role in tumor invasion and metastasis. However, we have established that there is a correlation between tumor CB activity and lung colonization potential of B16 melanoma variants, degradation of the extracellular matrix by B16 melanoma variants, spontaneous pulmonary metastasis by B16a and 3LL variants and the ability of B16a and 15091A cells and 15091A SSMV to induce platelet aggregation. This correlative evidence, in association with preliminary evidence that CB purified from murine B16a can degrade components of the basement membrane in vitro, suggests that tumor CB could be one of the proteinases active in a proteolytic metastatic cascade.

ACKNOWLEDGMENTS

We thank Drs. J.D. Crissman, A.S. Bajkowski and J.D. Taylor for their collaboration in part of the work presented in this chapter. We thank S.B. Makim, R. Ryan, J.G. Sadler and C. Evens for technical assistance. This work was supported in part by CA29997 and CA36481 from the National Institutes of Health and by a grant from Harper/Grace Hospitals.

REFERENCES

1. Barrett AJ. Fed. Proc. Fed. Am. Soc. Exp. Biol. 39:9-14, 1980.
2. Takio K, Towatari T, Katunuma N, Teller DC and Titani K. Proc. Natl. Acad. Sci. USA 80:3666-3670, 1983.
3. Suzuki K, Hayashi H, Hayashi T and Iwai K. FEBS Lett. 152:67-70, 1983.
4. Bajkowski AS and Frankfater A. J. Biol. Chem. 258:1645-1649, 1983.
5. Bajkowski AS and Frankfater A. J. Biol. Chem. 258:1650-1655, 1983.
6. Barrett AJ and McDonald JK. Mammalian Proteases, Academic Press, New York, Vol. 1, 1980.
7. Katunuma N and Kominami E. Curr. Topics Cell. Regulation 22:71-101, 1983
8. Mort JS, Recklies AD and Poole AR. Biochim. Biophys. Acta 614:134-143, 1980.
9. Aronson NN and Barrett AJ. Biochem. J. 171:759-765, 1978.
10. Bond JS and Barrett AJ. Biochem. J. 189:17-25, 1980.
11. Barrett AJ. Biochem. J. 131:809-822, 1973.
12. Schwartz WN and Bird JWC. Biochem. J. 167:811-820, 1977.
13. Noda T, Isogai K, Hayashi H and Katunuma N. J. Biochem. (Tokyo) 90:371-379, 1981.
14. McKay MJ, Offermann MK, Barrett AJ and Bond JS. Fed. Proc. Fed. Am. Soc. Exp. Biol. 42:1779, 1983.
15. Morrison RIG, Barrett AJ and Dingle JT. Biochim. Biophys. Acta 302:411-419, 1973.
16. Recklies AD and Poole AR. In: Liver Metastasis (Eds. Weiss L and Gilbert HA), G.K. Hall, Boston, pp. 77-95, 1982.
17. Burleigh MC, Barrett AJ and Lazarus GS. Biochem. J. 137:387-398, 1974.
18. Etherington DS and Evans PJ. Acta Biol. Med. Germ. 36:1555-1563, 1977.
19. Eeckhout Y and Vaes G. Biochem. J. 166:21-31, 1977.
20. Sylven B. Eur. J. Cancer 4:559-562, 1968.
21. Schwartz WN and Barrett AJ. Biochem. J. 191:487-497, 1980.
22. Kirschke H, Langner J, Wiederanders B, Ansorge S and Bohley P. Eur. J. Biochem. 74:293-301, 1977.

23. Kirschke H, Kembhavi AA, Bohley P and Barrett AJ. Biochem. J. 201:367-372, 1982.
24. Hathaway DR, Werth DK and Haeberle JR. J. Biol. Chem. 257:9072-9077, 1982.
25. Wheelock MJ. J. Biol. Chem. 257:12471-12474, 1982.
26. Yoshimura N, Kikuchi T, Sasaki T, Kitahara A, Hatanaka M and Murachi T. J. Biol. Chem. 258:8883-8889, 1983/
27. Malik MN, Fenko MD, Iqbal K and Wisniewski HM. J. Biol. Chem. 258:8955-8962, 1983.
28. Ishiura S. Life Sci. 29:1079-1087, 1981.
29. Adnot S, Poirier-Dupuis M, Franks DJ and Hamet P. J. Cyclic Nucleotide Res. 8:103-118, 1982.
30. Gates RE and King LE. Biochem. Biophys. Res. Commun. 113:255-261, 1983.
31. Nelson WJ and Traub P. Mol. Cell. Biol. 3:1146-1156, 1983.
32. Ishiura S, Nonaka I and Sugita H. In: Muscular Dystrophy (Ed. Ebashi S), Univ. of Tokyo Press, pp. 265-282, 1982.
33. Tsujinaka T, Sakon M, Kambayashi J and Kosaki G. Thromb. Res. 28:149-156, 1982.
34. Yoshida N, Weksler B and Nachman R. J. Biol. Chem. 258:7168-7174, 1983.
35. Liotta LA, Thorgeirsson UP and Garbisa S. Cancer Metastasis Rev. 1:277-288, 1982.
36. Hozumi M, Ogawa M, Sugimura T, Kakeuchi T and Umezawa H. Cancer Res. 32:1725-1728, 1972.
37. Kennedy AR and Little JB. Nature (London) 276:825-826, 1978.
38. Kennedy AR and Little JB. Cancer Res. 41:2103-2108, 1981.
39. Borek C, Miller R, Pain C and Troll W. Proc. Natl. Acad. Sci. USA 76:1800-1803, 1979.
40. Goetz IE, Weinstein C and Roberts E. Cancer Res. 32:2469-2474, 1972.
41. Schnebli HP and Burger MM. Proc. Natl. Acad. Sci. USA 69:3825-3827, 1972.
42. Burger MM. Nature (London) 227:170-171, 1970.
43. Rubin H. Science 167:1271-1272, 1970.
44. Langer R, Brem H, Falterman K, Klein M and Folkman J. Science 193:70-72, 1976.
45. Lee A and Langer R. Science 221:1185-1187, 1983.
46. Alexander B, Pechet L and Kliman A. Circulation 26:596-611, 1962.
47. Bosmann HB and Hall TC. Proc. Natl. Acad. Sci. USA 71:1833-1837, 1974.
48. Holmberg B. Cancer Res. 219:1386-1393, 1961.
49. Sylven B, Ottoson R and Revesz L. Br. J. Cancer 13:551-565, 1959.
50. Sylven B, Snellman O and Strauli P. Virchows Arch. B Cell Pathol. 17:97-112, 1974.
51. Dobrossy L, Pavelic ZP, Vaughn M, Porter N and Bernacki RJ. Cancer Res. 40:3281-3285, 1980.
52. Weiss L. Int. J. Cancer 22:196-203, 1978.
53. Sylven B and Malmgren H. Acta. Radiol. 154:1-124 (Suppl.), 1957.
54. Shamberger RJ and Rudolph G. Nature (London) 213:617-618, 1967.
55. Sloane BF, Honn KV, Sadler JG, Turner WA, Kimpson JJ and Taylor JD. Cancer Res. 42:980-986, 1982.
56. McLaughlin MEH, Liener IE and Wang N. Clin. Exp. Metastasis 1:359-372, 1983.
57. Olstein AD and Liener IE. J. Biol. Chem. 258:11049-11056, 1983.
58. Sloane BF, Dunn JR and Honn KV. Science 212:1151-1153, 1981.
59. Nakajima M, Irimura T, DiFerrante D, DiFerrante N and Nicolson GL. Science 220:611-613, 1983.
60. Bosmann HB, Bieber GF, Brown AE, Case KR, Gersten DM, Kimmerer TW and Lione A. Nature (London) 246:487-489, 1973.
61. Nicolson GL, Brunson KL and Fidler IJ. Acta Histochem. Cytochem. 10:114-133, 1977.

190

62. Dolbeare F, Vanderlaan M and Phares W. J. Histochem. Cytochem. 28:419-426, 1980.
63. Morgan RA, Inge KL and Christopher CW. J. Cell. Physiol. 108:55-66, 1981.
64. Pietras RJ, Szego CM, Roberts JA and Seeler BJ. J. Histochem. Cytochem. 29:440-450, 1981.
65. Burnett D, Crocker J and Vaughan ATM. J. Cell. Physiol. 115:249-254, 1983.
66. Miner KM, Kawaguchi T, Uba GW and Nicolson GL. Cancer Res. 42:4631-4638, 1982.
67. Welch DR and Nicolson GL. Clin. Exp. Metastasis 1:317-326, 1983.
68. Makim SB, Honn KV, Marnett LJ and Sloane BF. Submitted.
69. Reznikoff CA, Bertram JS, Brankow DW and Heidelberger C. Cancer Res. 33:3239-3249, 1973.
70. Poste G. In: Tumor Invasion and Metastasis (Eds. Liotta LA and Hart IR), Martinus Nijhoff, The Hague, pp. 147-171, 1982.
71. Meistrich ML, Grdina DJ, Meyn RE and Barlogie B. Cancer Res. 37:4291-4296, 1977.
72. Meistrich ML, Meyn RE and Barlogie B. Exp. Cell Res. 105:169-177, 1977.
73. Bauer KD, Keng PC and Sutherland RM. Cancer Res. 42:72-78, 1982.
74. Talmadge JE, Kay ME and Hart IR. Cancer Res. 41:1271-1280, 1981.
75. Graf M, Baici A and Strauli P. Lab. Invest. 45:587-596, 1981.
76. Recklies AD, Poole AR and Mort JS. Biochem. J. 207:633-636, 1982.
77. Labrosse KR and Liener IE. Mol. Cell. Biochem. 19:181-189, 1978.
78. Kirschke H, Langner J, Riemann S, Wiederanders B and Bohley P. In: Proteinases and Tumor Invasion. (Eds. Strauli P, Barrett AJ and Baici A), Raven Press:New York, pp. 69-79, 1980.
79. Honn KV, Cavanaugh P, Evens C, Taylor JD and Sloane BF. Science 217:540-542, 1982.
80. Cavanaugh PG, Sloane BF, Bajkowski A, Gasic GJ, Gasic TB and Honn KV. Clin. Exp. Metastasis 1:297-308, 1983.
81. Poole AR, Tiltman KJ, Recklies AD and Stoker TAM. Nature (London) 273:545-547, 1980.
82. Recklies AD, Tiltman KJ, Stoker TAM and Poole AR. Cancer Res. 40:550-556, 1980.
83. Rinderknecht J and Renner IG. N. Engl. J. Med. 303:462-463, 1980.
84. Pietras RJ, Szego CM, Mangan CE, Seeler BJ, Burtnett MM and Orevi M. Obstet. Gynecol. 52:321-327, 1978.
85. Pietras RJ, Szego CM, Mangan CE, Seeler BJ and Burtnett MM. Gynecol. Oncol. 7:1-17, 1979.
86. Perras J, Cramer J, Bishop R, Averette H and Sevin BU. Proc. Am. Assoc. Cancer Res. 24:130, 1983.
87. Recklies AD, Mort JS and Poole AR. Cancer Res. 42:1026-1032, 1982.
88. Sloane BF, Makim S, Dunn JR, Lacoste R, Theodorou M, Battista J, Alex R and Honn KV. In: Prostaglandins and Cancer (Eds. Bockman RS, Powles T, Honn KV and Ramwell P), Alan R. Liss:New York, pp. 789-792, 1982.
89. Mort JS, Leduc M and Recklies AD. Biochim. Biophys. Acta 662:173-180, 1981.
90. Mort JS, Leduc M and Recklies AD. Biochim. Biophys. Acta 755:369-375, 1983.
91. Macartney HW and Tschesche H. FEBS Lett. 119:327-332, 1980.
92. Pietras RJ and Roberts JA. J. Biol. Chem. 256:8536-8544, 1981.
93. Bohmer FD, Schmidt HE and Schon R. Acta Biol. Med. Germ. 41:883-890, 1982.
94. Gasic GJ, Catalfamo JL, Gasic TB and Avdalovic N. In: Malignancy and the Hemostatic System (Eds. Donati MB, Davidson JF and Garattini S), Raven Press:New York, pp. 27-35, 1981.
95. Gasic GJ, Boettiger D, Catalfamo JL, Gasic TB and Stewart GJ. Cancer Res. 38:2950-2955, 1978.
96. Poste G and Nicolson GL. Proc. Natl. Acad. Sci. USA 77:399-403, 1980.

97. Steven FS, Griffin MM, Itzhaki S and Al-Habib A. Br. J. Cancer 42:712-721, 1980.
98. Steven FS, Griffin MM and Itzhaki S. Eur. J. Biochem. 126:311-318, 1982.
99. Campbell EJ, Senior RM, McDonald JA and Cox DL. J. Clin. Invest. 70:845-852, 1982.
100. Bastida E, Ordinas A and Jamieson GA. Nature (London) 291:661-662, 1981.
101. Gasic GJ, Gasic TB and Jimenez SA. Lab. Invest. 36:413-419, 1977.
102. Hara Y, Steiner M and Baldini MG. Cancer Res. 40:1217-1222, 1980.
103. Karpatkin S and Pearlstein E. Ann. Intern. Med. 95:636-641, 1981.
104. Bastida E, Ordinas A, Giardina SL and Jamieson GA. Cancer Res. 42:4348-4352, 1982.
105. Jamieson GA, Bastida E and Ordinas A. In: Interaction of Platelets and Tumor Cells (Ed. Jamieson GA), Alan Liss:New York, pp. 405-413, 1982.
106. Pearlstein E, Ambrogio C, Gasic G and Karpatkin S. Cancer Res. 41:4535-4539, 1981.
107. Pearlstein E, Cooper L and Karpatkin S. J. Lab. Clin. Med. 93:332-344, 1979.
108. Pearlstein E, Salk PL, Yogeeswaran G and Karpatkin S. Proc. Natl. Acad. Sci. USA. 77:4336-4339, 1980.
109. Curatolo L, Colucci M, Cambini AL, Poggi A, Morasca L, Donati MB and Semeraro N. Br. J. Cancer 48:228-233, 1979.
110. Gordon SG and Cross BA. J. Clin. Invest. 67:1665-1671, 1981.
111. Dvorak HF, Quay SC, Orenstein NS, Dvorak AM, Hahn P, Bitzer P and Carvalho AC. Science 212:923-924, 1981.
112. Gordon SG. J. Histochem. Cytochem. 29:457-463, 1981.
113. Suzuki K, Tsuji S and Ishiura S. FEBS Lett. 136:119-122, 1981.
114. McGowan EB, Yeo K-T and Detwiler TC. Arch. Biochem. Biophys. 227:287-301, 1983.
115. Gasic GJ and Gasic TB. In: Interaction of Platelets and Tumor Cells (Ed. Jamieson GA), Alan Liss:New York, pp. 429-443, 1982.
116. Karpatkin S, Smerling A and Pearlstein E. J. Lab. Clin. Med. 96:994-1001, 1980.
117. Bajkowski AS, Marsh DM, Gasic TB, Gasic GJ, Sloane BF and Honn KV. Proc. Am. Assoc. Cancer Res., in press.
118. Starkey PM and Barrett AJ. Biochem. J. 131:823-831, 1973.
119. Sasaki M, Taniguchi K, Suzuki K and Imahori K. Biochem. Biophys. Res. Commun. 110:256-261, 1983.
120. Yamamoto RS, Umezawa H, Takeuchi T, Matsushima T, Hara K and Sugimura T. Proc. Am. Assoc. Cancer Res. 16:69, 1975.
121. Giraldi T, Nisi C and Sava G. Eur. J. Cancer 13:1321-1323, 1977.
122. Sutherland JHR and Greenbaum LM. Biochem. Biophys. Res. Commun. 110:332-338, 1983.
123. Umezawa H. Enzyme Inhibitors of Microbial Origin. (Tokyo:University of Tokyo Press), pp. 15-52, 1972.
124. Honn KV, Menter DG, Onoda JM, Taylor JD and Sloane BF. In: Cancer Invasion and Metastasis: Biologic and Therapeutic Aspects (Eds. Nicolson GL and Milas L), Raven Press:New York, pp. 361-388, 1984.

CHAPTER 13. ARACHIDONATE METABOLISM IN PLATELETS AND BLOOD VESSELS

ROBERT R. GORMAN

I. INTRODUCTION

Over fifty years have elapsed since Kurzrok and Lieb (1) made the original observation that human seminal plasma could contract uterine tissue. These studies were closely followed by the independent discoveries by Goldblatt (2) and von Euler (3) that extracts of human seminal plasma and of the vesicular gland of sheep produce a fall in blood pressure and contract smooth muscle. von Euler named the active agents "prostaglandins" and established some of the chemical properties of the compounds. Almost three decades passed between these initial studies and the isolation of crystalline compounds by Bergstrom and Sjovall (4). The actual structure of the compounds was determined by Bergstrom et al. (5) and Samuelsson (6). In 1964 a critical series of experiments established that essential fatty acids were precursors of prostaglandins (7-9). Dihomo-γ-linolenic acid is the precursor of "1" series prostaglandins; arachidonic acid is the precursor of "2" series prostaglandins and 5,8,11,14,17-eicosa-pentaenoate is the precursor of "3" series prostaglandins.

The initial discovery linking prostaglandins to thrombosis was made by Kloeze (1) who found that prostaglandin E_1 was a potent inhibitor of human platelet aggregation. The inhibitory activity of PGE_1 was subsequently associated with an elevation in platelet cyclic AMP levels (11). However, the key experiment, upon which all subsequent discoveries are based, was the isolation and characterization of two labile (half-life 5 min in aqueous solution) prostaglandin precursors. These endoperoxide molecules were called PGG_2 and PGH_2 by Hamberg, Samuelsson and their co-workers (12) or PGR_2 by Nugteren and Hazelhof (13). PGG_2 and PGH_2 are structurally identical with the exception that PGG_2 contains a hydroperoxy group at C-15, whereas PGH_2 has a hydroxyl group at C-15. Biologically the two endoperoxides have been found to have essentially identical profiles.

Coincident with the isolation of the endoperoxides, Willis and Kuhn (14) found that an unidentified "labile aggregation stimulating substance" (LASS) was formed in platelets during an arachidonic acid-induced platelet aggregation and that the synthesis of this activity could be blocked by aspirin. Smith and Willis (15) had already shown that aspirin inhibited prostaglandin synthesis in platelets and it was apparent that LASS was related in some way to prostaglandin synthesis. Hamberg et al. (18) later showed that both

PGH$_2$ and PGG$_2$ were potent inducers of human platelet aggregation and that LASS was actually a mixture of PGG$_2$ and PGH$_2$. In 1969, Piper and Vane (16) had found that sensitized guinea pig lungs released a rabbit aorta contracting substance (RCS) and the synthesis of this unknown material was also blocked by aspirin. Gryglewski and Vane (17) suggested that RCS was an endoperoxide intermediate in prostaglandin biosynthesis, but Hamberg et al. (12) were able to show the physical and chemical properties of RCS and endoperoxide were clearly different. Stimulated by these data, Hamberg et al. (18) pursued the metabolism of PGG$_2$ in human platelets and found that PGG$_2$ was converted to an unstable molecule with a half-life of 32 sec in aqueous solution. This molecule was called thromboxane A$_2$ (TXA$_2$) and it was found that the half-life and biological profile of RCS and TXA$_2$ were identical.

While extreme interest in TXA$_2$ was dominating the prostaglandin research area, another equally important discovery was being made, the discovery of "PGX" by Monocada et al. (19). PGX was found to be a product of PGH$_2$ metabolism in vascular tissue microsomes. In addition, PGX was found to induce vasodilation and to inhibit ADP-induced human platelet aggregation. The structural determination and total organic synthesis of PGX was achieved by Johnson et al. (20) and the previously unknown PGX-activity was then called prostacyclin or PGI$_2$. It should be mentioned that another group, working independently, was also very close to the discovery of PGX. Needleman et al (21) noted that arachidonic acid induced a relaxation response when added to bovine or human coronary artery strips. They also observed that the endoperoxides relaxed other arterial strips as well. The coronary arteries could continuously generate the vasodilator substance and these authors proposed that this pathway in bovine coronary arteries could function independently of endoperoxides released from platelets. Therefore, Needleman's group was also studying PGX, but without being aware that in addition to vasodilating, PGX was also a potent inhibitor of platelet aggregation. The importance of these findings was recently highlighted by the awarding of the Nobel Prize to Bergstrom, Samuelsson and Vane for their work in this area.

II. ARACHIDONATE METABOLISM

A. Phospholipase Activity

Regardless of the cell type, there is little or no intracellular free arachidonic acid. Therefore, synthesis of prostaglandins or thromboxane requires release of arachidonate, which is esterified mainly to cell phospholipids. Release is calcium dependent and can be accomplished by mechanical or biochemical stimulation. Most of the cellular arachidonic acid is stored in the 2' position of phospholipids and is released by specific phospholipase(s). Isakson et al. (22) and Bills et al. (23) have shown that phospholipases in the kidney and the platelet selectively liberate only arachidonic acid or dihomo-γ-linolenic acid (both prostaglandin precursors), even though the 2' position could be occupied by other fatty acids such as oleic acid. This indicates that there may be specificity with regard

194

to the fatty acid which the phospholipase liberates, as well as the hormone or perturbation that initiated the phospholipase activity. However, when changes in endogenous human platelet phospholipids are measured following stimulation with thrombin or calcium inophore A23187, the major decrease is in phosphatidylinositol (PI) (24). Platelet PI is particularly rich in arachidonic acid and it would appear to be a logical source of arachidonic acid for prostaglandin synthesis.

A current hypothesis is that thrombin stimulation of platelet results in transient accumulation of diglyceride by virtue of the action of a PI-specific phospholipase C (24). The fatty acid composition of the diglyceride is the same as that of platelet PI; thus the diglyceride may be assumed to be derived from PI. A diacylglycerol lipase, the activity of which has been demonstrated in human platelets, then cleaves arachidonate from the diglyceride. Bell et al. (25) postulated that phospholipase C converts phosphatidy-linositol into a 1,2-diglyceride which is then acted upon by diglyceride lipase, resulting in free arachidonic acid. An increase in platelet lysophosphatidylethanolamine following stimulation has also been reported (26). Due to the high content of arachidonate in platelet PE, these results would imply release of arachidonic acid by an alternate mechanism, such as a phospholipase A_2. A very similar picture of arachidonate mobilization is also observed in cultured human endothelial cells (27). In addition, the phospholipid sources of arachidonic acid may vary depending upon whether metabolism of endogenous or exogenous 20:4 is being studied. For example, thrombin stimulation of platelets labeled with radioactive arachidonate results in depletion of labeled phosphatidylcholine (23).

Since the phospholipase step is a possible point of pharmacological intervention for the control of arachidonic acid metabolism, there has been an extensive search for specific phospholipase inhibitors. There are two known ways to regulate phospholipase activity. First, an elevation in cyclic AMP will block arachidonate release in both human platelets and cultured vascular endothelial cells, presumably by an inhibition of the phospholipase step. However, in some cells cyclic AMP can actually stimulate arachidonate release which contrasts with the platelet and endothelial cell data. Second, phospholipase activity can be regulated through the use of anti-inflammatory steroids. Greaves and McDonald-Gibson (28) showed that glucocorticoids inhibit prostaglandin biosynthesis. Steroids were demonstrated to block the vasodilation that accompanies lipolysis in adipose tissue. These data were interpreted to indicate that anti-inflammatory steroids blocked release of prostaglandins from cells. More recently, it was shown that antiinflmmatory steroids control the availability of arachidonic acid by inhibiting its release (29). This concept was expanded by Flower et al. (30) who found that anti-inflammatory steroids stimulated synthesis of a "factor" that inhibited phospholipase activity. Synthesis of this "inhibitory factor" was blocked by puromycin, cycloheximide or actinomycin D, suggesting that it was a protein.

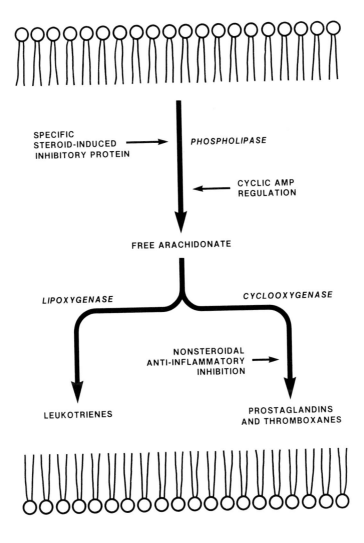

FIGURE 1. Arachidonate Release and Subsequent Formation of Oxygenated Products. Either chemical or mechanical stimulation of the cell rets in release of arachidonic acid from membrane phospholipids. The free arachidonate is subsequently processed by the cyclooxygenase and appropriate enzymes to prostaglandins and thromboxanes or by the lipoxygenase toward hydroxy fatty acids and/or leukotrienes. Sites of possible regulation by anti-inflammatory compounds and cyclic AMP are shown.

Hirata et al. (31) recently showed that in rabbit neutrophils glucocorticoids induce the synthesis of a specific protein(s) that inhibits the activity of a partially purified phospholipase A_2. These data support the earlier findings of Flower et al. (30)[2] and may represent a biochemical basis for the action of anti-inflammatory steroids.

A simplified scheme of arachidonic acid mobilization and subsequent synthesis of oxygenated products is shown in Figure 1. Following either chemical or mechanical stimulation of the cell, arachidonic acid is cleaved from phospholipids by a specific phospholipase(s). The free arachidonic acid is then metabolized by enzymes specific to that particular cell. The sites of possible regulation by cyclic AMP and/or anti-inflammatory agents are indicated.

B. Cyclooxygenase Activity

As mentioned above, the initial event in the synthesis of any molecule derived from arachidonic acid is the release of arachidonic acid from phospholipids. When arachidonic acid is released, it activates the cyclooxygenase. The cyclooxygenase (prostaglandin synthase) is really a group of enzymes that convert arachidonic acid or other 20-carbon unsaturated fatty acids into an endoperoxide configuration. The endoperoxides are the key precursor molecules for all subsequent prostaglandin, TXA_2 and PGI_2 cellular biosynthesis, including the platelet and endothelial cell. Since endoperoxides of exactly the same structure and stereochemistry are synthesized in all cell types, there appears to be no apparent heterogeneity in the cyclooxygenase enzyme, regardless of cell type.

The cyclooxygenase is a substrate-activated enzyme. The actual cyclization and oxygenation of arachidonic acid is shown in Figure 2. The enzymatic reaction has four basic requirements: one heme molecule per two subunits of cyclooxygenase, molecular oxygen, a hydroperoxide activator and free arachidonic acid. The first reaction is the oxygenation of C-11 of arachidonic acid. The formation of endoperoxide from 11-peroxy-5,8,12,14-eicosatetraenoic involves a series of concerted reactions. Another oxygen molecule is inserted at C-15, followed by isomerization of the Δ^{12}-double bond, the formation of a new carboncarbon bond between C-8 and C-12 (formation of cyclopentane ring) and finally an attack by the oxygen radical at C-9. The first product formed from arachidonate and O_2 is the 15-hydroperoxy endoperoxide PGG_2. However, the 15-hydroxy derivative PGH_2 is more abundant because the cyclooxygenase also possess peroxidase activity. Anggard and Samuelsson (32) found that in incubations using arachidonic acid and homogenates of guinea pig lung, both PGE_2 and $PGF_{2\alpha}$ were formed but the two prostaglandins were not interconvertible. This was really the first indication that prostaglandins shared a common precursor molecule. Labeled oxygen studies demonstrated that the two oxygens of the cyclopentane ring were either both ^{18}O or both ^{16}O. These data suggested both oxygens originated from the same molecule of O_2 and that the intermediate structure was a cyclic peroxide or endoperoxide. It should be

mentioned that this endoperoxide structure was postulated on the basis
of theoretical considerations by Beal et al. (9) in 1964.

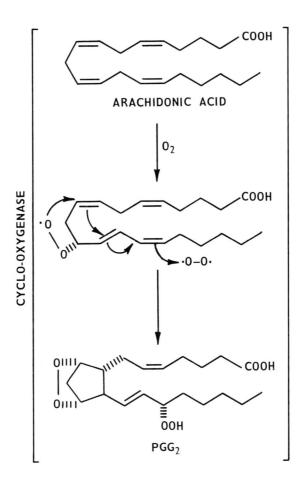

FIGURE 2. Endoperoxide Formation From Arachidonic Acid. In the
presence of molecular oxygen, the cyclooxygenase transforms essential
fatty acids (primarily arachidonic acid) into unstable endoperoxide
structures. The resulting endoperoxide is the key precursor for all
subsequent prostaglandin, thromboxane and prostacyclin synthesis (see
text for details).

The inhibition of cyclooxygenase activity by nonsteroidal anti-inflammatory drugs (NSAID) is one of the most important aspects of prostaglandin research. Vane (33) initially suggested that the mechanism of action of NSAIDs was inhibition of prostaglandin biosynthesis. The cyclooxygenase is inhibited by different NSAIDs in various ways. The cyclooxygenase reaction in platelets has important clinical implications, since nonsteroidal anti-inflammatory agents such as aspirin (ASA) inhibit the enzyme. ASA binds at the substrate site and irreversibly inactivates cyclooxygenase. This phenomenon is of significance in the platelet because platelets do not synthesize protein; therefore, inactivated enzyme cannot be replaced. Nucleated cells such as vascular endothelium are capable of synthesizing new protein and cyclooxygenase activity reappears within a few hours after aspirin treatment.

C. PGI_2 Synthase and Thromboxane A_2 Synthase

Once the endoperoxide is formed, the marked similarity of the synthetic process is lost. The endoperoxide can be converted into all of the various prostaglandins and thromboxanes. Subsequent synthetic steps are determined by the cell specific enzymatic profile. The cells of most importance to this discussion are the platelet, endothelial cell and underlying vascular elements including smooth muscle cells. In platelets, the endoperoxide is converted primarily into the pro-aggregatory and vasoconstrictive molecule TXA_2. In endothelial and smooth muscle cells the endoperoxide is converted primarily into the anti-aggregatory vasodilatory molecule PGI_2. The metabolic transformations of arachidonate in the platelet and vascular elements are summarized in Figure 3.

D. Arachidonate Lipoxygenation

Besides the metabolism of arachidonate by the cyclooxygenase, a whole series of lipoxygenases have been found. In contrast to the cyclooxygenase, the lipoxygenases are a heterogeneous group of enzymes. The lipoxygenation of arachidonic acid in human platelets results in a 12-OH arachidonate molecule (34,35). Turner et al. (36) originally demonstated that 12-OH arachidonate was a chemotactic molecule for polymorphonuclear cells (PMN). Later it was demonstrated that 12-OOH is also a potent chemotactic species for PMNs. Hydroperoxides such as those produced by the lipoxygenase pathway may serve as cyclooxygenase activators. It should be emphasized that on a quantitative basis, significant amounts of platelet arachidonate are converted to 12-HETE following stimulation and such transformation increases with time.

Interestingly, 12-OOH arachidonate (and other hydroperoxy fatty acids) inhibits the PGI_2 synthase in vascular endothelium (37). In addition, there has been one report that vascular tissue can actually synthesize 12-OH HETE. Thus, although no specific platelet or vascular function can be assigned to the 12-lipoxygenase pathway at present, it may be a fertile area for future research.

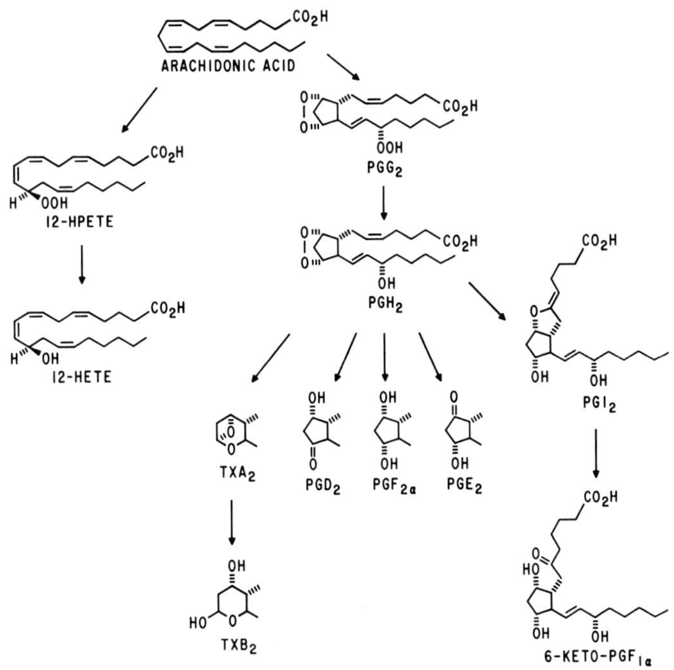

FIGURE 3. Pathways of Arachidonic Acid Metabolism in Human Platelets and Endothelial Cells. In the human platelet, arachidonic acid can be metabolized by two separate enzymatic pathways. The lipoxygenase pathway forms 12-hydroperoxyeicosatetraenoic acid (HPETE) and 12-hydroxyeicosatetraenoic acid (12-HETE). This enzyme is inhibited by 5,8,11,14-eicosatetraynoic acid (ETYA) but not by nonsteroidal anti-inflammatory compounds (e.g., aspirin). The platelet cyclooxygenase pathway forms the endoperoxide PGH_2, which can be converted to thromboxane A_2 and the various products shown. The endothelial cell also has a lipoxygenase that produces 12-HPETE and 12-HETE. However, endothelial cells produce primarily PGI_2 from the endoperoxide and all the other prostaglandins shown except thromboxane A_2.

Possibly the most important lipoxygenase products are formed by polymorphonuclear leukocytes (PMN). Borgeat and Samuelsson (38) elucidated the structure of several different oxygenated products of arachidonic acid in rabbit PMN cells. Arachidonic acid release in PMN's leads to the formation of 5-hydroperoxyeicosatetraenoic acid. The hydroperoxide is then converted either to a 5-hydroxy acid or to a 5(6)-oxido-7,9,11,14-eicosatetraenoic acid. This unstable epoxide then undergoes enzymatic hydrolysis to a 5,12-dihydroxy acid (leukotriene B$_4$) and other B$_4$ hydroxy fatty acids (38). This pioneering work together with recent data from several different laboratories has led to the elucidation of the structure of slow-reacting substances of anaphylaxis (SRS-A) or leukotriene D$_4$ (39,40). The synthesis and structures of leukotrienes are shown in Figure 4.

To date, no clear interactions between leukotrienes, platelets and the vascular wall have been reported. However, recent studies have shown that platelets and PMNs can interchange oxygenated arachidonate and add an additional OH group (41,42). The resulting 5S,12S-DiHETE molecules could have unknown biological importance and are being actively studied at the present time.

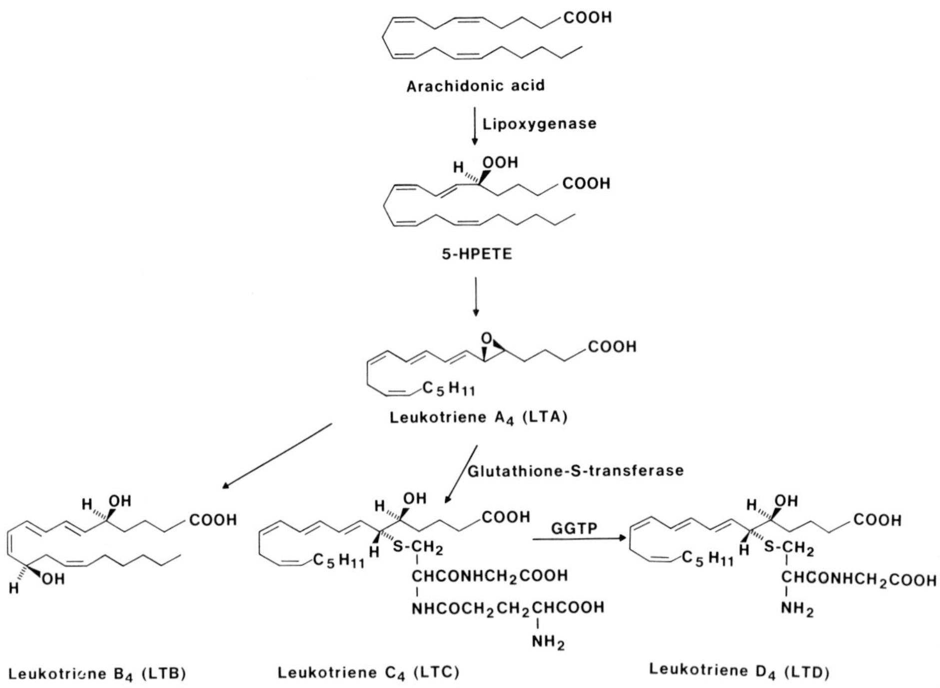

FIGURE 4. Leukotriene Synthesis from Arachidonic Acid. In polymorphonuclear cells, a lipoxygenase converts arachidonic acid into 5-hydroperoxy eicosatetraenoic acid. Then the hydroperoxide is converted into a 5(6)-oxido-eicosatetraenoic acid (leukotriene A). Leukotriene A is subsequently converted into either luekotriene B or C. Leukotriene C can then interact with a gamma-glutamyl trans-peptidase (GGTP) to form leukotriene D.

E. Metabolism of Prostaglandins and Thromboxanes

Regardless of the cell of origin, most prostaglandins have a half-life of approximately 5 to 10 min in circulation. Prostacyclin and thromboxane A_2 are inherently unstable molecules at physiological pH, but they are also metabolized by degradative enzymes as well. Most prostaglandins are metabolized during a single passage through the lungs. Prostacyclin is the only prostaglandin that is slowly metabolized by the lungs. The general sequence of prostaglandin and thromboxane metabolism is as follows:

1. Oxidation of the allylic alcohol group at C-15, catalyzed by 15-hydroxy-prostaglandin dehydrogenase. This enzyme is widespread but the lung, kidney and placenta are particularly rich sources (43,44). The enzyme is noncompetetively inhibited by 15-keto PGE_2 and 13,14-dihydro-15-keto-PGE_2. The enzyme reacts preferentially with compounds possessing a keto group at C-9 and a double bond at C-5 and bulky group substitution at or near C-15 usually yields an inactive substrate.

2. Oxidation at C-15 by the 15-hydroxy-prostaglandin dehydrogenase is usually followed by reduction of the 13,14-double bond. The reduction by the 15-keto-prostaglandin 13,14-reductase requires a carbonyl group at C-15. The 15-keto-prostaglandin reductase co-purifies with the 15-hydroxyprostaglandin dehydrogenase, and the activities of the two enzymes are difficult to separate. NADH is the preferred cofactor for the reductase, whereas NAD^+ is a competitive inhibitor and prostaglandin E_2 a noncompetitive inhibitor.

3. After oxidation of C-15 and reduction of the Δ^{13} double bond, the 13,14-dihydro-15-keto-prostaglandin can be β-oxidized or undergo ω-1 oxidation (45,46). The major urinary metabolite of PGE_2 in man is a 7α-hydroxy-5,11-diketo-tetranor-prosta-1,16-dienoic acid (47).

Studies of TXB_2 metabolism in man have shown that 2,3-dinor-thromboxane B_2 is the primary urinary metabolite (48). The presence of this metabolite indicates that TXB_2 undergoes a single step of β-oxidation. Studies of PGI_2 metabolism in man have suggested that 9,11-dihydroxy-6,15-diketo-1,2,19,20-tetranorprosta-3,18-dioic acid is the major urinary product (49). Figure 5 outlines the currently understood metabolism of PGE_2, TXB_2 and PGI_2.

III. MECHANISM OF ACTION OF TXA_2 AND PGI_2

Since this chapter is concerned with platelet-vessel wall arachidonate metabolism, I will use the human platelet as a model for the mechanism of action of prostaglandins, TXA_2 and PGI_2. The physiology and biochemistry of the platelet have been rigorously studied with respect to prostaglandins and thromboxanes, and the regulation of platelet adenylate cyclase by these agents well delineated.

Human platelet homeostasis is controlled by the "reciprocal regulation" of cyclic AMP levels by PGI_2 and TXA_2 (50). Agents that elevate cyclic AMP, such as PGE_1 or PGI_2, block primary (non-cyclooxygenase-dependent) and secondary (cyclooxygenase-dependent) aggregation. PGI_2 inhibits both primary and secondary aggregation regardless of the pro-aggregatory stimulus. The platelet inhibitor potency of prostaglandins can be directly correlated with their ability to stimulate platelet cyclic AMP levels.

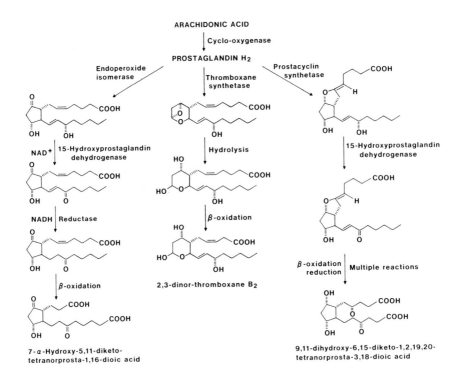

FIGURE 5. Metabolism of TXA_2, PGI_2 and PGE_2 in Human Tissues. PGI_2 and PGE_2 are dehydrogenated, reduced at the $\Delta^{13,14}$ double bond, and then β-oxidized to the primary urinary metabolites shown. TXA_2 is hydrolyzed to thromboxane B_2 (TXB_2) and TXB_2 is β-oxidized and excreted as 2,3-dinor-TXB_2. Of course many other metabolic sequences are possible.

TXA$_2$ is a strong inducer of human platelet aggregation. Like PGI$_2$, TXA$_2$ is formed from the endoperoxides of PGG$_2$ or PGH$_2$. In contrast to PGI$_2$, TXA$_2$ inhibits platelet adenylate cyclase. TXA$_2$ does not inhibit basal cyclic AMP levels in platelets. Such levels must be initially increased by PGE$_1$ or PGI$_2$ before the lowering effect of TXA$_2$ can be observed (50). This suggests that TXA$_2$ might block cyclic AMP indirectly.

Calcium is an integral part of the mechanism responsible for human platelet aggregation and it has even been suggested that prostaglandins and/or TXA$_2$ may act as calcium ionophores (51). Rodan and Feinstein (52) have shown that Ca^{2+} alone can inhibit PGE$_1$-stimulated cyclic AMP accumulation in human platelets. Thus it is logical to assume that Ca^{2+} might mediate the action of TXA$_2$. If TXA$_2$ can induce translocation of Ca^{2+} from the bound to the free state and can inhibit adenylate cyclase, then inhibition of adenylate cyclase by TXA$_2$ should be antagonized by agents that inhibit Ca^{2+} mobilization. An agent known as TMB-8 is a Ca^{2+} antagonist that is thought to block Ca^{2+} release from membranes. When TMB-8 was tested in the presence of PGI$_2$ and PGH$_2$ (TXA$_2$), the cylic AMP-lowering effect of TXA$_2$ was blocked, but the stimulatory activity of PGI$_2$ was not inhibited. In fact, in some instances the stimulation of cyclic AMP accumulation was enhanced by TMB-8 (53). Recently Hathaway and Adelstein (54) have demonstrated that the phosphorylation of platelet myosin kinase by a cyclic AMP-dependent protein kinase decreases myosin kinase activity. Phosphorylation decreases the ability of myosin kinase to bind calmodulin (which regulates the expression of Ca^{2+} effects). Therefore, an agent such as TXA$_2$ would stimulate Ca^{2+} mobilization (inhibiting adenylate cyclase), enhance the contraction of platelet actomyosin and induce platelet aggregation. Conversely, PGI$_2$ stimulation of cyclic AMP levels would enhance the phosphorylation of myosin kinase, favoring the unphosphorylated form of myosin and inhibition of platelet aggregation. Regardless of the exact mechanism(s) responsible for the PGI$_2$ inhibition of human platelet aggregation or TXA$_2$ stimulation of aggregation, it does appear that these two molecules oppose each other through the regulation of adenylate cyclase (50).

Prostacyclin also stimulates the adenylate cyclase of endothelial cells (55). The elevation in cyclic AMP attenuates subsequent PGI$_2$ biosynthesis but other systems may also be modulated. For example, the treatment of cultures of vascular endothelial cells with aspirin (which inhibits PGI$_2$ biosynthesis) reduces platelet adhesiveness to the endothelial cell monolayer (56). These data suggest that PGI$_2$ (presumably by elevating endothelial cell cyclic AMP levels) can influence platelet-endothelial cell interactions as well as platelet-platelet interaction. This observation may also be applicable to other systems. For example, PGI$_2$ may reduce metastasis by inhibiting tumor cell-platelet interactions as well as tumor cell-endothelial interactions (see chapter 14).

A somewhat oversimplified working model of platelet homeostasis is depicted in Figure 6. The blood vessel wall contains the enzyme prostacyclin synthase but not thromboxane synthase. The platelet contains a thromboxane synthase but not prostacyclin synthase. When platelets are stimulated they produce TXA_2 which stimulates the aggregation of other platelets and induces vasoconstriction. When vascular endothelium is stimulated (e.g., by thrombin), PGI_2 is produced which elevates cyclic AMP, inhibiting platelet aggregation and inducing vasodilation. It should be noted that the vasodilation induced by PGI_2 has also been shown to be associated with an elevation in cyclic AMP (57). However, there is no evidence of a TXA_2 inhibition of blood vessel adenylate cyclase. Thus the balance of the pro-aggregatory activity of TXA_2 and the anti-aggregatory activity of PGI_2 appears to control human platelet aggregation.

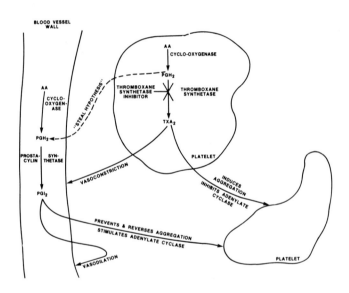

FIGURE 6. Model of Platelet and Vascular Homeostasis. Platelet aggregation and vascular tone are regulated by a balance between the pro-aggregatory and vasoconstricting actions of TXA_2 and the vasodilating and anti-aggregatory actions of PGI_2. The mechanism responsible for these activities is probably the reciprocal regulation of cAMP levels. TXA_2 lowers and PGI_2 stimulates cAMP levels.

Another interesting aspect of platelet-vessel wall interactions is the "steal hypothesis". It is believed that PGH_2 can migrate from the platelet to the vasculature and can be converted to PGI_2, that is, the vasculature steals endoperoxides from the platelets. Whether or not this occurs under normal physiological circumstances is debatable. However, there is no doubt that steal occurs in the presence of a thromboxane synthase inhibitor and this may prove to be the most beneficial aspect of a thromboxane synthase inhibitor (58).

IV. SUMMARY

The reciprocal regulation of cyclic AMP levels by PGI_2 and TXA_2 may not explain all of the actions of prostaglandins and thromboxanes but when thrombotic and metastatic diseases are discussed, cyclic AMP-regulated systems are clearly involved. In this chapter I have attempted to summarize the metabolism of arachidonate in platelets and vascular tissue and to relate these molecules to platelet aggregation and adhesion to vascular elements. Hopefully the mechanisms discussed in this chapter will help clarify the role of arachidonate metabolites in other chapters of this book which discuss vascular endothelium homeostasis and metastatic disease.

REFERENCES

1. Kurzrok R and Lieb CC. Proc. Soc. Exp. Biol. Med. 28:268–272, 1930.
2. Goldblatt MW. J. Physiol (London) 84:208–218, 1935.
3. von Euler US. J. Physiol (London) 88:208–218, 1935.
4. Bergstrom S and Sjovall J. Acta Chem. Scand. 14:1693–1699, 1960.
5. Bergstrom S, Ryhage R, Samuelsson B and Sjovall J. J. Biol. Chem. 238:3555–3561, 1963.
6. Samuelsson B. J. Am. Chem. Soc. 85:1878–1884, 1963.
7. Van Dorp DA, Beerthuis RK, Nugteren DH and Von Heman H. Biochim. Biophys. Acta 90:204–207, 1964.
8. Bergstrom S, Danielson H and Samuelsson B. Biochim. Biophys. Acta 90:207–212, 1964.
9. Beal PE, Fonken GS and Pike JE. The Upjohn Co., Belgium Patent 659,884, prior date U.S.A., February 19, 1964.
10. Kloeze J. In: Prostaglandins, Nobel Symposium 2. (Eds. Bergstrom S and Samuelsson B). pp. 241–252,, Interscience, New York, 1967.
11. Salzman EW and Levin L. J. Clin. Invest. 50:131–137, 1971.
12. Hamberg M, Svensson J, Wakabayashi T and Samuelsson B. Proc. Natl. Acad. Sci. USA 71:345–349, 1974.
13. Nugteren DH and Hazelhof E. Biochim. Biophys. Acta 326:448–461, 1973.
14. Willis AL and Kuhn DC. Prostaglandins 4:127–147, 1973.
15. Smith JB and Willia AL. Nature (London) 231:235–237, 1975.
16. Piper PJ and Vane JR. Nature (London) 223:29–31, 1969.
17. Gryglewski R and Vane JR. Br. J. Pharmacol. 45:37–44, 1972.
18. Hamberg M, Svensson J and Samuelsson B. Proc. Natl. Acad. Sci. USA 72:2994–2999, 1975.
19. Moncada S, Gryglewski R, Bunting S and Vane JR. Nature (London) 263:663–666, 1976.
20. Johnson RA, Morton DR, Kinner JH, Gorman RR, McGuire JC, Sun FF, Whittaker N, Bunting S, Salmon J, Moncada S and Vane JR. Prostaglandins 12:915–925, 1976.
21. Needleman P, Bryan B, Wyche A, Ronson SD, Eakins K, Ferrendelli JA and Minkes M. Prostaglandins 14:897–908, 1977.

206

22. Isakson PC, Raz A, Hsueh W and Needleman P. In: Advances in Prostaglandin and Thromboxane Research, (Eds. Samuelsson B and Paoletti R), pp. 113–120, Raven Press, New York, 1978.

23. Bills TK, Smith JB and Silver MJ. Biochim. Biophys. Acta 424:303–314, 1976.

24. Bell RL and Majerus PW. J. Biol. Chem. 255:1790–1792, 1980.

25. Bell RL, Kennerly DA, Stanford N and Majerus PW. Proc. Natl. Acad. Sci. USA 76:3238–3241, 1979.

26. Broekman MJ, Ward JW and Marcus AJ. J. Clin. Invest. 66:275–283, 1980.

27. Hong SL and Deykin D. J. Biol. Chem. 257:7151–7154, 1982.

28. Greaves MW and McDonald-Gibson W. Br. Med. J. 82:83–84, 1972.

29. Gryglewski RJ, Panczenko B, Korbut R, Grodzinska L and Ocetkiewicz P. Prostaglandins 10:343–355, 1975.

30. Flower RJ, Gryglewski RJ, Cedro HK and Vane JR. Nature (London) 238:104–106, 1972.

31. Hirata F, Schiffmann E, Venkatasubramanion K, Solomon D and Axelrod J. Proc. Natl. Acad. Sci. USA 77:2533–2536, 1980.

32. Anggard E and Samuelsson B. J. Biol. Chem. 240:3518–3521, 1965.

33. Vane JR. Nature (London) 231:233–235, 1971.

34. Nugteren DH. Biochim. Biophys. Acta 380:299–307, 1965.

35. Hamberg M, Svensson J and Samuelsson B. Proc. Natl. Acad. Sci. USA 71:3824–3838, 1974.

36. Turner SR, Tainer JA and Lynn WA. Nature (London) 257:680–681, 1975.

37. Gryglewski RJ, Bunting S, Moncada S, Flower RJ and Vane JR. Prostaglandins 12:685–713, 1976.

38. Borgeat P and Samuelsson B. J. Biol. Chem. 254:2643–2646, 1979.

39. Morris HR, Taylor GW, Piper PJ, Sirois P and Tippins JR. FEBS Lett. 87:203–206, 1978.

40. Murphy RC, Hammarstrom S and Samuelsson B. Proc. Natl. Acad. Sci. USA 76:4275–4279, 1979.

41. Borgeat P, Fruteau de Laclos B, Picard S, Drapeau J, Vallerand P and Corey EJ. Prostaglandins 23:713–720, 1982.

42. Marcus AJ, Broekman MJ, Safier LB, Ullman HL, Islam N, Serhan CN, Rutherford LE, Korchak HM and Weissman G. Biochem. Biophys. Res. Commun. 109:130–137, 1982.

43. Marrazzi MA and Matchinsky FM. Prostaglandins 1:373–388, 1972.

44. Jarabek J. Proc. Natl. Acad. Sci. USA 69:533–534, 1972.

45. Nakano J and Morsy HH. Clin. Res. 19:142–146, 1970.

46. Israelsson U, Hamberg M and Samuelsson B. Eur. J. Biochem. 11:390–394, 1969.

47. Hamberg M and Samuelsson B. J. Biol. Chem. 246:6713–6721, 1971.

48. Roberts LJ, Sweetman BJ, Payne NA and Oates JA. J. Biol. Chem. 252:7415–7417, 1977.

49. Fitzgerald GA. Personal communication, 1982.

50. Gorman RR, Fitzpatrick FA and Miller OV. In: Adv. in Cyclic Nucleotide Res., (Eds. George WJ and Ignarro LJ). Vol. 9, pp. 597–609, Raven Press, New York, 1978.

51. Gerrard JM, Butler AM and White JG. Prostaglandins 1:703–710, 1977.

52. Rodan GA and Feinstein MB. Proc. Natl. Acad. Sci. USA 73:1829–1833, 1976.

53. Gorman RR, Wierenga W and Miller OV. Biochim. Biophys. Acta 572:95–104, 1979.

54. Hathaway DR and Adelstein RS. Proc. Natl. Acad. Sci. USA 76:1653–1657, 1979.

55. Hopkins NK and Gorman RR. J. Clin. Invest. 67:540–546, 1981.

56. Czervionke RL, Hoak JC and Fry GL. J. Clin. Invest. 62:847–856, 1978.

57. Miller OV, Aiken JW, Hemker DP, Shebuski RJ and Gorman RR. Prostaglandins 18:915–925, 1979.

58. Aiken JW, Shebuski RJ, Miller OV and Gorman RR. J. Pharmacol. Expt. Ther. 219:299–308, 1981.

CHAPTER 14. PROSTACYCLIN/THROMBOXANES AND TUMOR CELL METASTASIS

KENNETH V. HONN, JAMES M. ONODA, DAVID G. MENTER, JOHN D. TAYLOR AND
BONNIE F. SLOANE

I. INTRODUCTION

The ability to metastasize is a characteristic which
distinguishes benign from malignant neoplasms. Metastasis can be
simply defined as a loss of contiguity between a tumor cell or a clump
of tumor cells and the primary tumor with successful transfer to, and
growth at, a spatially separate site. The overall process can be
regarded as a series of sequential events representing complex
interactions between the tumor cell and the host (Figure 1).

Carcinomas were once believed to metastasize via the lymphatics,
whereas malignant tumors of mesenchymal origin were believed to spread
via the hematogenous route. Hilgard et al. (1) noted that tumor cells
will reach the vascular system when injected initially into the
lymphatics. Similar conclusions have been reached by others (2,3) and
there is now substantial evidence that malignant cells can pass freely
between the lymphatics and blood vessels (4,5). Therefore, it can be
concluded that tumor cells disseminate via the hematogenous route at
some point in the metastatic cascade. Nevertheless, in humans there
is a reported lack of correlation between the presence of viable
circulating tumor cells and a poor prognosis (6,7). However, these
earlier studies are suspect because nonviable tumor cells and
megakaryocytes were incorrectly reported as viable tumor cells (6).
In animal models, large numbers of circulating tumor cells are
released from primary tumors. Butler and Gullino (8) determined that
3-4,000,000 cells/24 hr/g of tumor are shed from subcutaneous MTWG
mammary carcinomas. Liotta et al. (9) demonstrated that the number of
shed tumor cells increases with growth of the primary tumor. The
efficiency of tumor metastasis is also positively correlated with the
size of tumor cell aggregates (10) and the ability of tumor cells to
undergo homotypic aggregation (11). Glaves (12) recently investigated
whether there is a correlation between the numbers of circulating
tumor cells of Lewis lung carcinoma (3LL) and B16 melanoma and their
incidence of metastasis. The 3LL tumor cells form fewer lung colonies
following tail vein injection than the B16 cells. However,
subcutaneous 3LL tumors form a greater number of spontaneous pulmonary
metastases when compared to subcutaneous B16 tumors. Quantitation of
circulating tumor cells revealed that 3LL tumors shed four times more
cells into circulation than B16 tumors. Therefore, the low
colonization potential of the 3LL relative to the B16 is compensated

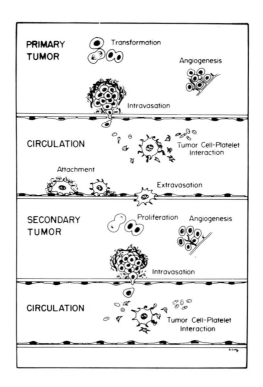

FIGURE 1. Overview of the Metastatic Cascade. The primary tumor is believed to be initiated by transformation (i.e., chemical, radiation or viral) of a normal cell which then proliferates until limited by blood supply and invasive properties of the tumor. As the tumor grows, the tumor cells release angiogenesis factors which induce neovascularization. To move to a secondary site, the tumor cells must be able to detach from the primary tumor and invade into the circulatory system (intravasate), wherein the tumor cells may interact with host platelets and neutrophils during transport. Tumor cells can induce platelet aggregation and this in turn is thought to facilitate attachment of tumor cells to the endothelium or to areas of exposed basement membrane. Dissolution of the basement membrane by proteolytic enzymes released from the tumor cell then may enable the cells to extravasate at a secondary site, at which the processes of proliferation, angiogenesis, invasion and metastasis (from a metastasis) can reoccur. [From Honn et al. (87) with permission.]

for during spontaneous metastasis by the increased number of circulating tumor cells (12). These results suggest that a quantitative prognostic relationship does exist between numbers of circulating tumor cells and incidence of metastasis.

The above mentioned studies report large numbers of circulating cancer cells in tumor-bearing animals. The actual number of metastases found in these animals is orders of magnitude lower than would be predicted by the number of circulating cells, suggesting that metastasis is an inefficent process (13). B16 amelanotic melanoma (B16a) tumor cells were temporarily arrested in the pulmonary microvasculature following intravenous injection into the tail vein of mice. These cells were then slowly released so that less than 5% of the original inoculum remained in the lung after 20 hr (Figure 2). Weiss and co-workers demonstrated that the majority of tumor cells initially arrested in the lung (14) of mice following tail vein injection, or arrested in the liver (15) following portal vein injection, are subsequently released as non-viable cells. They have suggested that metastatic inefficiency is due to the death of most circulating cancer cells in the first organ encountered after leaving the primary tumor (15). For example, bioassay data indicated that of 80,000 B16 cells released from the liver after portal vein injection of 100,000 cells, only 1% were delivered to the lung in a viable state (15). This suggests that metastasis to these "secondary organs" might be the result of cells released from metastases in the "first organ" as opposed to direct seeding from the primary tumor (metastasis from metastases, see Chapter 1). The mechanism for the killing of tumor cells following arrest in the first organ is unclear but may include mechanical trauma (16), attack by NK cells (17), macrophages (18) or neutrophils (19).

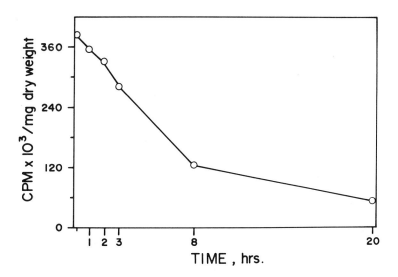

FIGURE 2. Time Dependent Loss of [125]IUdr Labeled B16a Cells from the Lungs of Syngeneic C57BL/6J Mice Following their Tail Vein Injection.

Once a tumor cell is in circulation it can undergo a variety of cell-cell interactions. Some of these interactions may be deleterious as suggested above. Others may facilitate tumor cell metastasis. It is intuitive that a circulating tumor cell must arrest in the microvasculature, form stable adhesions with the endothelium or basal lamina, and escape destruction by shear forces or cellular immune mechanisms in order to undergo extravasation. Several factors have been demonstrated to affect tumor cell adhesion to a variety of substrata. Most important are those which enhance tumor cell attachment to endothelium or basal lamina. In this regard, Nicolson and co-workers (20,21) have described a role for surface sialogalacto-proteins in tumor cell binding to endothelial cell monolayers, endothelial extracellular matrix and immobilized fibronectin. Cells treated with the antibiotic tunicamycin, which inhibits formation of asparagine-linked oligosaccharide chains on glycoproteins (22,23), demonstrate decreased adhesiveness to the above substrata as well as decreased lung colony formation in synegeneic mice (20). Liotta and co-workers demonstrated that metastatic tumor cells attach preferentially to type IV collagen (24). This attachment can be enhanced by laminin and blocked by anti-laminin antibody, but cannot be enhanced by fibronectin nor blocked by anti-fibronectin antibody (25). In addition, tumor cells that demonstrate laminin-enhanced attachment to type IV collagen produce more pulmonary tumor colonies in vivo. Lung colony formation can be decreased by anti-laminin antibody (25). Preferred attachment proteins may vary among tumor types (26). Schirrmacher et al. (27) have elegantly demonstrated that the metastatic capacity of a range of murine tumor cell lines is regulated by the degree of sialylation of two sugar moieties (D-galactose and N-acetylgalactosamine) found in animal cell membranes. Clearly, a number of tumor cell surface determinants may be involved in tumor arrest and adhesion to the vessel wall. In addition to these tumor cell surface determinants, the interaction of circulating tumor cells with host platelets is believed to facilitate metastasis. This may be due in part to platelet-enhanced tumor cell adhesion to the vessel wall.

II. PLATELETS, COAGULATION AND METASTASIS

Patients with malignant neoplasms often demonstrate abnormalities in their blood coagulability (28-30 and Chapter 22). These abnormalities include hyperaggregability of platelets (28), with resultant thrombocytopenia (31), and a reduction in fibrinogen concomitant with an increase in fibrin-fibrinogen degradation products (29,32,33). Tumor cells have been reported to possess both a platelet-activating material (34-37 and Chapters 10-12) and a pro-coagulant activity responsible for alterations in the fibrin-fibrinogen system (38-40 and Chapters 6 and 7) and possibly platelet aggregation (41).

The interaction of tumor cells with host platelets is believed to facilitate metastasis; however, the exact mechanism is, at this time, unknown. It is generally accepted that tumor cells become damaged during circulatory transport. This circulatory trauma may be due to humoral factors (i.e., macrophages, natural killer cells and antibody-mediated complement lysis) and physical factors (i.e., shear forces and mechanical trauma due to passage through the microvasculature). Tumor cells shielded within platelet thrombi may be protected from some or all of the above. In addition, platelets may enhance tumor cell adhesion to endothelial or de-endothelialized surfaces via platelet bridges. Finally, tumor cell survival and multiplication may be enhanced due to the release of platelet mitogenic factors [i.e., platelet-derived growth factor (Chapter 18)]. It is generally accepted that platelets enhance metastasis by facilitating processes that occur during tumor cell arrest and adhesion (42,43); whether that includes direct facilitation of adhesion and/or protection of arrested tumor cells from cellular immune destruction (44) is not certain. Injection of tumor cells i.v. has been observed to induce platelet aggregation (45). Thrombocytopenia induced by neuraminidase or antiplatelet antiserum results in decreased lung colony formation from tail vein-injected tumor cells (46) and spontaneous metastasis from s.c. tumors (47).

The above correlations have prompted the use of antiplatelet and anticoagulation drugs for the treatment of experimental (48-57) and human (58) metastasis. The results of these studies have been somewhat controversial. Indeed, several authors have proposed that the observed antimetastatic effect of anticoagulant and antiplatelet drugs is not due to their alterations of hemostasis (44,54-56).

III. PROSTACYCLIN, THROMBOXANES, PLATELETS AND METASTASIS

Compounds derived from arachidonic acid [prostacyclin (PGI_2) and thromboxane A_2 (TXA_2); Figure 3] have been demonstrated to have a profound but possibly not exclusive (59) role in platelet aggregation and normal hemostasis. Hamberg et al. (60) demonstrated the formation of TXA_2 from the endoperoxide intermediate prostaglandin H_2 (PGH_2) (Figure 3). Subsequently, platelet TXA_2 biosynthesis was found to be stimulated by numerous aggregating agents and thus believed to be an absolute requirement for platelet aggregation (61). This view has recently been challenged by the observations that in some cases the endoperoxide PGH_2 can initiate platelet aggregation independent of its conversion to TXA_2 (62,63).

One year following the discovery of TXA_2, Vane and co-workers (64) discovered PGI_2 as another transformation product of prostaglandin endoperoxides (Figure 3). PGI_2 is produced by vascular tissue of all species so far tested (65) and is the main product of arachidonic acid metabolism in isolated vascular tissue. It is the most potent endogenous inhibitor of platelet aggregation yet discovered, being 30 to 40 times more potent than prostaglandin E_1 (PGE_1; 66) and 1,000 times more potent than adenosine (67). In addition, PGI_2 can reverse secondary platelet aggregation in vitro (64,68) and in the circulatory system of man (69). It has been suggested that PGI_2 and TXA_2 play an antagonistic and pivotal role in the control of thrombosis centered upon their bidirectional (PGI_2 increases, TXA_2 decreases) effect on platelet cAMP levels. However, proaggregatory agents (i.e., 1-0-alkyl-2-0-acetyl-2sn-glyceryl-3-phosphorylcholine) in addition to TXA_2 should be considered for this pivotal role.

212

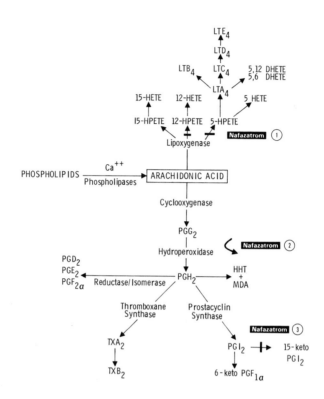

FIGURE 3. Arachidonic Acid Metabolism via the Lipoxygenase Pathway Resulting in Hydroperoxy Fatty Acids and Leukotrienes and via the Prostaglandin Endoperoxide Synthase (Cyclooxygenase plus Hydroperoxidase) Pathway Resulting in Prostaglandins (Including Prostacyclin) and Thromboxanes. Possible sites of action of nafazatrom include: (1) inhibition of lipoxygenase activity, (2) reducing co-factor for the hydroperoxidase of prostaglandin endoperoxide synthase and (3) inhibition of prostacyclin (PGI_2) degradation by 15-hydroxy-prostaglandin dehydrogenase. [From Honn et al. (87) with permission.]

Our working hypothesis (Figure 4) has been that the normal intravascular balance between PGI_2 and platelet arachidonic acid metabolism (i.e., TXA_2) is altered by tumor cells or products released from tumor cells. Although this hypothesis places emphasis on platelet-enhanced tumor cell adhesion it does not exclude other mechanisms (44). Given this hypothesis one can address a number of questions experimentally (Figure 5).

HYPOTHESIS

The primary tumor, circulating tumor cells and/or tumor cell shed membrane vesicles disrupt the relationship between arachidonic acid metabolites of the platelet and the vessel wall.

This alteration favors tumor cell-platelet thrombi formation, tumor cell adhesion to the vessel wall and ultimately metastasis.

FIGURE 4.

QUESTIONS

1. Is tumor cell induced platelet aggregation (TCIPA) dependent on the generation of platelet TXA_2?

2. Can TCIPA be inhibited by:
   a. cyclooxygenase inhibitors
   b. thromboxane synthase inhibitors
   c. prostacyclin
   d. calcium channel blockers
   e. calcium antagonists

3. Does a therapeutic synergism occur when the above drugs are combined?

4. Is prostacyclin an endogenous, natural deterrent to metastasis?

5. Do tumor cells produce substances which reduce the cancer patients ability to generate prostacyclin?

6. Would drugs which enhance endogenous prostacyclin production possess antimetastatic activity?

FIGURE 5.

A. Prostacyclin Effects in Vivo and in Vitro

1. Prostacyclin effects on tumor cell-induced platelet aggregation (TCIPA). Menter et al. (70) studied the effectiveness of PGI_2 for inhibition of TCIPA using four histologically distinct rodent tumors (amelanotic melanoma, carcinoma, adenocarcinoma and carcinosarcoma). Complete inhibition of TCIPA is achieved with PGI_2 (10 ng/ml) despite differences in the abilities of the various tumor lines to induce aggregation. Lerner et al. (71) have also found that PGI_2 inhibits platelet aggregation induced by a variety of human tumor cell lines in vitro (see also Chapter 11). These results suggest that the inhibitory effect of PGI_2 on TCIPA is not peculiar to tumor type. In contrast, inhibitors of TCIPA thought to be induced by ADP (72) or thrombin (73) do not exhibit generalized inhibition.

Comparison of the inhibitory effects of PGI_2 on TCIPA with that of other icosanoids reveals that the stable hydrolysis product of PGI_2 (6-keto-$PGF_{1\alpha}$) is essentially ineffective in inhibiting TCIPA, whereas PGE_1 and PGD_2 are 100-fold less potent than PGI_2 (70). Prostacyclin is also ten times more potent than 6-keto-PGE_1 or dibutyryl cAMP for inhibition of TCIPA (71). In addition to comparing the effects of PGI_2 with those of other icosanoids known to inhibit platelet aggregation (i.e., PGE_1 and PGD_2), Menter et al. (70) examined the interplay between PGI_2 and another icosanoid (i.e., PGE_2) which does not directly affect TCIPA. Prostaglandins, especially of the E series, have been shown to be elevated in a large number of human (74-77) and experimental tumors (78). These elevated levels of PGE_2 have been correlated with tumor growth (78), osteolysis (79), hypercalcemia (80) and immune incompetence of the tumor-bearing host (81). Rolland et al. (77) have suggested that PGE_2 levels in human breast cancer may serve as a marker for metastatic potential. In this regard, Bennett et al. (74) have reported that survival time after surgery for human breast cancer is inversely related to the tumor PGE_2 levels. PGE_2 would not be expected to reach detectable levels in circulation due to its rapid pulmonary metabolism. However, its enzymatic metabolite, 13,14-dihydro-15-keto-PGE_2, has been detected in circulation in rabbits bearing the VX_2 carcinoma (80) and in a series of patients with benign breast disease and breast cancer (82). Circulating levels of 13,14-dihydro-15-keto-PGE_2 are highest in patients with overt metastatic disease followed by patients with local malignant tumors and benign tumors (82). Menter et al. (70) found that in vitro both PGE_2 and its enzymatic metabolite, 13-14-dihydro-15-keto-PGE_2, reduce the inhibition of TCIPA by PGI_2. This reduced effectiveness may be due to these icosanoids interfering with PGI_2 binding to its platelet membrane receptor; one of the icosanoids tested (PGE_2) is known to bind to the platelet PGI_2 receptor (83). The relevance of the interaction between PGI_2 and PGE_2-like compounds in the formation of metastatic lesions is unknown. However, these in vitro results lead us to speculate that elevated levels of PGE_2 or 13,14-dihydro-15-keto-PGE_2 in vivo may facilitate metastasis by interfering with PGI_2's inhibition of tumor cell-platelet-vessel wall interactions.

Tumor cell-induced platelet aggregation occurs concomitantly with generation of TXA_2 (84). Nevertheless, the inhibition of TXA_2 production with selective thromboxane synthase inhibitors (TXSI) does not consistently results in inhibition of TCIPA even in the absence of measurable TXA_2 production (84 and unpublished observations). In fact, the only TXSI found to inhibit TCIPA are a series of endoperoxide analogs (85). Because of the close structural similarity between the endoperoxide analogs and the endoperoxide PGH_2, these effects may be ascribed to the blocking of PGH_2's interaction with the TXA_2 receptor by the endoperoxide analogs. The endoperoxide PGH_2 has been demonstrated to induce platelet aggregation (62,63). We have also tested aspirin (a cyclooxygenase inhibitor, Figure 3) for its inhibitory effect on TCIPA. Although aspirin completely blocked TXA_2 production during TCIPA, aggregation was only inhibited approximately 50% (unpublished observation). Since aspirin inhibition of cyclooxygenase would completely block TXA_2 and PGH_2 generation (Figure 3), we must conclude that TXA_2 production plays a role in TCIPA but it is not obligatory.

2. Prostacyclin effects on platelet-induced tumor cell adhesion in vitro. One proposed mechanism for platelet-facilitated metastasis is that platelets enhance tumor cell arrest in the microvasculature (via formation of platelet-tumor cell emboli) or that platelets, in some yet undefined way, enhance the adhesion of tumor cells to the endothelium or subendothelium. We have investigated platelet-facilitated tumor cell adhesion to a variety of substrata under both aggregatory and non-aggregatory conditions. Hara et al. (86) reported that tumor cells will not aggregate washed platelets. However, the addition of a small amount (2% v/v) of platelet poor plasma (PPP) restores a full aggregation response, suggesting an absolute requirement for a plasma factor during TCIPA (70,86). We have previously demonstrated that platelet-tumor cell adhesion can occur in the absence of overt platelet aggregation and that this interaction results in alterations of the tumor cell surface topology (87). We, therefore, explored the possibility that platelets could enhance the adhesion of W256 cells under non-aggregatory (no PPP) and aggregatory (> 0.1% PPP, v/v) conditions.

The adhesion of W256 cells to plastic plates, normal endothelial cells derived from rat cerebral microvasculature (primary cultures) and to their virally transformed counterparts (RCE-T1; 88) was enhanced by platelets (Figure 6). This increase varied with platelet preparation but ranged between 100-200% under non-aggregatory conditions (Figure 6). An even larger increase (200-300%) was observed if tumor cells were allowed to aggregate (addition of > 0.1% PPP) with platelets (Figure 6). In a representative scanning electron micrograph (Figure 7), the physical association between platelets and tumor cells during rat platelet facilitated W256 tumor cell adhesion to rat mesothelial cells is demonstrated. In this study and virtually all of the experiments examined thus far (87), the tumor cell does not appear to be engulfed by platelets. When attachment occurs, it seems to be between a limited number of platelets and tumor cells. Generally, attachment is followed by activation of surrounding

216

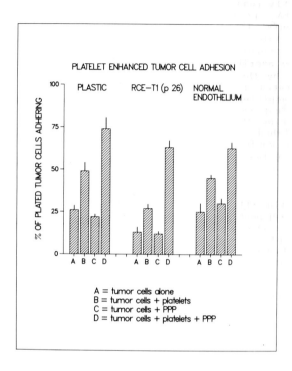

FIGURE 6. Effects of Rat Platelets on W256 Tumor Cell Adhesion to Plastic, Normal Rat Endothelial Cells Derived from Cerebrovasculature and their Virally Transformed Counterparts (RCE-T1; Passage 26) under Aggregatory and Non-aggregatory Conditions.

platelets with the formation of aggregates. This mechanism does not preclude, of course, that preformed platelet aggregates may also attach to tumor cells. If the attachment of a limited number of platelets to the tumor cells is a selective process, heterogenous platelet populations may exist. Indeed, there are some recent studies that indicate that functionally heterogenous platelet populations do exist (89,90). The above results suggest that the physical shielding of tumor cells by platelets is not a consistent feature of tumor cell-platelet interactions and cannot explain all of the observed antimetastatic effects of antiplatelet agents as has been suggested (44).

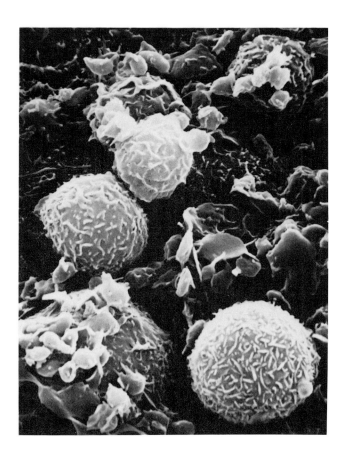

FIGURE 7. Scanning Electron Micrograph Demonstrating the Physical Interactions among Rat Platelets, W256 Tumor Cells and Rat Mesothelial Cells.

Fantone et al. (91) have demonstrated that the adherence of W256 cells to plastic plates or nylon fibers can be stimulated by the tumor promotor phorbol myristate acetate and the chemotactic peptide f-Met-Leu-Phe. Prostacyclin directly inhibits this increased adhesion; however, it has no effect on basal (unstimulated) W256 cell adhesion (91). We examined the effects of PGI_2 on platelet-facilitated adhesion to a variety of substrata. The addition of 30 μg/ml PGI_2 completely abrogates the platelet-facilitated adhesion of W256 cells to plastic (87). The effect is dose-dependent both in the presence and absence of PPP; a 40% decrease is observed at 1 μg/ml PGI_2. Prostacyclin had no effect on basal (unstimulated) W256 cell adhesion (87). Exogenous PGI_2 also limited W256 tumor cell adhesion to rat aortic endothelial cells (unpublished observation). These _in vitro_ results suggest that platelets may increase tumor cell adhesion to endothelium _in vivo_ and PGI_2 may limit the formation of a stable tumor cell-endothelial cell interaction. Support for this concept can also be derived from the experiments of Marcum _et al_. (92) in which rabbit aortic segments in a standard Baumgartner perfusion chamber are used to study tumor cell (HUT 20)-platelet-endothelial cell and subendothelial interactions. Tumor cells and platelets are perfused in the presence of PGE_1 (30 μg/ml) or PGI_2 (50 ng/ml). Both agents totally inhibit TCIPA and the deposition of both tumor cells and platelets on the vascular surface. Interestingly, perfusion of HUT 20 cells with whole blood deficient in factor VIII/von Willebrand factor (found in normal platelet α granules) resulted in a > 97% inhibition of tumor cell adherence to endothelial and de-endothelialized surfaces, suggesting a role for this platelet protein in tumor cell metastasis.

3. Prostacyclin effects on metastasis in vivo. We have previously reported that bolus i.v. injection of PGI_2 into mice reduces lung colony formation from tail vein-injected B16a cells by greater than 70%; in combination with a phosphodiesterase inhibitor (theophylline), PGI_2 reduces such formation by > 93% (49,50; Figure 8). Prostaglandins E_2 and $F_{2\alpha}$ and the stable hydrolysis product of PGI_2, 6-keto-$PGF_{1\alpha}$, are ineffective (49,50). PGD_2 is also antimetastatic as reported by Stringfellow and Fitzpatrick (93); however, we find PGD_2 to be less than 1/3 as effective as PGI_2 (49). These results correlate well with the effects of these various icosanoids on TCIPA (see above).

Willmott et al. (94) recently reported that treatment of animals with the antiplatelet drug RA233 prior to tail vein injection of S-180 sarcoma cells enhances extrapulmonary tumor formation. We demonstrated that PGI_2 does not significantly alter tumor cell distribution patterns using $^{125}IUdr$-labeled tumor cells. The data in Figure 9 shows both the loss of $^{125}IUdr$-labeled B16a cells from the lungs and liver of C57BL/6J mice with and without PGI_2 pretreatment. Prostacyclin has no effect on the initial entrapment of tumor cells in the lungs following i.v. injection (Figure 9); a decrease might have been expected if the PGI_2 effect is due to vasodilation. However, by 20 hr the PGI_2 treated animals retain fewer B16a cells in their lungs than the controls (Figure 9). The number of B16a cells arrested in the liver at 30 min is greater in the PGI_2-treated group than controls (Figure 9). However, at 20 hr there are no detectable tumor cells in the liver of PGI_2 treated animals whereas tumor cells were present in the untreated controls (Figure 9). These results suggest that although some alteration of tumor cell distribution may occur in the presence of PGI_2, once released from the lung these cells are not retained in the organ of secondary arrest (liver, spleen, etc.). Similar findings have been observed by Weiss and collaborators (14,15) in their experiments on metastatic inefficiency.

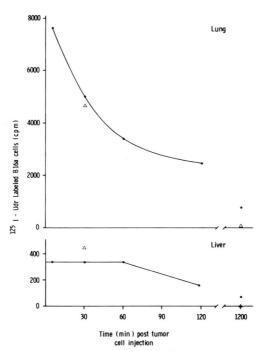

FIGURE 8.   Dose Dependent Inhibition of Lung, Liver and Spleen Colony Formation by PGI_2 Following Tail Vein Injection of B16a Cells (49).

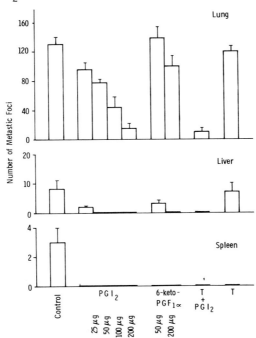

FIGURE 9.   Effect of PGI_2 on the Retention of ^{125}IUdr Labeled B16a Cells in the Lungs and Liver of C57BL/6J Mice (49).   Solid circles = control; triangles = PGI_2 treated.

4. <u>Role of endogenous PGI$_2$ in tumor metastasis.</u> The above results with PGI$_2$ demonstrate its efficacy as an antimetastatic agent. We have also proposed that the production of PGI$_2$ by the vascular endothelium is a natural deterrent to metastasis (49). To test this hypothesis, we perfused mice with a lipoxygenase product of arachidonic acid, 15-hydroperoxyeicosatetraenoic acid (15-HPETE), prior to tail vein injection of B16a tumor cells. Hydroperoxy fatty acids in general are potent inhibitors (K$_1$ $\sim$ 0.1 μM) of prostacyclin synthase (95). Little structural specificity is evident in the inhibition, since a number of isomeric hydroperoxides are equally effective (95). If mice are treated with 15-HPETE (100-200 μg/animal) approximately 20 min prior to tail vein injection of B16a cells, 300-500% more pulmonary metastatic lesions are observed 26 da later (Figure 10). Increased macroscopic tumors are also found in the liver and spleen of 15-HPETE-treated animals (Figure 10). Infusion of 15-HPETE followed by PGI$_2$ plus theophylline significantly reduces the number of metastases compared to 15-HPETE infusion alone (Figure 10). Collectively, these results suggest that endogenous PGI$_2$ production may function as a natural deterrent to metastasis, possibly by limiting tumor cell-platelet-vessel wall interactions.

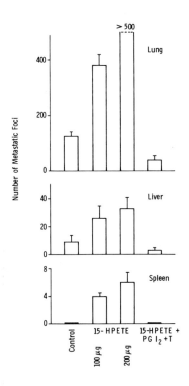

FIGURE 10. Increased Lung Colony Formation of B16a Cells by Prior Administration of the PGI$_2$ Synthase Inhibitor, 15-HPETE. Exogenous PGI$_2$ reverses this effect. T = theophylline. [From Honn <u>et al</u>. (87) with permission.]

5. <u>Effect of agents that stimulate or synergize with endogenous PGI$_2$ production</u>. The use of PGI$_2$ as a clinical therapeutic entity is still in its infancy (96), although several studies report that PGI$_2$ infusion has therapeutic efficacy in advanced atherosclerotic lower limb peripheral vascular disease (97), peripheral artery disease (98), idiopathic pulmonary artery hypertension (99), coronary artery disease and unstable angina (100). Nevertheless, infusion of PGI$_2$ is impractical for clinical use as an antimetastatic agent. We had originally proposed that long-lived analogs of PGI$_2$ could be used as antimetastatic agents (49). Numerous analogs have been developed (100-104). Although some of these analogs have interesting and promising biological effects (103), none is more potent than native PGI$_2$ and the most effective of these must be administered by vascular infusion. We, therefore, propose that agents that stimulate endogenous PGI$_2$ production or inhibit its metabolism may be clinically useful as antimetastatic agents.

a. Agents that alter PGI$_2$ metabolism. One compound that alters PGI$_2$ metabolism may represent the prototype of a new class of pharmacologically active agents - nafazatrom (Bay g 6575; 2,4-dihydro-5-methyl-2[2-(napthyloxy)ethyl]-3H-pyrazol-3-one). Seuter <u>et al.</u> (105) first reported significant antithrombotic activity of nafazatrom in several rat and rabbit models of thrombosis. These authors reported that nafazatrom is devoid of direct effects on platelet TXA$_2$ production, aggregation <u>in vitro</u> and <u>ex vivo</u> and ADP- and collagen-induced platelet aggregation. Recently, Buchanan <u>et al.</u> (106) reinvestigated the antithrombotic effects of nafazatrom and reported that it has no effect on venous thrombosis and yet inhibits arterial thrombosis. Differences in the model systems used for venous thrombosis could account for this discrepancy. In addition, Buchanan <u>et al.</u> (106) reported that nafazatrom inhibits ADP-induced platelet aggregation <u>in vivo</u> and prolongs platelet survival time. Fiedler (107,108) has recently reported that nafazatrom reduces canine coronary artery thrombosis and reduces the size of ligature-induced myocardial infarcts in the conscious rat.

The relationship between the pharmacokinetics and the anti-thrombotic effects of nafazatrom is complex. Nafazatrom is rapidly and almost completely absorbed after oral administration (109). However, the plasma levels of unchanged nafazatrom are very low, suggesting an extensive metabolism during the first passage through the liver (109). Following intravenous injection, plasma nafazatrom concentration decreases with a half-life of 3.5 hr for the first 4 hr. Thereafter, up to 24 hr post administration, plasma nafazatrom decreases with a half-life of 8 hr (109). Thus the plasma levels of nafazatrom may only indirectly reflect its effective concentration at its site of action. Nafazatrom is a highly lipophilic compound (109) and thus should freely pass into the cell membrane. In fact, nafazatrom may localize in the vessel wall (W. Seuter personal communication). Localization of nafazatrom in the vessel wall would be consonant with its proposed mechanism(s) of action.

The mechanism(s) responsible for the antithrombotic effects of nafazatrom is a matter of current debate which centers on nafazatrom's ability to stimulate vascular wall PGI_2 production, prolong its biological half-life or protect PGI_2 synthase (Figure 3). Vermylen et al. (110) first presented evidence for increased PGI_2 production. Plasma obtained from human volunteers after they ingested a single dose (1.2 g) of nafazatrom stimulates PGI_2 release from slices of rat aorta. Subsequently Carreras et al. (111) and Chamone et al. (112) investigated the effects of nafazatrom on PGI_2 production in normal and diabetic rats. Aortas were excised from animals (normal and diabetic) pretreated with nafazatrom or solvent control, cut into 1 mm rings and incubated in vitro. Aortic rings isolated from both normal and diabetic rats treated with nafazatrom release significantly more PGI_2 than aortic rings from untreated control or diabetic rats. Finally, nafazatrom has been reported to enhance arachidonic acid-stimulated PGI_2 production by ram seminal vesicle microsomes (113,114).

Despite the above findings, nafazatrom administration to male human volunteers produces no effect on platelet aggregation ex vivo or on 6-keto-$PGF_{1\alpha}$ (stable hydrolysis product of PGI_2) levels in vivo (115). This raises the possibility that nafazatrom does not directly stimulate basal PGI_2 production by vessel wall endothelium, but rather it may enhance or prolong PGI_2 production "on demand." Such demand for PGI_2 production could occur during an acute thrombotic incident such as platelet-tumor cell-vessel wall interactions. Support for the hypothesis that nafazatrom increases PGI_2 production on demand comes from the work of Deckmyn et al. (116). These authors developed an experimental model designed to study local prostaglandin production by platelets and the vessel wall following stimulation in vivo. In this model a thin nylon thread is inserted into the external jugular vein of rabbits. The thread stimulates platelet activation but not an occluding thrombus. Blood samples are taken immediately distal to the stimulus and assayed for TXB_2 and 6-keto-$PFG_{1\alpha}$ levels. Thromboxane values rise and remain elevated for at least 4 hr whereas 6-keto-$PGF_{1\alpha}$ levels immediately increase and then return to basal levels within 3 hr. This loss of PGI_2 synthetic ability in the presence of a continual stimulus is attributed to "exhaustion of the endothelial cells" (116). However, if the animals are pretreated with nafazatrom, TXB_2 levels are unaltered whereas PGI_2 production is sustained over the 4 hr observation period (116), suggesting that nafazatrom protects the endothelial cells from "exhaustion."

This endothelial cell exhaustion may be due to alterations in their "peroxide tone" during arachidonic acid oxidative metabolism by prostaglandin endoperoxide synthase (cyclooxygenase and hydro-peroxidase; Figure 3). Weksler et al. (117) demonstrated that endothelial cell monolayers stimulated first with arachidonic acid respond poorly to a subsequent stimulation by thrombin. Two likely explanations for this observation are: 1) product-mediated negative feedback and 2) inactivation of the enzymes responsible for PGI_2 biosynthesis. Brotherton et al. (118) have demonstrated that a cAMP-mediated negative feedback mechanism is not involved in the short term regulation of endothelial cell PGI_2 biosynthesis. However, considerable evidence exists for the inactivation of the cyclooxygenase component of prostaglandin endoperoxide synthase and PGI_2 synthase by peroxidized fatty acids and free radicals. Lands and co-workers (119,120) were the first to demonstrate that a certain ambient level of hydroperoxides are required for cyclooxygense activity and that they actually stimulate the enzyme. Endoperoxide PGG_2 formed by the bis-dioxygenation of arachidonic acid can serve as such a hydroperoxide stimulant. However, higher levels of hydroperoxide generated during the continuous oxygenation of arachidonic acid will lead to irreversible inactivation of cyclooxygenase (120). Prostacyclin synthase is similarily inactivated by hydroperoxides as discussed above. Kent et al. (121) studied arachidonate metabolism in rabbit aortas in response to a continuous infusion of arachidonic acid. They concluded that there is a close correlation between total arachidonate metabolism and the inhibition of both cyclooxygenase and PGI_2 synthase. Both enzymes are inactivated by the metabolism of endogenous arachidonic acid, however, there is a preferential inactivation of cyclooxygenase. Similar results have been obtained by Brotherton et al. (122). Kent et al. (121) also demonstrated that the inhibitory effects of oxidizing intermediates (hydroperoxy fatty acids) supplied exogenously are opposite to those found for endogenous oxidizing intermediates (i.e., greater inhibition of PGI_2 synthase vis a vis cyclooxygenase). In this regard the results of Mehta and co-workers (see Chapter 15) are particularly interesting. They examined the in vitro PGI_2 biosynthetic capability of vessels removed from patients with osteogenic sarcoma and of vessels removed from patients without cancer. Both basal and arachidonic acid-stimulated PGI_2 production are lower in vessels removed from cancer patients. It is tempting to speculate that the PGI_2 synthase from these vessels is inactivated. The nature of any inhibitory substance(s) is not known. However, tumor derived hydroperoxy fatty acids are one possible factor. We have shown (see above) that the i.v. injection of hydroperoxy fatty acids significantly increases lung colony formation by tail vein-injected B16a cells. Furthermore, animal tumor cells can synthesize hydroperoxy fatty acids from arachidonic acid (123; Figure 11).

The above results suggest that agents which "regulate" hydroperoxide levels during arachidonic acid metabolism by endothelial cells could influence PGI_2 production by protecting cyclooxygenase and/or PGI_2 synthase from hydroperoxy fatty acid and/or free radical inactivation. The results of Deckmyn et al. (116) suggest such a role for nafazatrom. Three biochemical mechanisms have been proposed to explain the PGI_2-enhancing effects of nafazatrom. These mechanisms are depicted in Figure 3. First, nafazatrom may inhibit cytosolic lipoxygenase (generation of HPETE) of B16a cells (123) and Lewis lung carcinoma cells (Figure 11) as well as that of human and rabbit neutrophils (124). Since vascular endothelial cells have been found to produce 12-HPETE by lipoxygenation of arachidonic acid (125), hydroperoxy fatty acid has been proposed as an endogenous regulator of PGI_2 biosynthesis. Nafazatrom may interfere with inhibition of PGI_2 synthase and/or cyclooxygenase by lipoxygenase-derived hydroperoxy fatty acids. Second, nafazatrom may act as a reducing co-factor for the hydroperoxidase activity of prostaglandin endoperoxide synthase

224

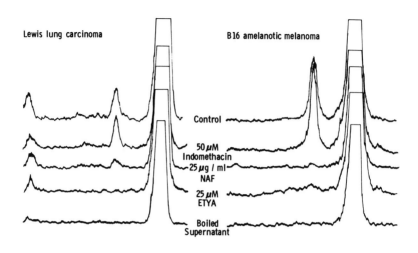

Lewis lung carcinoma

B16 amelanotic melanoma

Control

50 μM
Indomethacin

25 μg / ml
NAF

25 μM
ETYA

Boiled
Supernatant

FIGURE 11. Effects of Indomethacin, Nafazatrom (NAF) and ETYA on Lipoxygenase Enzyme Production of a Hydroperoxy Fatty Acid (i.e., 12-HPETE) from Arachidonic Acid by Microsomal Supernatants of Lewis Lung Carcinoma and B16 Amelanotic Melanoma. No inhibition is observed with indomethacin indicating that the product is not cyclooxygenase-derived.

(113,114). Nafazatrom may reduce the ambient level of hydroperoxy fatty acid generated during PGG_2 to PGH_2 conversion (Figure 3). Marnett et al. (114) have demonstrated that nafazatrom does not stimulate PGI_2 synthase conversion of PGH_2 to PGI_2 but rather protects PGI_2 synthase from hydroperoxy fatty acid inactivation. Nafazatrom can effect the reduction of hydroperoxy fatty acids to their corresponding alcohols (114), which do not inhibit PGI_2 synthase or cyclooxygenase. In addition, nafazatrom is an extremely sensitive free radical scavenger (126). All of the above are consonant with a mechanism whereby nafazatrom enhances PGI_2 production "on demand." Third, nafazatrom may inhibit the enzymatic degradation of PGI_2 to 15-keto-PGI_2 by 15-hydroxy-prostaglandin dehydrogenase (127). This is the major route of PGI_2 catabolism in the cat (128) and man (129). Any or all of the above mechanisms would increase endogenous PGI_2 levels.

Nafazatrom has been evaluated for its antimetastatic activity against elutriated B16a and 3LL tumor cells injected intravenously (tail vein). It inhibits lung colony formation by > 70% (52). In addition, this compound significantly reduces spontaneous pulmonary metastasis from subcutaneous B16a and 3LL tumors (52). Ambrus et al. (130) have also reported antimetastatic activity of nafazatrom in three of four tumor lines tested. Collectively, these results point to significant antimetastatic properties of this PGI$_2$-enhancing agent.

b. Thromboxane synthase inhibitors. Thromboxane synthase inhibitors result in decreased platelet adhesion to injured vascular wall (131) and increased platelet sensitivity to PGI$_2$ inhibition (132), presumably because the lower the platelet TXA$_2$ biosynthetic capability the lower the dose of PGI$_2$ required for inhibition of aggregation (133). In addition, TXSI have been reported to reorient platelet endoperoxide (PGH$_2$, Figure 12) metabolism towards PGI$_2$ biosynthesis by the vessel wall (134). This hypothesis was originally termed the "steal hypothesis" when first proposed by Gryglewski et al. (135). It

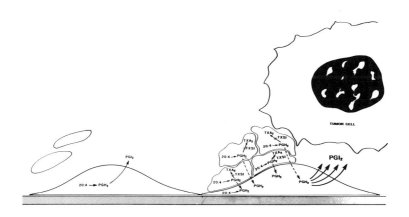

FIGURE 12. Schematic Illustration Demonstrating PGI$_2$ Production by the Vessel Wall from Platelet-Derived PGH$_2$ in the Presence of a Thromboxane Synthase Inhibitor ("Steal Hypothesis").

states that under conditions in which aggregating platelets are juxtaposed to the endothelium (in a narrow vessel lumen), platelet PGH_2 may be utilized by vessel wall PGI_2 synthase to augment basal PGI_2 production (Figure 12). These results are consistent with the work of Needleman et al. (136), which suggested that normally the "steal" of precursor by the vessel wall may not be an important pathway for PGI_2 biosynthesis. However, under conditions of a strong stimulus for platelet aggregation (i.e., circulating tumor cells), the selective blockade of TXA_2 synthase could drive platelet PGH_2 metabolism into PGI_2 biosynthesis by the vessel wall (Figure 12). In vivo evidence for the "steal hypothesis" has been provided by the experiments of Aiken et al. (133). Recently, Deckmyn et al. (116) convincingly demonstrated in their rabbit model that the TXSI dazoxiben significantly increases PGI_2 production as a result of platelet PGH_2 being reoriented to and utilized by the vessel wall.

We had proposed that TXSI, in addition to PGI_2, would also fuon as antimetastatic agents (49). This prediction was based on the working hypothesis that circulating tumor cells disrupt the intravascular balance between PGI_2 and TXA_2. We initially investigated a series of endoperoxide analogs that were TXSI. One endoperoxide analog TXSI, U54701 (9,11-iminoepoxy-prosta-5,13-dienoic acid), completely inhibits TXA_2 production by human platelets in response to elutriated Lewis lung carcinoma cells concomitant with an inhibition of platelet aggregation (84). However, W256 TCIPA is only inhibited 25% by a comparable dose of U54701, even though TXA_2 biosynthesis is almost completely inhibited (84). Furthermore, TXSI that are imidazole derivatives [i.e., 1-(7-carboxyheptyl)imidazole] do not inhibit TCIPA in vitro even in the presence of inhibited platelet TXA_2 production. These unexpected results suggest that tumor cells can initiate platelet aggregation by a mechanism independent of TXA_2 biosynthesis. Nevertheless, both endoperoxide analogs and imidazole derivatives possess antimetastatic activity in vivo (50).

We propose that the discrepancy between lack of consistent inhibition of TCIPA by TXSI in vitro and their antimetastatic activity in vivo is due to the operation of the "steal hypothesis" in vivo. In vitro, TCIPA may proceed by pathways independent of TXA_2 biosynthesis. Thus, the antimetastatic activity of TXSI in vivo may ultimately be due to augmented PGI_2 biosynthesis. In addition, we have found that TXSI sensitize platelets to the inhibitory effects of PGI_2. The TXSI compound U63557A at a dose that completely inhibited TXA_2 biosynthesis did not inhibit 3LL TCIPA (Figure 13). However, the combination of this dose of U63557A with a suboptimal dose of PGI_2 elicited a synergistic inhibition of TCIPA (Figure 13). It is not known if such synergistic inhibition occurs in vivo.

IV. CONCLUSIONS

It is intuitive that for hematogenous metastasis to occur, the tumor cell must arrest in the microvasculature and attach to the vessel wall prior to extravasation and growth into a metastatic focus. Indirect evidence supports the concept that tumor cells interact with platelets during this process as discussed above. We propose that the metabolism of arachidonic acid in the tumor cell, the platelet and the vessel wall plays an essential role in the sum total of these interactions.

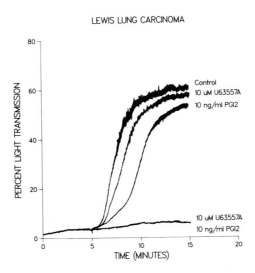

FIGURE 13. Synergistic Inhibition of Platelet Aggregation Induced by Lewis Lung Carcinoma by Suboptimal Doses of the Thromboxane Synthase Inhibitor, U63557A, and PGI_2.

ACKNOWLEDGEMENTS

Investigations in the authors laboratories were supported by grant numbers CA29405 and CA29997 awarded by the National Cancer Institute, Department of Health and Human Services and by American Cancer Society Grant BC-356, Miles Institute for Preclinical Pharmacology and Bayer AG. The excellent technical assistance of Marjorie Carufel, John Dunn, Deborah Moilanen, Gregory Neagos and Kim Pampalona is appreciated.

REFERENCES

1. Hilgard P, Beyerle L, Hohage R, Hiemeyer V and Kubler M. Eur. J. Cancer 8:347-352, 1972.
2. del Regato JA. Semin. Oncol. 4:33-38, 1977.
3. Fisher ER and Fisher B. Arch. Pathol. 83:321-324, 1967.
4. Fidler IJ, Gersten DM and Hart I. Adv. Cancer Res. 28:149-250, 1978.
5. Weiss L. Semin. Oncol. 4:5-17, 1977.
6. Cole WH, Robert SS, Webb RS, Strehl FW and Oates GD. Ann. Surg. 161:753-768, 1965.
7. Salsbury AJ. Cancer Treat. Rev. 2:55-72, 1975.
8. Butler TP and Gullino PM. Cancer Res. 35:512-516, 1975.
9. Liotta LA, Kleinerman J and Saidel GM. Cancer Res. 34:997-1004, 1974.
10. Liotta LA, Kleinerman J and Saidel GM. Cancer Res. 36:889-894, 1976.
11. Lotan R and Raz A. Cancer Res. 43:2088-2093, 1983.
12. Glaves D. Br. J. Cancer 48:665-673, 1983.
13. Weiss L. In: Tumor Invasion and Metastasis (Ed. Liotta LA and Hart IR), Martinus Nijhoff, The Hague, pp. 81-98, 1982.
14. Weiss L. Int. J. Cancer 25:385-392, 1980.
15. Weiss L, Ward PM and Holmes JC. Int. J. Cancer 32:79-83, 1983.
16. Sato H and Suzuki M. In: Fundamental Aspects of Metastasis (Ed. Weiss L), American Elsevier:New York, pp. 311-317, 1976.
17. Hanna N. Cancer Metastasis Rev. 1:45-64, 1982.
18. Fidler IJ, Barnes Z, Fogler WE, Kirsh R, Bugelski P and Poste G. Cancer Res. 42:496-501, 1982.
19. Glaves D. Invasion Metastsis 3:160-173, 1983.
20. Irimura T, Gonzalez R and Nicolson GL. Cancer Res. 41:3411-3418, 1981.
21. Irimura T and Nicolson GL. J. Supramol. Struct. Cell. Biochem. 17:325-336, 1981.
22. Takacz JS and Lampen JO. Biochem. Biophys. Res. Commun. 65:248-257, 1975.
23. Takatsuki A, Kohno K and Tamura G. Agr. Biol. Chem. 39:2089-2091, 1975.
24. Murray JC, Liotta L, Rennard SI and Martin GR. Cancer Res. 40:347-351, 1980.
25. Terranova VP, Liotta LA, Russo RG and Martin GR. Cancer Res. 42:2265-2269, 1982.
26. Vlodavsky I and Gospodarowicz D. Nature (London) 289:304-306, 1981.
27. Shirrmacher V, Altervogt P, Fogel M, Dennis J, Walker CA, Barz D, Schwartz R, Cheingsong-Popov R, Springer G, Robinson PJ, Nebe T, Brossmer W, Vlodavsky I, Paweletz N, Zimmermann HP and Uhlenbrach G. Invasion Metastasis 2:313-360, 1982.
28. Zacharski LR, Rickles FR, Henderson WG, Martin JF, Forman WB, van Eeckhout JP, Cornell CJ and Forcier RJ. Am. J. Clin. Oncol. 5:593-609, 1982.
29. Rickles FR and Edwards RL. Blood 62:14-31, 1983.
30. Laghi F, DiRoberto PF, Panici PB, Margariti PA, Scribano D, Cudillo L, Villani L and Bizzi B. Tumori 69:349-353, 1983.
31. Brain MC, Azzopardi JG, Baker LRI, Pinco GF, Roberts PD and Dacic JV. Br. J. Haematol. 18:183-190, 1970.
32. Donati MB and Poggi A. Br. J. Haematol. 44:173-182, 1980.
33. Harker LA and Slichter SJ. N. Eng. J. Med. 287:999-1005, 1972.
34. Gasic GJ, Boettiger D, Catalfamo JL, Gasic TB and Stewart GJ. Cancer Res. 38:2950-2955, 1978.
35. Karpatkin S, Smerling A and Pearlstein E. J. Lab. Clin. Med. 96:994-1001, 1980.
36. Pearlstein E, Cooper LB and Karpatkin S. J. Lab. Clin. Med. 93:332-344, 1979.
37. Pearlstein E, Salk PL, Yogeeswaran G and Karpatkin S. Proc. Natl. Acad. Sci. USA 77:4336-4339, 1980.

38. Curatolo L, Colucci M, Cambini AL, Poggi A, Morasca L, Donati MB and Sejeraro N. Br. J. Cancer 40:228-233, 1979.
39. Gordon SG and Cross BA. J. Clin. Invest. 67:1665-1671, 1981.
40. Gordon SG, Franks JJ and Lewis B. Thromb. Res. 6:127-137, 1975.
41. Cavanaugh PG, Sloane BF, Bajkowski AS, Gasic TB, Gasic GJ and Honn KV. Clin. Exp. Metastasis 4:297-307, 1983.
42. Fidler IJ. Eur. J. Cancer 9:223-227, 1973.
43. Liotta LA, Kleinerman J and Saidel GM. Cancer Res. 36:889-894, 1976.
44. Gorelik E, Berc WW and Herberman RB. Int. J. Cancer 33:87-94, 1984.
45. Gastpar H. J. Med. 8:103-114, 1977
46. Gasic GJ, Gasic TB and Stewart CC. Proc. Natl. Acad. Sci. USA 61:46-52, 1968.
47. Sindelar WR, Tralka TS and Ketcham AS. J. Surg. Res. 18:137-161, 1975.
48. Gasic GJ, Gasic TB, Galanti N, Johnson T and Murphy S. Int. J. Cancer 11:704-718, 1973.
49. Honn KV, Cicone B and Skoff A. Science 212:1270-1272, 1981.
50. Honn KV. Clin. Exp. Metastasis 1:103-114, 1983.
51. Honn KV, Busse WD and Sloane BF. Biochem. Pharmacol. 32:1-11, 1983.
52. Honn KV, Meyer J, Neagos G, Henderson T, Westley C and Ratanatharathorn V. In: Interaction of Platelets and Tumor Cells (Ed. Jamieson GA), Alan R. Liss:New York, pp. 295-331, 1982.
53. Lione A and Bosmann HB. Cell Biol. Int. Rep. 82:81-86, 1978.
54. Maat B and Hilgard P. J. Cancer Res. Clin. Oncol. 101:275-283, 1981.
55. Colucci M, Delnini F, DeBelles Vitti G, Locati D, Poggi A, Semeraro N and Donati MB. Biochem. Pharmacol. 32:1689-1691, 1983.
56. Maniglia CA, Tudor G, Gomez J and Sartorelli AL. Cancer Lett. 16:253-260, 1982.
57. Gasic GJ, Viner ED, Budzynski AZ and Gasic GP. Cancer Res. 43:1633-1636, 1983.
58. Zacharski LR, Henderson WG, Rickles FR, Forman WB, Cornell Jr. CJ, Forcier RJ, Harrower HW and Johnson RO. Cancer 44:732-741, 1979.
59. Vargaftig BB, Chignard M and Benveniste J. Biochem. Pharmacol. 30:263-271, 1981.
60. Hamberg M, Svensson J and Samuelsson B. Proc. Natl. Acad. Sci. USA 72:2994-2998, 1975.
61. Gorman RR. Fed. Proc. Fed. Am. Soc. Exp. Biol. 38:83-88, 1979.
62. Heptinstall S, Bevan J, Cockbill SR, Hanley SP and Parry MJ. Thromb. Res. 29:219-230, 1980.
63. Rybicki JP and LeBreton GC. Thromb. Res. 30:407-414, 1983.
64. Moncada S, Gryglewski RJ, Bunting S and Vane JR. Nature (London) 263:663-665, 1976.
65. Moncada S and Vane JR. In: Advances in Prostaglandin and Thromboxane Research (Eds. Samuelsson B, Ramwell PW and Paoletti R), Raven Press:New York, Vol. 6, pp. 43-60, 1980.
66. Moncada S and Vane JR. In: Biochemical Aspects of Prostaglandins and Thromboxanes (Eds. Kharasch N and Fried J), Academic Press:New York, pp. 155-177, 1977.
67. Mullane KM, Dusting GJ, Salmon JA, Moncada S and Vane JR. Eur. J. Pharmacol. 54:217-228, 1979.
68. Moncada S, Gryglewski RJ, Bunting S and Vane JR. Prostaglandins 12:715-733, 1976.
69. Szczeklik A and Gryglewski RJ. In: Clinical Pharmacology of Prostacyclin (Eds. Lewis PJ and O'Grady J), Raven Press:New York, pp. 159-167, 1981.
70. Menter DG, Onoda JM, Taylor JD and Honn KV. Cancer Res. 44:450-456, 1984.
71. Lerner WA, Pearlstein E, Ambrogio C and Karpatkin S. Int. J. Cancer 31:463-469, 1983.

72. Bastida E, Ordinas A, Giardina SL and Jamieson GA. Cancer Res. $\underline{42}$:4348-4352, 1982.
73. Pearlstein E, Ambrogio C, Gasic G and Karpatkin S. Cancer Res. $\underline{41}$:4535-4539, 1981.
74. Bennett A, Berstock DA, Raja B and Stamford IF. Br. J. Pharmacol. $\underline{66}$:415P, 1979.
75. Bennett A, DelTacca M, Stamford IF and Zebro T. Br. J. Cancer $\underline{35}$:881-884, 1977.
76. Feller N, Malachi T and Halbrecht I. J. Cancer Res. Clin. Oncol. $\underline{93}$:275-280, 1979.
77. Rolland PH, Martin PM, Jacquemier J, Rolland AM and Toga M. J. Natl. Cancer Inst. $\underline{64}$:1061-1070, 1980.
78. Humes JL and Strausser HR. Prostaglandins $\underline{5}$:183-197, 1974.
79. Dowsett M, Easty GS, Powles TJ, Easty DM and Neville AM. Prostaglandins $\underline{11}$:447-460, 1976.
80. Tashjian AH, Voekel EF and Levine L. Prostaglandins $\underline{14}$:309-317, 1977.
81. Plescia DJ, Smith AN and Grinwich K. Proc. Natl. Acad. Sci. USA $\underline{72}$:1848-1851, 1975.
82. Powles TJ, Coombes RC, Munro-Neville A, Ford H and Gazet JC. Lancet $\underline{2}$:138, 1977.
83. MacIntyre DE. $\underline{In}$: Platelets in Biology and Pathology (Ed. Gordon JL), Elsevier/North Holland:Amsterdam, Vol. 2, pp. 211-247, 1981.
84. Honn KV, Menter D, Cavanaugh PG, Neagos G, Moilanen D, Taylor JD and Sloane BF. Acta Clin. Belg. $\underline{38}$:53-67, 1983.
85. Fitzpatrick F, Bundy G, Gorman R, Honohan T, McGuire J and Sun F. Biochim. Biophys. Acta $\underline{573}$:238-244, 1979.
86. Hara Y, Steiner M and Baldini MG. Cancer Res. $\underline{40}$:1217-1222, 1980.
87. Honn KV, Menter DG, Onoda JM, Taylor JD and Sloane BF. $\underline{In}$: Cancer Invasion and Metastasis: Biologic and Therapeutic Aspects (Eds. Nicolson GL and Milas L), Raven Press:New York, pp. 361-368, 1984.
88. Diglio CA, Grammas P, Giacomelli F and Weiner J. Lab. Invest. $\underline{46}$:544-563, 1982.
89. George JW, Thoi LL and Morgan RK. Thromb. Res. $\underline{23}$:69-77, 1981.
90. Thompson CB, Eaton K, Princiotta SM, Rushin CA and Valleri CR. Br. J. Haematol. $\underline{50}$:509-519, 1982.
91. Fantone JC, Elgas LJ, Weinberger L and Varani J. Oncology $\underline{40}$:421-426, 1983.
92. Marcum JM, McGill M, Bastida E, Ordinas A and Jamieson GA. J. Lab. Clin. Med. $\underline{96}$:1048-1053, 1980.
93. Stringfellow DA and Fitzpatrick FA. Nature (London) $\underline{282}$:76-78, 1979.
94. Willmott N, Malcolm A, McLeod T, Gracie A and Calman KC. Invasion Metastasis $\underline{3}$:32-51, 1983.
95. Salmon JA, Smith DR, Flower RS, Moncada S and Vane JR. Biochim. Biophys. Acta $\underline{523}$:250-262, 1978.
96. Moncada S. Br. J. Pharmacol. $\underline{76}$:3-31, 1982.
97. Szczeklik A, Nizankowski R, Skawinski S, Szczeklik J, Gluszko P and Gryglewski RJ. Lancet $\underline{1}$:1111-1114.
98. Szczeklik A, Gryglewski RJ, Nizankowski R, Musial J, Pieton R and Mruk J. Pharmacol. Res. Commun. $\underline{10}$:545-556, 1978.
99. Watkins WD, Peterson MB, Crone RK, Shannon DC and Levine L. Lancet $\underline{1}$:1083, 1980.
100. Hall RJC and Dewar HA. Lancet $\underline{1}$:949, 1981.
101. Morton DR and Brokow FC. J. Org. Chem. $\underline{44}$:2880-2887, 1979.
102. Nishiyama H and Ohno K. Tetrahed. Lett. $\underline{36}$:3481-3484, 1979.
103. Whittle BJR, Moncada S, Whiting F and Vane JR. Prostaglandins $\underline{19}$:605-627, 1980.

104. Pike JE and Bundy GL. In: Prostaglandins and Cancer (Eds. Powles TJ, Bockman RS, Honn KV and Ramwell P), Alan R. Liss:New York, pp. 67-77, 1982.
105. Seuter F, Busse WD, Meng F, Hoffmeister F, Moller E and Horstmann H. Arzneim.-Forsch./Drug Res. 29:54-59, 1979.
106. Buchanan MR, Blajchman M and Hirsch J. Thromb. Res. 28:157-170, 1982.
107. Fiedler VB. Basic Res. Cardiol. 78:266-280, 1983.
108. Fiedler VB. Eur. J. Pharmacol. 88:263-267, 1983.
109. Philipp E, Ritter W and Patzschke K. Thromb. Res. Suppl. 4:129-133, 1983.
110. Vermylen J, Chamone DAF and Verstraete M. Lancet 1:518-520, 1979.
111. Carreras LO, Chamone DAF, Klerckx P and Vermylen J. Thromb. Res. 19:663-670, 1980.
112. Chamone DAF, van Damme B, Carreras LO and Vermylen J. Haemostasis 10:297-303, 1981.
113. Eling TE, Honn KV, Busse WD, Seuter F and Marnett LJ. In: Prostaglandins and Cancer (Eds. Powles TJ, Bockman RS, Honn KV and Ramwell P), Alan R. Liss:New York, pp. 783-787, 1982.
114. Marnett LJ, Siedlik PH, Ochs R, Das M, Honn KV, Warnock R, Tainer B and Eling TE. Mol. Pharmacol., in press.
115. Fischer S, Struppler M and Weber PC. Biochem. Pharmacol. 32:2231-2236, 1983.
116. Deckmyn H, van Houtte E, Verstraete M and Vermylen J. Biochem. Pharmacol. 32:2757-2762, 1983.
117. Weksler BB, Ley LW and Jaffe EA. J. Clin. Invest. 62:923-930, 1978.
118. Brotherton AFA, Macfarlane DE and Hoak JC. Thromb. Res. 28:637-647, 1982.
119. Hemler ME, Cook HW and Lands WEM. Arch. Biochem. Biophys. 193:340-345, 1979.
120. Hemler ME and Lands WEM. J. Biol. Chem. 255:6253-6261, 1980.
121. Kent RS, Diedrich SL and Whorton AR. J. Clin. Invest. 72:455-465, 1983.
122. Brotherton AFA and Hoak JC. J. Clin. Invest. 72:1255-1261, 1983.
123. Honn KV and Dunn JR. FEBS Lett. 139:65-68, 1982.
124. Busse WD, Mardin M, Grutzmann R, Dunn JR, Theodoreau M, Sloane BF and Honn KV. Fed. Proc. Fed. Am. Soc. Exp. Biol. 41:1717, 1982.
125. Herman AG, Claeys M, Moncada S and Vane JR. Prostaglandins 18:439-452, 1979.
126. Sevilla MD and Marnett LJ. Biochem. Biophys. Res. Commun. 115:800-806, 1983.
127. Wong PY-K, Chao P H-W and McGiff JC. J. Pharmacol. Exp. Ther. 223:757-760, 1982.
128. Machleidt C, Forstermann U, Anhut H and Hertting G. Eur. J. Pharmacol. 74:19-26, 1981.
129. Rosenkranz B, Fischer C, Weimer KE and Frolich JC. J. Biol. Chem. 255:10194-10198, 1980.
130. Ambrus JL, Ambrus LM, Gastpar H and Williams C. J. Med. 13:35-47, 1982.
131. Hall ER, Chen YC, Ho T and Wu KK. Thromb. Res. 27:501-511, 1982.
132. Bertele V, Falanga A, Roncaglioni MC, Cerletti C and de Gaetano G. Thromb. Haemostasis 47:294, 1982.
133. Aiken JW, Shebuski RJ, Miller OV and Gorman RR. J. Pharmacol. Exp. Ther. 219:299-308, 1981.
134. Defreyn G, Deckmyn H and Vermylen J. Thromb. Res. 26:389-400, 1982.
135. Gryglewski RJ, Bunting S, Moncada S, Flower RJ and Vane JR. Prostaglandins 12:685-713, 1976.
136. Needleman P, Wyche A and Raz A. J. Clin. Invest. 63:345-349, 1979.

CHAPTER 15. EVIDENCE FOR ALTERED ARACHIDONIC ACID METABOLISM IN TUMOR METASTASIS

PAULETTE MEHTA

I. INTRODUCTION

The major challenge in the treatment of cancer is control of metastasis. In most instances, a tumor can be managed initially with chemotherapy, radiation therapy and/or surgery. In many cases, however, tumor cells escape from the primary site, traverse the vascular beds and may adhere to the vascular endothelium at distant sites. Subsequently growth and proliferation of the tumor occurs resulting in clinical metastasis. There is evidence that tumor cell-platelet-vessel wall interactions are important in the process of metastasis. Several platelet-, vessel wall- and tumor cell-generated prostaglandins (PG) are important in these interactions. The purpose of this paper is to review the current information on the role that these prostaglandins may have in the regulation of tumor metastasis (see also Chapter 14).

II. NORMAL PLATELET AND VESSEL WALL ACTIVITY

Platelets play an important role in hemostasis and in the maintenance of normal vascular integrity (1 and Chapters 9 and 13). Platelets circulate through an undamaged vasculature without adhering to the vessel wall or altering in function. Damage to the vascular lining results in exposure of the subendothelial collagen which stimulates platelets. Stimulated platelets adhere to the damaged vasculature and undergo the release reaction. During the release reaction numerous vasoactive peptides, prostaglandins and other substances are released. These products cause irreversible platelet aggregation, vasoconstriction and eventually formation of a platelet thrombus adhering to the vessel wall. Thromboxane A_2 (TXA_2) is the most potent endogenous PG vasoconstrictor and platelet proaggregatory agent.

Vascular endothelial cells counteract platelet thrombus formation at the site of injury by release of heparin-like polymucosaccharides, prostaglandins and a variety of anti-coagulant factors. Vessel wall-generated prostacyclin (PGI_2) inhibits platelet aggregation and possesses vasodilator activity.

The opposing actions of TXA_2 and PGI_2 are necessary for regulation of physiologic vascular tone and unimpeded blood flow. An increase in TXA_2 or a decrease in PGI_2 has been proposed to favor thrombus formation, vasoconstriction and impedance of blood flow. These opposing activities may also be important in tumor metastasis (2). There is evidence that some tumor cells metastasize only after interaction with platelets and formation of a thrombus consisting of tumor cells and platelets. Adhesion of these thrombi to vascular beds may be a critical step in the genesis of metastasis. This abnormal interaction may be mediated by disturbances in vessel wall and platelet-generated prostaglandins (see Chapter 14).

III. PLATELETS AND TUMOR GROWTH

The importance of thrombus function in the trapping of tumor cells and their subsequent deposition at sites distant from the primary tumor has been recognized since the early 1960's (3,4). Electron microscopy revealed that platelets were an important constituent of the thrombus forming around tumor cells (5-7).

Subsequent studies in animal models demonstrated that the injection of certain tumor cells resulted in the formation of a dense platelet thrombus as an initial step in the deposition of tumor cells on the vessel wall (6,7), and in the stabilization of this attachment (7). These studies suggest that the nature of the deposition of the platelet-tumor cell aggregate varies with the continuity of the endothelial lining (5). Attachment of the platelet-tumor cell mass to an intact endothelium results in a weak attachment to the vessel wall. In contrast, attachment of this mass to the disrupted endothelium is associated with a thick layer of fibrin around the platelet-tumor cell aggregate and a firm adhesion of this mass to the subendothelial layers (7).

Trapping of platelets around the tumor cells is confirmed by occurrence of thrombocytopenia within hours of intravenous injection of tumor cells (8). Thrombocytopenia has been shown to correlate to preferential trapping of platelets in the lungs in mice (9). Certain tumor cell lines directly stimulate aggregation of platelets (10-14). The degree to which platelets are stimulated by rat renal sarcoma cells correlates to the metastatic potential of the tumor (15). The factor responsible for promoting platelet aggregation in vivo by transformed mouse fibroblasts has been identified as an urea-extractable sialic acid residue, named "platelet aggregating material" by Karpatkin (13 and Chapter 11).

After attachment to the vessel wall, platelets may promote the passage of tumor cells through the vessel wall and their subsequent growth (see Chapter 18). Products of the platelet release reaction such as platelet-basic protein (15), platelet-derived permeability factor (16), histamine, serotonin and perhaps β -thromboglobulin and platelet factor-4 increase vascular permeability (15,17). It has also been proposed that platelet-derived growth factors may directly stimulate growth of tumor cells (18-20 and Chapter 18).

Certain prostaglandins by virtue of their role in platelet aggregation (21) may also participate in tumor deposition (2,22).

IV. PRODUCTION OF PROSTAGLANDINS BY TUMOR CELLS

A large number of studies indicate that tumor cells produce prostaglandins. In most of the early studies, release of prostaglandins of the E and F series was evaluated. More recently, some investigators have examined the synthesis of TXA_2 and PGI_2. Many of these studies have been fraught with methodological problems. For example, early studies relied on measurements obtained by bioactivity rather than on direct measurement of prostaglandins or their metabolites. Most studies have been conducted in animal models of tumors under conditions which do not mimic the human situation. The studies in patients have been fraught with difficulties in interpretation. Plasma concentrations of metabolites of prostaglandins do not necessarily reflect prostaglandin synthesis by the tumor mass alone since blood vessels, platelets and other body tissues also generate prostaglandins. In addition, small but significant local release of prostaglandins may not be reflected in the peripheral blood. The ex vivo studies have, however, suggested abnormalities in prostaglandin synthesis by tumor tissues and by blood vessels in the tumor area as well as those distant from the primary site. The data obtained point to alterations in prostaglandin synthesis or release which indicate a pathophysiologic role of icosanoids in the systemic manifestation of certain tumors as well as in the progression of tumor metastasis.

A wide variety of animal and human tumor cell lines have been associated with abnormal prostaglandin release (Tables 1 and 2). Prostaglandin release may be greater from the tumor tissue than from the adjacent non-tumor tissue. Bennett et al. (23) identified PGE_2 release from breast carcinoma which was higher than that from the adjacent tissue. Similarly, sarcomas of the hind limb induced by Moloney virus were shown to produce more prostaglandin E and F compared to normal tissue from the contralateral limb (24). Prostaglandin production, viability of the tumor cells and malignant potential of some tumor cells were correlated to one another in one study (25). In this same study (25), human colon carcinoma cells were shown to generate both prostaglandins E_2 and $F_{2\alpha}$. With replacement of tumor cells by fibroblasts in vitro, the production of these prostaglandins declined, suggesting a selective production of these prostaglandins by the tumor cells. In another study (26), hamster fibroblasts upon transformation into neoplastic cells by polyoma virus generated increased amounts of prostaglandins E_2 and $F_{2\alpha}$, suggesting a relationship of increased prostaglandin generation to the malignant potential of these cells. Some reports have recently appeared on production of prostaglandin D_2 and TXA_2 from histiocytosis-X cells (27), melanoma cells (28) and carrageenin-induced granuloma cells (29). Findings of abnormal TXA_2 production may be important since this icosanoid has been implicated in the regulation of tumor metastasis (2,30).

A major goal of many of the studies shown in Tables 1 and 2 was to clarify the relationship to prostaglandins of "idiopathic" hypercalcemia associated with cancer. In 1970, Tashjian et al. (31) demonstrated that transplantable tumors in mice were associated with

Table 1. Animal Tumors Associated with Prostaglandin E_2 and/or $F_2\alpha$ Release.

I. NATURALLY OCCURRING TUMORS:

    Mouse
          Ascites BP8
          Neuroblastoma
          $HSDM_1$ Fibrosarcoma
          S180 Tumor
          Ehrlich Tumor

    Rat
          Hepatoma 223
          Glioma

    Rabbit
          VX_2 Carcinoma

    Dog
          Melanoma

II. EXPERIMENTALLY INDUCED TUMORS:

    Mouse
          Methylcholanthrene Transformed
          Moloney Virus Induced Sarcoma

    Rat
          7,12 Dimethylbenzanthracine Induced Mammary Tumors

    Hamster
          Polyoma Virus Transformed Fibroblasts

---

enhanced production of prostaglandins, hypercalcemia and bone resorption. Thereafter, Powles and his colleagues (32) quantitated the bone resorbing ability of breast cancer cells and correlated this activity to release of prostaglandin E_2. It was, therefore, reasonable to assume that the prostaglandins released from the tumor cells may be responsible for the hypercalcemia seen in some patients. It has been speculated by this group, but not proved, that the bone lytic lesions induced by prostaglandins may precede and facilitate subsequent metastasis. In support of this speculation Dowsett et al. (33) showed a correlation in patients with breast cancer between the ability of tumor cells to stimulate bone resorption in vitro and metastasis occurring concurrently or subsequently.

Table 2.   Human Tumors Associated with Prostaglandin E_2 and/or $F_{2\alpha}$ Release.

Neuroblastoma
Pheochromocytoma
Medullary Carcinoma of the Thyroid
Insulinoma
Islet Cell Carcinoma
Kaposi's Sarcoma
Renal Cell Carcinoma
Breast Carcinomas
Squamous Cell Carcinoma of Lung and Bronchus
Oat Cell Carcinoma of Lung
Undifferentiated Carcinoma of Lung
Colon and Rectal Carcinomas
Hodgkin's Disease
Squamous Cell Carcinoma of Skin, Gingiva

V.   ROLE OF PROSTAGLANDINS IN PROMOTING TUMOR METASTASIS BY EFFECTS ON PLATELETS AND VESSEL WALLS

Platelet activity has been shown to relate to tumor metastasis in some instances. This activity appears to be critical in forming platelet-tumor cell aggregates and in causing these aggregates to adhere to the vessel wall as discussed earlier. Thromboxane A_2 and PGI_2 are the most potent icosanoids known to affect platelets and vascular tone (21). These icosanoids have been implicated in modulating tumor growth (2,30).

Thromboxane A_2 is a potent platelet aggregatory agent and vasoconstrictor, while PGI_2 is anti-aggregatory and a vasodilator. These effects are believed to be mediated through their regulation of intracellular cyclic AMP and Ca^{++}. Certain tumors produce TXA_2 which may facilitate tumor growth (34). Gonzalez-Cuissi et al. (27) reported high concentrations of TXB_2 in histiocytosis-X cells in lungs and lymph nodes from a single patient. Chang et al. (29) noted significant production of TXA_2 in carrageenin-induced granuloma cells. On the other hand, a decrease in PGI_2 production or a stabilization of PGI_2 production (35-38) could result in tumor metastasis by altering TXA_2-PGI_2 "balance" (see Chapter 14).

In our laboratory, we have examined arachidonic acid metabolites in a variety of patients with cancer. In a series of representative patients with malignant bone tumors, plasma concentrations of the stable metabolite of TXA_2 (TXB_2) were within normal limits (Figure 1). However, concentrations of a metabolite of PGI_2 (6-keto-$PGF_{1\alpha}$) were markedly less than those of control subjects (Figure 2). In contrast, patients with lymphoid and reticulo-endothelial cancer (i.e., leukemia, lymphoma, neuroblastoma and histiocytosis-X) had normal

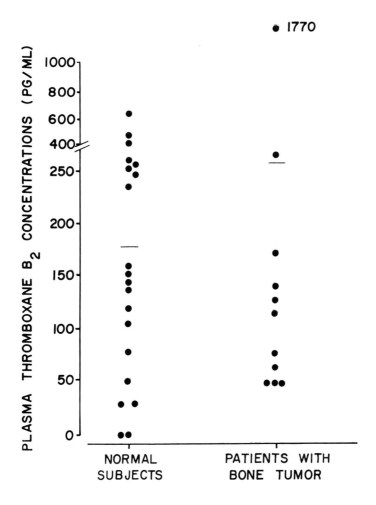

FIGURE 1.   Plasma Concentrations of Thromboxane B_2 (stable metabolite of thromboxane A_2) in Normal Subjects and Patients with Malignant Bone Tumors.   There was no significant difference between these groups.

concentrations of metabolites of TXA_2 and of PGI_2. These data suggest that a decrease in PGI_2 occurs in some patients with cancer and that this decrease may be related to the metastatic capability of different tumor types.   However, measurement of circulating concentrations of 6-keto-$PGF_{1\alpha}$ may not adequately reflect actual vessel wall production at a particular site.   Therefore, we evaluated PGI_2 release from arteries obtained from patients with bone tumors.   Release of PGI_2 (measured as RIA detectable 6-keto-$PGF_{1\alpha}$) from arteries in or near

238

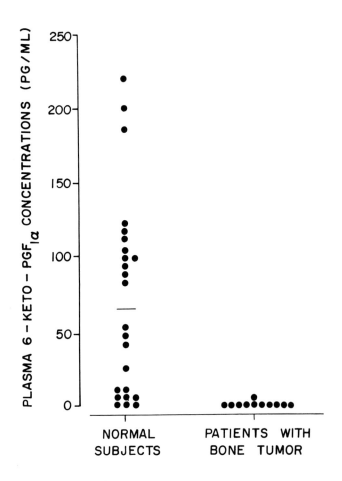

FIGURE 2. Plasma Concentrations of 6-keto-PGF$_{1\alpha}$ (stable hydrolysis product of prostacyclin) in Normal Subjects and in Patients with Malignant Bone Tumors. Plasma 6-keto-PGF$_{1\alpha}$ concentrations were significantly less in patients with malignant bone tumors than in normal subjects.

the tumor bed of patients with cancer was significantly less than that in control femoral or splenic arteries, but was similar to that in internal mammary arteries (Figure 3). These arteries were taken from patients with advanced atherosclerosis. Atherosclerosis of vessels has been previously shown to be associated with decreased capacity to generate PGI$_2$. After stimulation of the arteries with exogenous arachidonic acid, the amount of PGI$_2$ released from all arteries increased. However, the stimulated levels of PGI$_2$ from arteries of patients with cancer remained significantly less than that of control vessels. Stimulated PGI$_2$ release from the arteries in the tumor bed was less than that from arteries away from the tumor.

PGI₂ RELEASE FROM ARTERIES FROM PATIENTS WITH AND WITHOUT TUMORS

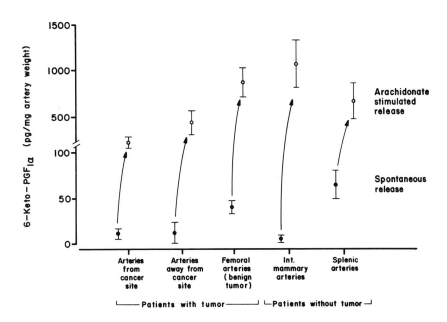

FIGURE 3. Arterial Generation of Prostacyclin in Patients with Malignant Bone Tumors and in Control Subjects. Prostacyclin release in vessels stimulated (o) or not stimulated (●) with arachidonic acid is shown.

Decreased production of PGI_2 in patients with bone tumors may relate to the high risk of metastasis in these patients. The decreased amounts of PGI_2 could facilitate the deposition of tumor cell-platelet aggregates and facilitate subsequent extravasation.

We have also observed abnormalities in activity of PGI_2 in plasma of patients with bone tumors (37). Authentic PGI_2 incubated in plasma of patients with tumors was found to be less stable than PGI_2 incubated in normal plasma. We evaluated stabilization of PGI_2 activity by incubating authentic PGI_2 in plasma of patients and control subjects for 1, 15 and 30 min. Biological activity of PGI_2 was then evaluated by measuring inhibition of normal platelet aggregation. Prostacyclin incubated in the plasma from patients with bone tumors maintained biological activity for significantly less time compared to that in plasma from normal subjects (Table 3). A representative example of PGI_2 activity after its incubation in plasma of a normal subject or of a patient with osteogenic sarcoma is shown in Figure 4. Prostacyclin incubated in patient plasma demonstrated a rapid loss of platelet antiaggregatory activity compared to that seen in the normal subject.

240

Table 3. Platelet Aggregation Inhibition (%) by PGI_2 Incubated in PPP of Normal Subjects and Patients with Tumors.

Incubation Time	Normal Subjects (n = 22)	Patients (n = 7)	P Value
1	71 ± 3	37 ± 10	< 0.05
15	54 ± 5	33 ± 8	< 0.05
30	34 ± 6	14 ± 6	< 0.05

Abbreviations: PGI_2 = prostacyclin; PPP = platelet poor plasma

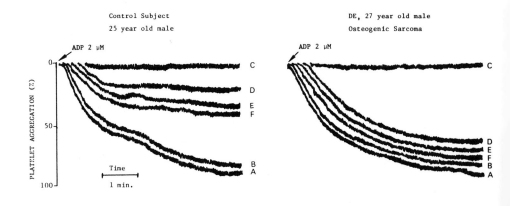

A-PRP + NS; B-PRP + PPP; C-PRP + PPP (No ADP); D- PRP + PGI_2 in PPP (incubation time 1 min.); E-PRP + PGI_2 in PPP (incubation time 15 min.); F-PRP + PGI_2 in PPP (incubation time 30 min.)

FIGURE 4. Bioactivity of Prostacyclin Incubated in Normal Plasma (left panel) and Patient Plasma (right panel). Note rapid loss of prostacyclin antiplatelet activity in patient plasma. This patient had osteogenic sarcoma.

Decreased stabilization of PGI_2 has recently been recognized as a potential mechanism of in vivo thrombus formation. Chen et al. (39) described a 39 year old man with chronic thrombotic thrombocytopenic purpura. Exogenous PGI_2 incubated in his plasma demonstrated anti-platelet aggregatory activity which lasted for less than one minute; in contrast anti-aggregatory activity was present for over 15 min when PGI_2 was incubated in normal plasma. This patient was treated with plasma exchange and demonstrated a marked improvement in stabilization of PGI_2 as well as in clinical course. This defect was also corrected when normal plasma was mixed with the patient's plasma in vitro. Prolongation of PGI_2 activity in this patient by normal plasma suggested that the deficiency of "prostacyclin stabilizing factor" in his plasma may have predisposed to severe thrombotic tendency.

Decreased stabilization of PGI_2 in plasma of patients with cancer in association with decreased PGI_2 production could result in a similar "thrombotic" tendency in which tumor cells adhere to the vessel walls. Thereafter, growth, proliferation and spread of tumor cells could occur.

VI. SUMMARY

The results of the studies cited here support the hypothesis (2,22,30) that products of arachidonic acid metabolism modulate tumor metastasis by their effects on platelets and the vessel walls (see Chapter 14). This hypothesis is presented schematically in Figure 5. The primary tumor may promote platelet activation and generation of TXA_2 and other vasoactive substances. These products by their pro-aggregatory and vasoconstrictor actions could predispose to the formation of platelet-tumor cell aggregates. Platelet activity could also result in increased release of platelet-derived factors which facilitate tumor growth.

The primary tumor may generate prostaglandins, which mediate some of the clinical manifestations in patients with cancer. Prostaglandin E_2 has potent immuno-suppressive actions and could, therefore, cause decreased surveillance of tumor cells. Thus, tumor cells could be released into the circulation and metastasize without being detected. The tumor may cause direct physical or chemical injury to the vessel wall, resulting in decreased production of PGI_2. Decreased PGI_2 production would leave platelet aggregation and actions of TXA_2 unopposed, thereby promoting the formation of platelet-tumor cell aggregates and their deposition on the vessel wall.

These concepts are speculative at this time. More studies will be needed to further delineate the interrelationships of platelets, prostaglandins and tumors. The role of other prostaglandins and related substances such as leukotrienes also needs to be determined.

242

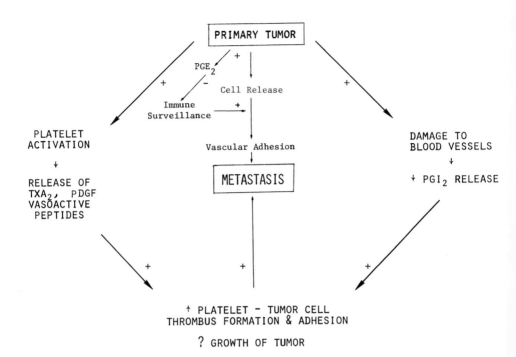

FIGURE 5. Schematic Diagram of Proposed Interrelationships of Platelets, Prostaglandins and Tumors.

REFERENCES

1. Weiss HJ. N. Engl. J. Med. 293:531-580, 1975.
2. Honn KV, Cicone B and Skoff A. Science 212:1270-1272, 1981.
3. Wood S, Jr., Holyoke ED and Yardley JH. Proc. Can. Cancer Res. Conf. 4:167-223, 1961.
4. Wood S, Jr. Bull. Schweiz. Akad. Med. Wiss. 20:92-121, 1964.
5. Warren BA and Vales O. Br. J. Exp. Pathol. 53:301-313, 1972.
6. Jones DS, Wallace AC and Fraser EF. J. Natl. Cancer Inst. 46:493-504, 1971.
7. Sindelar WF, Tralica TS and Ketcham AS. J. Surg. Res. 18:137-161, 1975.
8. Gasic GJ, Gasic TB, Galanti N, Johnson T and Murphy S. Int. J. Cancer 11:704-718, 1973.
9. Gasic G, Gasic T and Stewart CC. Proc. Natl. Acad. Sci. USA 61:46-53, 1968.
10. Hilgard P, Heller H and Schmidt CG. Z. Krebsforsch. 86:243-250, 1976.

11. Pearlstein E, Salk PL, Yogeeswaran G and Karpatkin S. Proc. Natl. Acad. Sci. USA 77:4336-4339, 1980.
12. Gasic GJ, Boettiger D, Catalfamo JL, Gasic TB and Stewart GJ. Cancer Res. 38:2950-2955, 1978.
13. Pearlstein E, Cooper LB and Karpatkin S. J. Lab. Clin. Med. 93:332-334, 1979.
14. Honn KV, Cavanaugh P, Evens C, Taylor JD and Sloane BF. Science 217:540-542, 1982.
15. Paul D, Niewiarowski S, Kodungallore GV, Rucinski B, Rucker S and Lange E. Proc. Natl. Acad. Sci. USA 77:5914-5918, 1980.
16. Nachman RL, Weksler B and Ferris B. Annu. Rev. Med. 30:119-134, 1979.
17. Holmsen H and Weiss HJ. Annu. Rev. Med. 30:119-134, 1979.
18. Kohler N and Lipton A. Proc. Am. Assoc. Cancer Res. 18:244A, 1977.
19. Cowan DH and Graham J. Proc. Am. Assoc. Cancer Res. 22:56A, 1981.
20. Witoski E, Kapner N, Jefferson LS and Lipton A. Proc. Am. Assoc. Cancer Res. 22:57A, 1981.
21. Moncada S and Vane JR. N. Engl. J. Med. 300:1142-1147, 1979.
22. Honn KV, Busse WD and Sloane BF. Biochem. Pharmacol. 32:1-11, 1983.
23. Bennett A, Berstock DA, Harris M, Raja B, Rowe DJF, Stanford F and Wright JE. Adv. Prostaglandin Thromboxane Res. 6:595-600, 1980.
24. Humes JL, Cupo JJ, Jr. and Strausser HR. Prostaglandins 6:463-473, 1974.
25. Jaffe BM, Philpott GW, Hampricht B and Parker CW. Adv. Biosci. 9:179, 1973.
26. Hammarstrom S, Samuelsson B and Bjursel G. Nature (London) New Biol. 243:50-51, 1973.
27. Gonzalez-Crussi F, Hsueh W and Wiederhold MD. Am. J. Clin. Pathol. 75:243-253, 1981.
28. Fitzpatrick FA and Stringfellow DA. Proc. Natl. Acad. Sci. USA 76:1765-1769, 1979.
29. Chang WC, Muroto S and Tsurufuji S. Prostaglandins 13:17-25, 1977.
30. Honn KV, Meyer J, Neagos G, Henderson T, Westley C and Ratanatharathorn V. In: Interactions of Platelets and Tumor Cells (Ed. Jamieson GA), Alan Liss, New York, pp. 295-331, 1982.
31. Tashjian AH, Jr., Voelkel EF, Levin L and Goldhaver P. J. Exp. Med. 136:1329-1343, 1972.
32. Powles TJ, Clark SA, Easty DM, Easty GC and Neville A. Br. J. Cancer 28:316-321, 1973.
33. Dowsett M, Easty GC, Powles TJ, Easty DM and Neville AM. Prostaglandins 11:447-460, 1976.
34. Honn KV and Meyer J. Biochem. Biophys. Res. Commun. 102:1122-1129, 1981.
35. Mehta P, Gross S and Ostrowski N. Am. J. Pediat. Hematol. Oncol. (in press), 1983.
36. Mehta P, Springfield D and Ostrowski N. Cancer (Philadelphia) (in press), 1983.
37. Mehta P, Gross S, Ostrowski N and Brigmon L. Blood (Suppl):218A, 1982.
38. Mehta P. Blood (in press), 1983.
39. Chen YC, McLeod B, Hall EE and Wu KK. Lancet 2:267-269, 1981.

CHAPTER 16. CALCIUM CHANNEL BLOCKERS: INHIBITORS OF TUMOR CELL-PLATELET-ENDOTHELIAL CELL INTERACTIONS

JAMES M. ONODA, BONNIE F. SLOANE, JOHN D. TAYLOR AND KENNETH V. HONN

I. CALCIUM CHANNEL BLOCKERS

The movement of calcium ions across cellular membranes (e.g., plasma membrane, endoplasmic or sarcoplasmic reticulum) can serve as a molecular messenger that modulates biochemical processes appropriate to the specific cell type. Calcium antagonists by preventing release of Ca^{2+} from intracellular stores, by preventing influx of external Ca^{2+} or by inhibiting the effects of Ca^{2+} through interactions with Ca^{2+}-binding proteins such as calmodulin can interfere with these biochemical functions. The primary action of one subgroup of calcium antagonists is to interact with the channels in the cell membrane through which calcium enters the cells. This class of compounds originally described by Fleckenstein has been called by a variety of names including Ca^{2+}-channel blockers, Ca^{2+}-entry blockers, Ca^{2+}-channel inhibitors and slow-channel blockers (for review see 1-3). We will use the terminology calcium channel blockers (CCB) in this chapter.

Four chemical classes of organic CCB are currently known: 1. dihydropyridine (nimodipine), 2. phenylalkylamine (verapamil), 3. diphenylalkylamine (prenylamine) and 4. benzothiazepine (diltiazem). The chemical structure for a representative of each of these classes is presented in Figure 1. In a recent study of receptor binding by CCB, Murphy et al. (4) demonstrated that the phenylalkylamines, diphenylalkylamines and benzothiazepines all act at a single site on the membrane which is allosterically linked to the dihydropyridine receptor. Diphenylalkylamines and phenylalkylamines decrease the affinity of dihydropyridines for their receptor whereas benzothiazepines increase the affinity (4). At least one study has shown that phenylalkylamines may act at a site on the inside of the plasma membrane (5). Calcium channels seem to exist in three distinct states: resting, open and inactivated and the chemical classes of CCB differ in their ability to block Ca^{2+} channels in these three states. Phenylalkylamines such as verapamil block Ca^{2+} channels in the open or inactivated state (5). Benzothiazepines such as diltiazem bind primarily in the inactivated state (6). Dihydropyridines such as nitrendipine block Ca^{2+} channels in both their resting and open states (6). The phenylalkylamine verapamil and the benzothiazepine diltiazem have been described as exhibiting a greater use-dependence than do dihydropyridines, i.e., their Ca^{2+} blocking activity is more dependent upon the frequency of stimulation. Presumably this could be due to

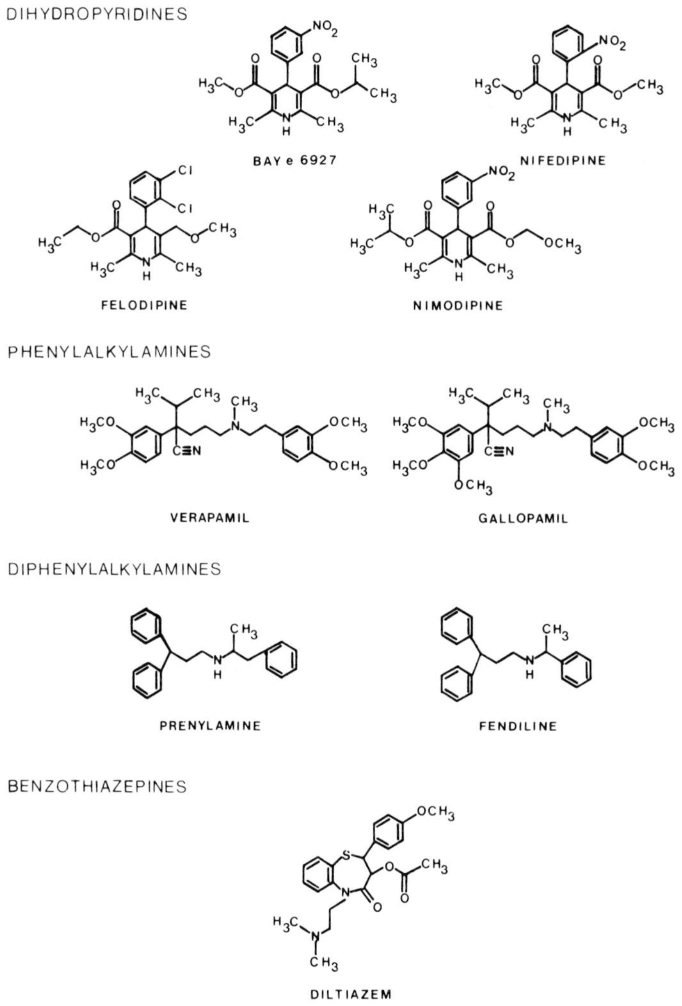

DIHYDROPYRIDINES

BAY e 6927

NIFEDIPINE

FELODIPINE

NIMODIPINE

PHENYLALKYLAMINES

VERAPAMIL

GALLOPAMIL

DIPHENYLALKYLAMINES

PRENYLAMINE

FENDILINE

BENZOTHIAZEPINES

DILTIAZEM

FIGURE 1. Structure of Calcium Channel Blockers Representative of Each of the Four Known Chemical Classes.

differences in binding sites and/or to dihydropyridines binding to Ca^{2+} channels in their resting state rather than in their inactivated state.

There also seems to be specificity among the chemical classes of CCB for Ca^{2+} channels in different cell types. However, the mechanisms for the differential effects of CCB on vascular smooth muscle and on cardiac muscle have not been definitively established. Vascular smooth muscle contraction is more dependent upon entry of extracellular Ca^{2+} than is cardiac muscle contraction. Dihydropyridine receptors in smooth and cardiac muscle membranes are high affinity sites. However, in intact cardiac muscle cells the binding sites seem to be low affinity (7). Although the reasons for differential Ca^{2+}-blocking activities in different tissues are not clear, these differences are reflected in the therapeutic efficacies of CCB. Due to their inhibition of Ca^{2+} entry in vascular smooth muscle and thus their inhibition of contraction (vasodilation) CCB are used in the treatment of vasospasms and of hypertension. Dihydropyridines are particularly useful clinically because they inhibit Ca^{2+} entry into vascular smooth muscle cells at much lower concentrations than they do Ca^{2+} entry into cardiac muscle. Thus, they can be used to treat vasospasm or hypertension without causing a reduction in myocardial contractility. These compounds have already received widespread used in the treatment of cardiovascular disease in Europe (8,9) and are now in clinical use (verapamil, diltiazem, nifedipine) or in clinical trials for use in the USA (nimodipine).

CCB seem to have effects on tissues other than muscle, e.g., brain, platelets, tumor cells. High affinity binding sites for dihydropyridines have been found in brain membranes (10), but dihydropyridine receptors have not been found in platelets (11). Recently CCB have been found to enhance conventional antitumor therapy. CCB of the phenylalkylamine and benzothiazepine classes enhanced the cytotoxicity of drug resistant lines derived from several murine solid tumors to standard chemotherapeutic agents such as adriamycin, vincristine and vinblastine (12,13). In addition, verapamil has been demonstrated to selectively increase (> 50%) blood flow to a murine adenocarcinoma at levels which did not significantly alter arterial blood pressure (14). As previously discussed, at low concentrations CCB reduce the transmembrane transport of extracellular Ca^{2+}. However, at higher concentrations these agents can also affect cellular mobilization of Ca^{2+} (15). The effects of CCB on platelets and on tumor cells may be due to inhibition of intracellular Ca^{2+} mobilization rather than to inhibition of Ca^{2+} entry.

II. ROLE OF PLATELETS IN TUMOR METASTASIS

Interactions between tumor cells and platelets are thought to facilitate metastasis by enhancing tumor cell arrest in the microvasculature or tumor cell adhesion to the blood vessel wall (16). Although the mechanisms by which platelets might enhance metastasis are not yet fully delineated, several laboratories have demonstrated that both human and animal tumor cells can induce platelet aggregation in vitro (17-19) and that i.v. injection of tumor cells results in thrombocytopenia in vivo (20,21). Gasic et al. (20,22) reported that in the presence of thrombocytopenia (induced by neuraminidase or antiplatelet antiserum) the number of lung colonies produced upon tail vein injection of TA3 ascites tumor cells was reduced. In this "experimental metastasis" model the concomitant infusion of platelets prevented the thrombocytopenia-induced decrease in number of lung colonies (20,21). We have shown that prostacyclin (PGI_2), the most potent platelet antiaggregatory agent known, is also a potent inhibitor of platelet aggregation induced by rodent tumor cells in vitro (23,24). Lerner et al. (25) have demonstrated that PGI_2 can also inhibit platelet aggregation induced by several human tumor cell lines. We have demonstrated that a number of agents which inhibit platelet aggregation [exogenous and endogenous PGI_2, PGI_2 stimulating agents (nafazatrom) and thromboxane (TX) synthase inhibitors] are antimetastatic in animal tumor models (16,26,27). Recently we have suggested that overt platelet aggregation may not be required in order for platelet-tumor cell interactions to enhance metastasis (16) and that the critical event in the hematogenous phase of the metastatic cascade may be tumor cell arrest and formation of stable adhesions to the endothelium or de-endothelianized surfaces. Therefore, we have been exploring the possibility that interactions among tumor cells, platelets and endothelial cells facilitate tumor cell arrest and adhesion (16,26). In a homologous system we found that rat platelets enhanced the adhesion of rat W256 carcinosarcoma cells to plastic substratum and to both normal endothelial cells derived from rat cerebral microvasculature and to their virally transformed counterparts. Adhesion was enhanced both in the absence and presence of overt platelet aggregation and PGI_2 inhibited this platelet-enhanced tumor cell adhesion (16).

III. RATIONALE FOR USE OF CALCIUM CHANNEL BLOCKERS AS ANTIMETASTATIC
       AGENTS

Both intracellular and extracellular Ca^{2+} seem to be required for irreversible platelet aggregation (28,29). Thromboxane A_2 is a platelet proaggregatory agent which may act in part by releasing intracellular stores of Ca^{2+} in the platelet (30,31), whereas PGI_2, a platelet antiaggregatory agent, acts in part by increasing intracellular sequestration of Ca^{2+} in the platelet (28). CCB, which prevent the influx of extracellular Ca^{2+} in several cell types (3,32,33), have recently been shown to inhibit ADP-, epinephrine- and collagen-induced platelet aggregation in vitro (34-36), perhaps due to inhibition of intracellular Ca^{2+} mobilization (37). In humans with coronary heart disease administration of nifedipine, a dihydropyridine class CCB, has been shown to decrease ADP- and collagen-induced aggregation of platelets ex vivo and to increase bleeding time (38). The ability of CCB to inhibit platelet aggregation in vitro and ex vivo, in conjunction with our previous studies indicating that antiplatelet agents are antimetastatic, suggested that CCB might be effective inhibitors of tumor cell-platelet-endothelial cell interactions in vitro and in turn of metastasis in vivo.

248

IV. ANTIPLATELET EFFECTS OF CALCIUM CHANNEL BLOCKERS

A. Platelet Aggregation Induced by Chemical Agonists

There have been numerous reports that CCB can inhibit aggregation in vitro of citrated platelet rich plasma (PRP) from humans, rabbits and cats (34-36,39,41-45) and can affect platelet function in vivo in humans and rats (36,38,40). The CCB employed in these studies represented three classes of CCB (dihydropyridine, phenylalkylamine and benzothiazepine). The ability of the CCB to inhibit platelet aggregation was not consistent from species to species. For example, nifedipine and nimodipine did not inhibit ADP-induced aggregation of cat citrated PRP (35), yet did inhibit ADP-induced aggregation of human citrated PRP (34) and human heparinized PRP. Although it is difficult to compare these reports due to differences in the agonist employed, to differences in the concentration of agonist employed and to the failure to provide IC_{50} values, some consistencies are evident. For example, verapamil inhibited platelet function in vitro and in vivo in all species studied (34-37,40-43). However, the IC_{50} values reported for the inhibition of ADP-induced aggregation of human citrated PRP by verapamil seem to be dependent on the strength of the stimulus; the IC_{50} for stimulation with 1 μM ADP was 163 μM (44) and with 9 μM ADP was 500 μM (34). Diltiazem also seemed to consistently inhibit aggregation of human PRP or rabbit PRP in vitro (34,39,45).

In our laboratories we have tested four CCB in vitro for inhibition of ADP- and thrombin-induced platelet aggregation of heparinized human PRP. By using heparinized PRP we were able to study the antiplatelet effects of CCB in the presence of normal plasma concentrations of Ca^{2+}. The four CCB tested represented three chemical classes: dihydropyridines (nimodipine and nifedipine), phenylalkylamines (verapamil) and benzothiazepines (diltiazem). All of the CCB inhibited, in a dose-dependent manner, both ADP- and thrombin-induced platelet aggregation. The IC_{50} values for inhibition of platelet aggregation induced by 10 μM ADP were 200, 480, 550 and 650 μM for nimodipine, diltiazem, verapamil and nifedipine, respectively. The IC_{50} values for inhibition of platelet aggregation induced by 20 NIH units/ml thrombin were 110, 200, 550 and 650 μM for diltiazem, nimodipine, verapamil and nifedipine, respectively. This dose of thrombin (20 NIH units/ml) was consistently able to induce aggregation of heparinized PRP. Diltiazem was a more effective inhibitor of thrombin-induced than ADP-induced aggregation whereas the other three CCB had the same relative potency in both systems. We did observe that the IC_{50} value for any one of the CCB could vary by up to 25% depending on platelet donor. Therefore, the IC_{50} values reported here represent the means of triplicate determinations with PRP from 2 to 4 separate donors. Our IC_{50} values agree with those reported by Ono and Kimura (34) for inhibition of aggregation of human citrated PRP by 9 μM ADP; their IC_{50} for diltiazem was 500 μM and for verapamil 500 μM. In contrast, we determined an IC_{50} value for inhibition by nifedipine of 650 μM whereas Ono and Kimura (34) determined an IC_{50} of 100 μM. We cannot account for this discrepancy.

Platelet thromboxane production from endogenous arachidonic acid in response to ADP, epinephrine or collagen has been shown to be inhibited by nifedipine, verapamil and diltiazem (37,43,45). We demonstrated that the CCB we tested were able to inhibit, in a dose dependent manner, platelet thromboxane production from endogenous arachidonic acid in response to either ADP or thrombin. However, the order of potency for inhibition of TXA_2 production did not correspond to that for inhibition of platelet aggregation. In response to ADP the order of potency was nimodipine = nifedipine > diltiazem $\geq$ verapamil and in response to thrombin was nimodipine = diltiazem $\geq$ nifedipine > verapamil.

Representatives of three chemical classes of CCB have been shown to inhibit aggregation of both citrated and heparinized PRP. However, the concentrations of CCB required for inhibition in heparinized plasma (i.e., in the presence of normal plasma concentrations of Ca^{2+}) are supra-pharmacological and probably cannot be achieved in vivo. For example, an 80 mg oral dose of verapamil in humans results in a peak one hour plasma level of 100-200 μM (46) and an oral nifedipine dose of 10 mg results in an one hour plasma level of 64 nM (47). Nifedipine and verapamil have been shown to affect platelet function in vivo in humans and rats at peak plasma levels well below those reported to inhibit platelet aggregation (14,36,38,43). These discrepancies suggest that platelets in vivo may be more sensitive to the antiaggregatory effects of CCB. One possible explanation is that in vivo CCB may act in concert with endogenous antiaggregatory agents such as PGI_2.

Ikeda et al. (41) demonstrated that a combination of PGI_2 and verapamil resulted in a synergistic inhibition of aggregation. The dose of PGI_2 employed did not inhibit aggregation of human PRP to a variety of stimuli (ADP, epinephrine, A23187) and that of verapamil was also suboptimal. In contrast, Mehta et al. (45) observed that PGI_2 did not synergize with diltiazem in the inhibition of ADP- or epinephrine-induced aggregation of human PRP. However, the dose of PGI_2 employed in this latter study was able to inhibit platelet aggregation by 50%. We have demonstrated that when both nimodipine and PGI_2 are utilized at suboptimal doses (< 10% inhibition of aggregation in response to ADP or to thrombin in the same PRP) the combination results in a synergistic inhibition of ADP- and thrombin-induced aggregation. ADP-induced aggregation was inhibited 59% and thrombin-induced aggregation 42%. In contrast, PGI_2 when tested at a dose that inhibited platelet aggregation $\geq$ 50% did not enhance the inhibition due to nimodipine alone. Concentrations of nimodipine alone or PGI_2 alone which minimally inhibited TXA_2 production in response to either ADP or thrombin resulted in a synergistic inhibition of TXA_2 production in response to either ADP or thrombin when tested in combination. Thromboxane synthase inhibitors do not inhibit platelet aggregation in vitro possibily because the precursor to TXA_2, PGH_2, may at high concentrations mimic the actions of TXA_2 (48). We have demonstrated that a suboptimal dose of nimodipine in combination with the TX synthase inhibitor U63557A (at a dose which does not affect platelet aggregation in vitro) resulted in a synergistic inhibition of ADP- and thrombin-induced aggregation.

250

The dose of U63557A used inhibited TXA$_2$ production in response to ADP by 80% and in response to thrombin by 90%, whereas nimodipine alone resulted in a minimal inhibition of TXA$_2$ production. The combination of U63557A plus nimodipine produced only a slight potentiation of the inhibition of TXA$_2$ production by U63557A alone (in response to either ADP or thrombin).

The results of our study utilizing heparinized PRP (49) and previous studies utilizing citrated PRP (11,34,35,41,43,45) suggest that the concentration of CCB necessary to inhibit platelet aggregation induced by a variety of stimuli in vitro is higher than could be achieved therapeutically. Nevertheless, several CCB have been shown to alter platelet function in vivo. We suggest that the ability of CCB to alter platelet function in vivo may be related to their synergism with endogenous antiaggregatory agents like PGI$_2$.

B. Platelet Aggregation Induced by Tumor Cells

Elutriated murine B16 amelanotic melanoma (B16a) and rat Walker 256 carcinosarcoma (W256) cells induce irreversible aggregation of human PRP in vitro and elutriated rat W256 cells induce irreversible aggregation of rat PRP in vitro. Two CCB of the dihydropyridine class (nimodipine and nifedipine) were shown to inhibit, in a dose-dependent manner, the induction of platelet aggregation by B16a cells and by W256 cells (Figure 2). In both cases nimodipine was the more effective inhibitor of tumor cell-induced platelet aggregation. The IC$_{50}$ for inhibition by nimodipine of B16a-induced platelet aggregation was 85 μM and of W256-induced platelet aggregation was 900 μM. For inhibition by nifedipine the IC$_{50}$'s were 400 μM (B16a) and 1450 μM (W256). Nimodipine was also inhibitory in a homologous system consisting of rat tumor cells (W256) and rat PRP prepared from heparinized blood; the IC$_{50}$ was 25 μM. Recently we have demonstrated that representatives of two other classes of CCB (phenylalkylamine and benzothiazepine) can inhibit B16a-induced platelet aggregation (Figure 3). The IC$_{50}$ for inhibition of B16a-induced platelet aggregation by diltiazem was 350 μM and by verapamil was 340 μM. The degree of inhibition by the CCB was inversely related to the strength of the aggregating stimulus (tumor cell concentration) and varied with platelet donor. Platelet thromboxane production from endogenous arachidonic acid in response to tumor cells (data not shown) was also inhibited by the three chemical classes of CCB tested (dihydropyridine, phenylalkylamine and benzothiazepine).

The ability of calcium channel blockers to inhibit platelet aggregation induced by ADP or thrombin was enhanced by PGI$_2$ or by a TX synthase inhibitor (see above). Therefore, we tested for possible synergistic inhibition of platelet aggregation induced by tumor cells. We tested representatives of the dihydropyridine class of calcium channel blockers in combination with PGI$_2$ or a TX synthase inhibitor using concentrations of the dihydropyridines, PGI$_2$ and the TX synthase inhibitors which inhibited platelet aggregation induced by B16a or

TUMOR CELL INDUCED PLATELET AGGREGATION

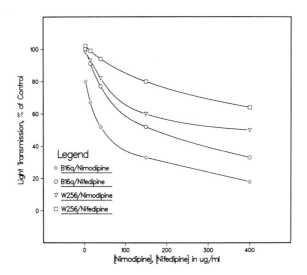

FIGURE 2. Dose-Response Curve for Inhibition of Tumor Cell-Induced Platelet Aggregation by Dihydropyridine Class Calcium Channel Blockers (52).

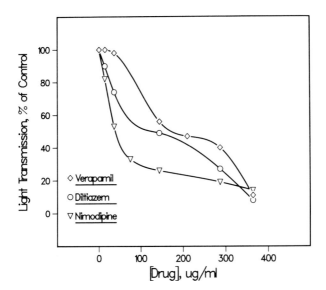

FIGURE 3. Dose-Response Curve for Inhibition of B16a Tumor Cell-Induced Platelet Aggregation by Three Chemical Classes of Calcium Channel Blockers.

W256 tumor cells by ≤ 10%. All combinations tested resulted in a synergistic inhibition of platelet aggregation. Representative examples of this synergistic inhibiton are illustrated in Figures 4 and 5.

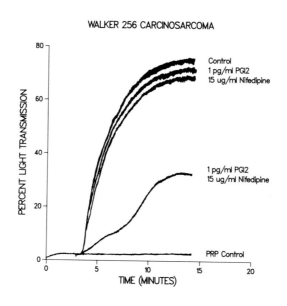

FIGURE 4. Synergistic Inhibition by Nifedipine and Prostacyclin of W256 Tumor Cell-Induced Platelet Aggregation.

C. Platelet-Enhanced Adhesion of Tumor Cells to Endothelium

We have reported that platelets enhance the adhesion of W256 cells to monolayers of normal endothelial cells (derived from rat cerebral microvasculature) under non-aggregatory and aggregatory conditions (50). This enhancement of adhesion does not require overt platelet aggregation yet is potentiated if platelet aggregation is allowed to occur. Platelet-enhanced adhesion of W256 cells to both normal and transformed endothelial cells seems to be quantitatively similar (50). Using a homologous system of rat W256 tumor cells, washed rat platelets (WRP) and monolayers of transformed endothelial cells from rat cerebral microvasculature we demonstrated that adhesion of W256 cells to endothelial cells was increased in the presence of platelets: 100% under non-aggregatory conditions [absence of platelet poor plasma (PPP)] and 385% under aggregatory conditions (presence of 0.1% PPP). Previous studies (18) have demonstrated that a variety of tumor cell lines require a plasma factor (PPP) to induce aggregation of washed platelets. Two CCB of the dihydropyridine class were tested

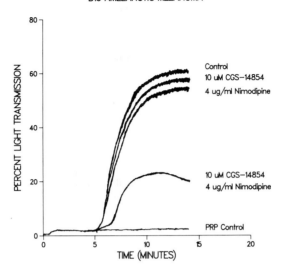

FIGURE 5. Synergistic Inhibition by Nimodipine and a Thromboxane Synthase Inhibitor (CGS-14854) of B16a Tumor Cell-Induced Platelet Aggregation.

for their abilities to inhibit the platelet-enhanced W256 cell adhesion to endothelium. Nimodipine at a dose of 100 µM inhibited platelet-enhanced W256 cell adhesion under both non-aggregatory and aggregatory conditions (Figure 6). In contrast nifedipine at a dose of 100 µM did not significantly inhibit platelet-enhanced W256 cell adhesion under non-aggregatory conditions but did inhibit adhesion by 38% under aggregatory conditions. We have recently demonstrated that representatives of the phenylalkylamine and benzothiazepine classes of CCB also inhibit platelet-enhanced tumor cell adhesion to endothelium.

V. ANTIMETASTATIC EFFECTS OF CALCIUM CHANNEL BLOCKERS

Since we have previously demonstrated that compounds which inhibit interactions among tumor cells, platelets and endothelial cells in vitro have antimetastatic properties when administered in vivo (23,26,27), we tested CCB for antimetastatic activity in vivo using spontaneous and "experimental" metastasis models (51,52). The "experimental" metastasis model, using intravenously injected tumor cells, enabled us to examine the effects of CCB on the interactions among tumor cells (circulating), platelets and endothelial cells.

254

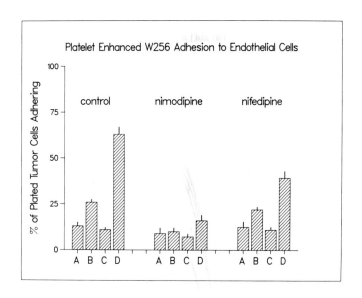

FIGURE 6. Inhibition of Platelet-Enhanced Tumor Cell Adhesion to Confluent Monolayer of Virally (Rous Sarcoma) Transformed Rat Cerebral Microvascular Endothelial Cells. Bars represent $\bar{x}$ ± SEM, n = 6. A = tumor cells (TC), B = TC + WRP, C = TC + PPP, D = TC + WRP + PPP (52).

Results obtained in the "experimental" metastasis model were then confirmed by daily administration of CCB in a spontaneous model (metastasis from a subcutaneous tumor) in which the drugs may exert multiple effects, i.e., on the primary tumor as well as on circulating tumor cells or on host cells (platelets).

A single administration of nimodipine (10 mg/kg body wt, p.o.) one hour prior to and one hour post intravenous injection of elutriated B16a tumor cells resulted in a 57% decrease in lung colony formation whereas nifedipine at the same dose decreased lung colony formation by 33% (52). In additional studies employing lower drug concentrations (0.1 to 4.0 mg/kg body wt), nimodipine was also a more effective inhibitor of lung colony formation than was nifedipine. The antimetastatic effects of felodipine were only tested at the lowest drug concentration (0.1 mg/kg body wt). At this dose the ability of felodipine to inhibit lung colony formation (43% decrease) was not significantly different than that of nimodipine (34% decrease) (52) . In our most recent study, verapamil at 1 mg/kg body wt (p.o.) did not significantly inhibit lung colony formation by B16a tumor cells whereas nifedipine at the same dose inhibited lung colony formation by 28% (Figure 7).

EXPERIMENTAL METASTASIS

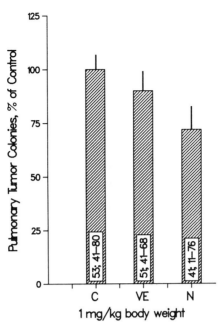

FIGURE 7. Inhibition of Pulmonary Tumor Colony Formation by Calcium Channel Blockers. Mean number of control metastases was 57 ± 4. Bars represent x̄ ± SEM (as % of control); n = 12.

Daily administration of dihydropyridine class CCB (10 mg/kg body wt, p.o.) to mice bearing subcutaneous B16a tumors resulted in a 72% reduction in the number of pulmonary metastases by nimodipine and a 40% reduction by nifedipine (52). Nimodipine and nifedipine did not significantly reduce either the wet weight or the volume of the primary subcutaneous tumors. Daily administration of either verapamil or nifedipine at a lower concentration (1 mg/kg body wt, p.o.) resulted in a slight but insignificant reduction (19%) by verapamil and a significant reduction (41%) by nifedipine of pulmonary metastases (Figure 8).

We have demonstrated that three chemical classes of CCB inhibit tumor cell-induced platelet aggregation and platelet-enhanced tumor cell adhesion to endothelial cells in vitro and tentatively suggest that their antimetastatic effects in vivo may be related to inhibition of tumor cell-platelet-endothelial cell interactions. However, we do not exclude the possibility that the CCB may be antimetastatic in vivo due to their effects on hemodynamic parameters (53), to inhibition of phosphodiesterase (54), to inhibition of calmodulin (55) or to

256

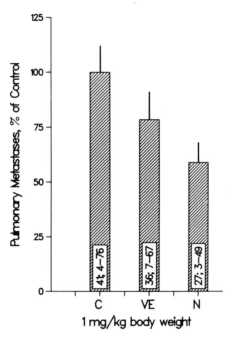

SPONTANEOUS METASTASIS

FIGURE 8. Inhibition of Spontaneous Pulmonary Metastasis by Calcium Channel Blockers. Mean number of control metastases was 41 ± 5. Bars represent x̄ ± SEM (as % of control); n = 12.

stimulation of PGI$_2$ production by pulmonary endothelial cells (56). Inhibition of phosphodiesterase or of calmodulin and stimulation of PGI$_2$ would, of course, all result in inhibition of platelet aggregation. We have previously shown that PGI$_2$ inhibits tumor cell-induced platelet aggregation and platelet- enhanced tumor cell adhesion in vitro and lung colony formation in vivo (16,26,27). Phosphodiesterase inhibitors have been reported to be antimetastatic in vivo although Maniglia et al. (57) suggested that the antimetastatic effects of the phosphodiesterase inhibitor 2,6-bis (diethanolamino)-4-piperidinopyrimido[5,4-d]-pyrimidine (RA233) were due to inhibition of primary tumor growth not to antiplatelet activity. In our studies the dihydropyridines exhibited antimetastatic effects in the absence of effects on primary tumor growth.

VI. SUMMARY

We propose that CCB may represent a new generic class of antimetastatic agents. This proposal is attractive in that CCB: 1. have been selected for low chronic toxicity due to their intended long term use in cardiovascular patients, 2. can be administered orally, 3. are currently in clinical trial or have been approved for use for cardiovascular disease in the USA and, therefore, could be readily available for Phase I clinical trials in cancer if efficacy in animal models can be demonstrated, 4. may synergize with PGI_2-stimulating agents and thromboxane synthase inhibitors (which lower platelet intracellular Ca^{2+}), compounds which are currently under development as antimetastatic agents and 5. may, at the same time, enhance conventional cytotoxic chemotherapy and radiation therapy.

REFERENCES

1. Fleckenstein A. Annu. Rev. Pharmacol. Toxicol. 17:149–166, 1977.
2. Janis RA and Triggle RJ. J. Med. Chem. 26:775–785, 1983.
3. Braunwald E. N. Engl. J. Med. 307:1618–1627, 1982.
4. Murphy KMM, Gould RJ, Largent BL and Snyder SH. Proc. Natl. Acad. Sci. USA 80:860–864, 1983.
5. Nayler WG and Grinwald P. Fed. Proc. Fed. Am. Soc. Exp. Biol. 40:2855–2861, 1981.
6. Lee KS and Tsien RW. Nature (London) 302:790–794, 1983.
7. Janis RA and Scriabine A. Biochem. Pharmacol. 32:3499–3507, 1983.
8. Wellens D, Goossens T and Reyntjens A. Angiology 12:821–827, 1980.
9. Conti CR. J. Fl. Med. Assoc. 68:883–886, 1981.
10. Murphy KMM and Synder SH. Eur. J. Pharmacol. 77:201–202, 1982.
11. Motulsky HJ, Snavely MD, Hughes RJ and Insel PA. Circ. Res. 52:226–231, 1983.
12. Tsuruo T, Iida H, Tsukagoshi S and Sakurai Y. Cancer Res. 43:2267–2272, 1983.
13. Tsuruo T, Iida H, Nojiri M, Tsukagoshi S and Sakurai Y. Cancer Res. 43:2905–2910, 1983.
14. Kaelin WG, Shrivastav S, Shand DG and Jirtle RL. Cancer Res. 42:3944–3949, 1982.
15. Winquist RJ, Webb RC and Bohr DF. Fed. Proc. Fed. Am. Soc. Exp. Biol. 40:2852–2854, 1981.
16. Honn KV, Menter DG, Onoda JM, Taylor JD and Sloane BF. In: Cancer Invasion and Metastasis (Eds. Nicolson GL and Milas L), Raven Press:New York, pp. 361–388, 1984.
17. Bastida E, Ordinas A and Jamieson GA. Nature (London) 291:661–662, 1981.
18. Hara Y, Steiner M and Baldini MG. Cancer Res. 40:1217–1222, 1980.
19. Karpatkin S, Smerling A and Pearlstein E. J. Lab. Clin. Med. 96:994–1001, 1980.
20. Gasic GJ, Gasic TB and Stewart CC. Proc. Natl. Acad. Sci. USA 61:46–52, 1968.
21. Gastpar H, Ambrus J and Thurber LE. J. Med. 8:53–56, 1977.
22. Gasic GJ, Gasic TB, Galanti N, Johnson T and Murphy J. Int. J. Cancer 11:704–718, 1973.
23. Honn KV, Busse WD and Sloane BF. Biochem. Pharmacol. 32:1–11, 1983.
24. Menter DG, Onoda JM, Taylor JD and Honn KV. Cancer Res. 44:450–456, 1984.

25. Lerner WA, Pearlstein E, Ambrogio C and Karpatkin S. Int. J. Cancer 31:463–469, 1983.
26. Honn KV. Clin. Exp. Metastasis 1:103–114, 1983.
27. Honn KV, Cicone B and Skoff A. Science 212:1270–1272, 1981.
28. Owen NE, Feinberg H and LeBreton GC. Am. J. Physiol. 239:H483–H488, 1980.
29. Owen NE and LeBreton GC. Am. J. Physiol. 241:H613–H619, 1981.
30. Miller OV, Johnson RA and Gorman RR. Prostaglandins 13:599–609, 1977.
31. Gorman RR. Fed. Proc. Fed. Am. Soc. Exp. Biol. 38:83–88, 1979.
32. Fleckenstein A. Arzneim.Forsch./Drug Res. 20:1317–1322, 1970.
33. Godfraind T. Fed. Proc. Fed. Am. Soc. Exp. Biol. 40:2866–2871, 1981.
34. Ono H and Kimura M. Arzneim.Forsch./Drug Res. 31:1131–1134, 1981.
35. Schmunk GA and Lefer AM. Res. Commun. Chem. Pathol. Pharmacol. 35:179–187, 1982.
36. Ribeiro LGT, Brandon TA, Horak JK, Ware JA, Miller RR and Solis RT. J. Cardiovas. Pharmacol. 4:170–173, 1982.
37. Han P, Boatwright C and Ardlie NG. Thromb. Haemostas. 50:513–517, 1983.
38. Dale J, Landmark KH and Myhre E. Am. Heart J. 105:103–105, 1983.
39. Shinjo A, Sasaki Y, Inamasu M and Morita T. Thromb. Res. 13:941–955, 1978.
40. Okamatsu S, Peck RC and Lefer AM. Proc. Soc. Exp. Biol. Med. 166:551–555, 1981.
41. Ikeda Y, Kikuchi M, Toyama K, Wantanabe K and Ando Y. Thromb. Haemostasis 45:158–161, 1981.
42. Addonizio VP, Fisher CA, Strauss JF and Edmunds LH. Thromb. Res. 28:545–556, 1982.
43. Mehta J, Mehta P, Ostrowski N and Crews F. Thromb. Res. 30:469–475, 1983.
44. MacIntyre DE and Shaw AM. Thromb. Res. 21:833–844, 1983.
45. Mehta P, Mehta J, Ostrowski N and Brignon L. J. Lab. Clin. Med. 102:332–339, 1983.
46. Schomerus M, Spiegelhalder B, Stevens B and Eichelbaum K. Cardiovas. Res. 10:605–612, 1976.
47. Foster TS, Hamann SR, Richards VR, Bryant PJ, Graves DA and McAllister RG. J. Clin. Pharmacol. 23:161–170, 1983.
48. Rybicki JP and LeBreton GC. Thromb. Res. 30:407–414, 1983.
49. Onoda JM, Sloane BF and Honn KV. Submitted.
50. Honn KV, Onoda JM, Diglio CA, Carufel MM, Taylor JD and Sloane BF. Clin. Exp. Metastasis, in press.
51. Honn KV, Onoda JM, Diglio CA and Sloane BF. Proc. Soc. Exp. Biol. Med. 174:16–19, 1983.
52. Honn KV, Onoda JM, Pampalona K, Battaglia M, Neagos G, Taylor JD, Diglio CA and Sloane BF. Submitted.
53. Gerold M, Eigenmann R and Haeusler G. J. Cardiovas. Pharmacol. 4:419–429, 1982.
54. Norman JA, Ansell J and Phillips MA. Eur. J. Pharmacol. 93:107–112, 1983.
55. Bostrum SL, Ljung B, Mardh S, Forsen S and Thulin E. Nature (London) 292:777–778, 1981.
56. Srivastava KC and Awasthi KK. Prostaglandins Leukotrienes Med. 10:411–417, 1983.
57. Maniglia CA, Tudor G, Gomez J and Sartorelli AC. Cancer Lett. 16:253–260, 1982.

CHAPTER 17. EVIDENCE FOR THE ANTIMETASTATIC EFFECTS OF COUMARIN DERIVATIVES

PETER HILGARD

I. BACKGROUND

The first morphological evidence for an association of intravascular cancer cells with thrombotic material was found at the beginning of this century (1). However, not until more than 50 yr later was the possible pathogenic significance of this phenomenon recognized. Observing the fate of intravascular tumor cells in vivo in the Hopkins rabbit ear chamber, Wood (2) found that a tumor cell embolus was rapidly surrounded by microthrombi shortly after its initial attachment to the vascular endothelium. By time-lapse cinematography the investigator was able to document how these intravascular cancer cells, sheltered by their surrounding thrombus, penetrated the vessel wall into the perivascular tissue where they started to proliferate into a "secondary" tumor. From these observations Wood concluded that the activation of the coagulation system at the site of tumor cell lodgment was of significance in the initial phase of the hematogenous spread of malignant tumors.

II. EXPERIMENTAL MODELS

Most of our present knowledge of the interrelationships between blood coagulation and metastasis formation was derived from experiments in rodents. Two basic models were employed in studies of tumor metastases:

A. Lung Colonies

Viable tumor cell suspensions were injected into the blood stream of experimental animals and their fate in the capillary bed was observed. When animals were left to survive, tumor nodules developed in various organs which, with appropriate techniques, could be quantitatively and qualitatively evaluated. Most commonly the experimental tumor cells were injected intravenously which resulted in intrapulmonary "metastatic" tumor growth ("lung colonies"). Morphological studies employing conventional and/or electron microscopy had shown that the activation of the coagulation system at the site of arrest of a tumor cell was a very early event of short duration. Fibrin or fibrin-like material as well as platelets could easily be identified in association with tumor cells within the first

15 min, but after 6 hr the thrombotic material had disappeared, although most tumor cells were still intravascular (3).

B. Spontaneous Metastases

Some intramuscularly or subcutaneously transplanted tumors (e.g., B16 melanoma, Lewis lung carcinoma) metastasize spontaneously to other organs during their growth. This experimental approach is obviously more physiological and resembles the clinical situation more closely. Spontaneous metastases from transplanted tumors can be evaluated with respect to their number and size. In addition, after surgical removal or irradiation of the primary tumor, the survival of the animals represents a biological parameter for the extent of tumor dissemination.

III. ANTICOAGULANTS AND TUMOR METASTASES

Investigations into the role of blood coagulability in the metastatic process have focussed on the use of anticoagulants in the experimental models described above. The intravenous injection of viable experimental tumor cell suspensions into animals with altered blood coagulability gave fairly constant results. In general, drug-induced hypocoagulability or induction of fibrinolysis were found to exert "antimetastatic" effects whereas hypercoagulability or inhibited fibrinolysis resulted in an increase of lung colonies (4). In contrast, studies of spontaneous metastases from transplanted solid tumors gave conflicting results and most anticoagulants or fibrinolytic drugs failed to reproducibly influence the spontaneous spread of experimental tumors (5). Although this discrepancy may be partially explained by the difficulty of maintaining rodents in a long term state of anticoagulation, the main reason for the poor reproducibility of antimetastatic effects with anticoagulants in a spontaneous metastasis model was probably intrinsic differences in the model systems employed in these studies. Furthermore, many anticoagulants also interact with biological systems other than the coagulation cascade and additional pharmacological effects might have influenced the lodgment and subsequent growth of metastatic tumor cells.

IV. COUMARIN DERIVATIVES

Although a definite pathogenic link between drug-induced hypocoagulability and diminished tumor spread is not yet fully established, coumarin anticoagulants have emerged from these investigations as potent antimetastatic agents. They constitute a good example of the complexity of factors involved in experimental studies into the metastatic process. Oral anticoagulants of the coumarin type were widely used to investigate the effects of hypocoagulability on tumor dissemination in the models described above (sections IIA and B). A comparative evaluation of the literature on anticoagulants and experimental metastases revealed that only coumarin derivatives consistently produced a reduction of spontaneous metastasis in experimental animals, whereas all other anticoagulants (heparin, snake venoms, fibrinolytic enzymes) gave variable results (5). Apart from antimetastatic effects, inhibition of primary tumor growth by coumarin anticoagulation was reported (6) and in cancer patients oral anticoagulants improved the survival, even in disseminated disease (7). These observations suggested that coumarin anticoagulants may possess unique and exceptional properties as antitumor drugs.

A. Pharmacology and Toxicology of Coumarins

Besides their effects on the biosynthesis of vitamin K-dependent clotting factors, coumarin anticoagulants have a variety of pharmacological and toxicological properties which have to be considered in the present context. Alterations in blood vessel permeability and cardiovascular effects are well documented (8,9). In addition, some 4-hydroxy-coumarin derivatives appear to possess analgesic and antiinflammatory properties (10). Furthermore, coumarins inhibit the growth of bacteria (11). Other studies have suggested an important role for vitamin K in cell metabolism through its participation in mitochondrial oxidative phosphorylation (12). Closely related to the general pharmacology of coumarin anticoagulants is their toxicity and it should be remembered that 4-hydroxy-coumarin derivatives are potent rodenticides (13).

B. Antitumor Effects of Coumarins

In therapeutic doses coumarins are not cytotoxic. Preincubation of Lewis lung carcinoma cells with phenprocumon prior to implantation did not alter the kinetics of tumor growth (6). Coumarin anticoagulation throughout the growth of the lymphoid leukemia L1210 in DBA/2 mice did not influence the mean survival time of these animals (6) and short-term warfarin therapy was ineffective on primary or metatatic L1210 leukemia and adenocarcinoma 755 (14). In contrast, high doses of warfarin led to an inhibition of thymidine and uridine uptake into the DNA and RNA of L1210 leukemia cells (15). Kirsh and coworkers (16) showed that warfarin even at low concentrations inhibited cell replication of malignant human glial cells in culture. In accordance with this latter finding anticoagulation with warfarin selectively inhibited cancer cell motility in the rabbit ear chamber in vivo, an effect which could be reversed by the administration of vitamin K (17). Although coumarins apparently do not possess a major cytotoxic effect, the above data indicate that they can indirectly interfere with certain cellular functions which in turn might be of importance in the biology of malignant tumors.

C. Antimetastatic Effects of Coumarin Derivatives

Long term anticoagulation of animals bearing the subcutaneouly transplanted Lewis lung carcinoma resulted in a significant reduction of the number and incidence of spontaneous metastases to the lungs (6). Under identical experimental conditions neither heparin nor ancrod was effective, although the hypocoagulability induced by these two agents was comparable to that in the phenprocumon-treated group (5). These findings suggested that the therapeutic benefit of oral anti-coagulation was independent of the drug-induced coagulation effect. Further experiments revealed, however, that phenprocumon exhibited antitumor and antimetastatic effects only if a well controlled, continuous state of anticoagulation was achieved. In contrast, deliberate interruption of short term coumarin treatment did not influence primary and metastatic tumor growth (18). From a series of experiments with a methylcholanthrene-induced sarcoma in mice Hoover et al. (19) concluded that full anticoagulation in the range of 2.5 to 3 times the normal prothrombin time was required for a maximal antimetastatic effect and that there was a clear-cut dose response relationship for warfarin in these experiments.

To further elucidate the mechanism by which oral anticoagulants affect metastasis formation from blood-borne cancer cells, several experiments were carried out using the "lung colony assay." In accordance with the real events outlined above (see section IIA) the pharmacological prevention of microthrombosis requires hemostatically effective therapy at the time of and during a short period following tumor cell challenge. Pretreatment of C57BL mice with various anticoagulants followed by the intravenous injection of a suspension of viable Lewis lung carcinoma cells consistently resulted in a reduction in lung colonies, independent of the anticoagulant used. However, if anticoagulation with heparin, ancrod and urokinase was initiated 24 hr after the tumor cell challenge under otherwise identical experimental conditions, no influence whatsoever on the subsequent development of lung colonies was observed (20). In contrast, warfarin treatment was as effective as in the previous experiment. In the same experimental model the coumarin-induced coagulation defect was restored by the administration of prothrombin complex, yet, the "antimetastatic" effects were not abolished (20).

D. Vitamin K Deficiency and Experimental Metastases

The above experiments clearly indicated that coumarin treatment did not exert its mode of action through altered blood coagulability but that other mechanisms must account for the pronounced antitumor and antimetastatic effects. Poggi et al. (21) confirmed that the antimetastatic properties of racemic warfarin in the Lewis lung carcinoma, and further studies with its two enantiomers revealed that the effects were accounted for by the biologically active S(-)-warfarin isomer; R(+)-warfarin had no influence on the number and incidence of metastases. These observations indicated in connection with the data described above that the antimetastatic effects of coumarin anticoagulants were not related to a direct action of these compounds but required the impairment of vitamin K-availability (see Chapter 17). It could be shown that diet-induced vitamin K deficiency was as effective as coumarin anticoagulation in diminishing tumor colonies after i.v. tumor cell challenge (18) as well as in preventing spontaneous metastases from transplanted solid tumors (22). These experiments ruled out a direct drug effect and suggested that the mode by which coumarin anticoagulants act as antimetastatic agents was likely to involve vitamin K metabolism.

The role of vitamin K in protein synthesis has only recently been elucidated and it has become evident that this vitamin is not a unique coagulation vitamin but that it also takes part in the biosynthesis of a variety of other proteins with hitherto mostly unknown biological functions (23). Vitamin K is required for the postribosomal carboxylation of glutamic acid in these proteins, all of which subsequently exhibit high affinity for calcium and phospholipids. Hypothetically, reduction of these calcium and/or phospholipid binding sites on the cell membrane through vitamin K antagonists might profoundly influence the function of tumor cells or certain host target cells.

V. THE VITAMIN K DEPENDENT CANCER PROCOAGULANT

Although the host's coagulability appears to be of minor importance, the coagulation mechanism might be involved in the antimetastatic and antitumor effects of coumarin derivatives at a cellular level. Numerous enzymatic activities have been described in association with malignant cells and a factor X-activating enzyme, which appears to be present in many human and experimental neoplastic cells, is of particular interest in this context (24). The biological characteristics of this procoagulant activity were distinctly different from the factor VII-dependent thromboplastic activity of other cellular sources. Since this enzymatic activity appeared in serum-free media of fibroblasts after chemical transformation to the malignant phenotype, it was suggested that it might even represent a marker of malignancy (25). Further analysis indicated that the enzyme is a cysteine endopeptidase, thus being also chemically different from the other known factor X-activating serine proteinases (26 and Chapters 6 and 12). It was suggested that in the presence of malignancy an alternative cellular pathway exists in the initiation of blood clotting which bypasses the classical intrinsic and extrinsic mechanisms (27). The factor X-activating enzyme (cancer procoagulant A) appears to be actively secreted by the tumor cells because it can be detected in appreciable amounts in culture media as early as 2 hr after the addition of viable tumor cells (28). Furthermore, this enzyme activity is significantly decreased in tumors of animals treated with vitamin K antagonists indicating that its biosynthesis is vitamin K-dependent (28). Colucci et al. (29) confirmed the vitamin K-dependency of this enzyme and correlated the antimetastatic activity of coumarin anticoagulation to the levels of this vitamin K-dependent enzyme. Again, the systemic coagulation defect appeared of no significance since the administration of mouse prothrombin complex concentrate, although reversing the coagulation defect, did not alter the reduced cancer cell procoagulant activity. Further studies into the vitamin K-dependent cancer procoagulant might ultimately provide an explanation for the substantial antitumor effects of vitamin K antagonists.

VI. COUMARIN DERIVATIVES AND MACROPHAGES

Oral anticoagulants of the coumarin type can also alter host factors; this is suggested by the observation of their effects on peritoneal macrophages in mice. Although coumarin derivatives do not directly interact with macrophages, they can significantly enhance their sensitivity to activation by appropriate stimuli (18). The in vivo finding that macrophage poisons such as silica and carrageenin totally abolished the antimetastatic effect of warfarin in the Lewis lung carcinoma and in the B16 melanoma of mice provides evidence for an involvement of the macrophage system in the antitumor effects of these drugs (30)

VII. CONCLUSION

Independent of their relationship to or the validity of the microthrombosis concept, coumarin anticoagulants are potent antimetastatic drugs with well established activity in numerous experimental systems. Their evaluation in the clinic as antimetastatic drugs faces a major difficulty: the fundamental difference between the experimental and the clinical situation in relation to the time of diagnosis and treatment. Since most malignant human tumors will already be disseminated at the time of diagnosis, the efficacy of antimetastatic treatments is almost impossible to assess (see also Chapter 1). However, the profound effects of coumarin anticoagulants on established experimental tumors could be verified in the clinic and preliminary evidence suggests that such an approach is not only feasible but might also be successful (see Chapter 25).

REFERENCES

1. Schmidt MB. Die Verbreitungswege der Carcinome und die Beziehung generalisierter Sarkome zu den leukamischen Neubildungen. Fisher, Jena, 1903.
2. Wood S, Jr. Arch. Pathol. 66:550–568, 1958.
3. Hilgard P. In: The Thromboembolic Disorders (Eds. van de Loo J, Prentice CRM and Beller FK), Schattauer Verlag, Stuttgart, pp. 457–470, 1983.
4. Hilgard P and Thornes RD. Eur. J. Cancer 12:755–762, 1976.
5. Maat B and Hilgard P. J. Cancer Res. Clin. Oncol. 101:275–283, 1981.
6. Hilgard P, Schulte H, Wetzig G, Schmitt G and Schmidt CG. Br. J. Cancer 35:78–85, 1977.
7. Thornes RD. Cancer (Philadelphia) 35:91–97, 1975.
8. Matis P, Konold P, Mayer W and Liebaldt G. Thromb. Diath. Haemorrh. Suppl. 15:109–121, 1964.
9. Jindal MN and Shah DS. Arzneim.-Forsch./Drug Res. 16:878–881, 1966.
10. Fontaine L, Grand M, Quentin Y and Merle S. Med. Pharmacol. Exp. 13:137–154, 1965.
11. Goth A. Science 101:383, 1945.
12. Martius C and Nitz-Litzow D. Biochim. Biophys. Acta 12:134–140, 1953.
13. McGirr JL and Papworth DS. Vet. Rec. 67:124–131, 1955.
14. Higashi H and Heidelberger C. Cancer Chemotherp. Rep. Part I 55:29–33, 1971.
15. Chang JC and Hall TC. Oncology 28:232–236, 1973.

16. Kirsh WM, Schulz D, van Buskirk JJ and Young HE. J. Med. 5:69-75, 1974.
17. Thornes RD, Edlow DW and Wood S, Jr. Johns Hopkins Med. J. 123:305-324, 1968.
18. Hilgard P. In: Malginancy and the Hemostatic System (Eds. Donati MB, Dvaidson JF and Garattini S), Raven Press, New York, pp. 103-111, 1981.
19. Hoover HD, Jr., Jones D and Ketcham AS. Surgery 879:625-6730, 1976.
20. Hilgard P and Maat B. Eur. J. Cancer 15:183-187, 1979.
21. Poggi A, Mussoni L, Kornblihtt L, Ballabio E, de Gaetano G and Donati MB. Lancet 1:163-164, 1978.
22. Hilgard P. Br. J. Cancer 35:891-892, 1977.
23. Stenflo J. J. Biol. Chem. 251:355-363, 1976.
24. Gordon SG, Franks JJ and Lewis B. Thromb. Res. 6:127-131, 1975.
25. Gordon SG, Franks JJ and Lewis BJ. J. Natl. Cancer Inst. 62:773-778, 1979.
26. Gordon SG and Cross BA. J. Clin. Invest. 67:1665-1671, 1981.
27. Semeraro N and Donati MB. In: Malignancy and the Hemostatic System (Eds. Donati MB, Davidson JF and Garattini S), Raven Press, New York, pp. 65-81, 1981.
28. Hilgard P and Whur P. Br. J. Cancer 41:642-643, 1980.
29. Colucci M, Delaini F, de Bellis Vitti G, Locati D, Poggi A, Semeraro N and Donati MB. Biochem. Pharmacol. 32:1689-1691, 1983.
30. Maat B. Br. J. Cancer 41:313-316, 1980.

CHAPTER 18. MITOGENIC STIMULATION OF TUMOR CELLS BY PLATELET DERIVED GROWTH FACTORS

ALLAN LIPTON, CHERYL CANO AND KIM LEITZEL

I. INTRODUCTION

There is evidence that platelets are involved in the hematogenous spread of malignant tumors. Certain tumor cells aggregate platelet in vitro (1-4) and an intimate relationship between platelets and tumor cells is further suggested by ultrastructural studies in vivo which show arrested tumor emboli surrounded by platelets (5-8). Certain tumor lines also induce thrombocytopenia in vivo (1,5,9). The reasons for this close platelet-tumor cell relationship are speculative at present. Possibilities include: 1) protection by platelets of the tumor cell against immune destruction, 2) enhanced tumor cell transit of the vascular endothelium via platelet adherence or 3) tumor cell survival and multiplication due to release of platelet mitogenic factors.

The concept that platelets contain mitogenic factors developed from the observation by Balk (10) that chicken plasma was less effective than chicken serum for promoting the growth of chicken fibroblasts. He postulated either that the serum mitogenic factors are released from precursors in plasma or from thrombocytes when blood is clotted during the preparation of serum. Kohler and Lipton (11) and Ross et al. (12) extended this observation and actually demonstrated that platelets contain growth factor.

II. PLATELET-DERIVED GROWTH FACTOR FOR MESENCHYMAL CELLS (PDGF$_1$)

Extracts of frozen-thawed or thrombin treated platelets contain growth factor activity. This platelet-derived growth factor (PGDF$_1$) can stimulate the multiplication of fibroblasts (11,13), smooth muscle cells (12) and glial cells (14). It does not promote the growth of arterial endothelial cells or cells of epithelial origin.

Purification of a platelet-derived growth factor (PDGF$_1$) was facilitated by the observation that this molecule withstood heating for 10 minutes at 100°C and was a basic protein with an isoelectric point of about 9.8. This polypeptide growth factor that stimulates the proliferation of connective tissue cells has been purified by several groups. It is a protein with a molecular weight of approximately 30,000 daltons. PDGF$_1$ consists of two chains of approximately 17,000 and 14,000 molecular weight joined by disulfide bonds. Retention of the disulfide bonds in the native configuration is necessary for activity (14-17). A class of high-affinity receptors for $PDGF_1$ has been demonstrated on responsive cells using ^{125}I-ligand (14). The receptor is specific for $PDGF_1$ in the sense that other growth factors such as epidermal growth factor, fibroblast growth factor or insulin do not compete with [125]I-$PDGF_1$ for binding (14). In addition, various unresponsive cells such as those of epithelial origin show no significant specific binding of [125]I-$PDGF_1$. The cell surface receptor for $PDGF_1$ has been estimated to have a molecular weight of 164,000 daltons (20).

$PDGF_1$ has been localized subcellularly to the platelet α granules. It is released along with other α-granule constitutents (platelet factor 4, beta thromboglobulin and platelet fibrinogen) following stimulation with thrombin, arachidonic acid or collagen (21,22). Megakaryocytes are platelet precursors in the bone marrow that are known to be active in protein synthesis. Growth factor activity as determined by the stimulation of ^{3}H-thymidine incorporation into DNA of quiescent 3T3 cells in culture has recently been found in guinea pig bone marrow. Quantitative dilution studies demonstrated that, of the cells present in the guinea pig bone marrow, only the magakaryocyte possessed significant amounts of activity similar to $PDGF_1$ (23). The amount of activity present in one megakaryocyte was equivalent to that present in 1,000-5,000 platelets, approximately the number of platelets shed from a single megakaryocyte (23). Thus $PDGF_1$ appears to have its origin in the bone marrow megakaryocyte.

$PDGF_1$ plays a critical role in the cell cycle of nontransformed fibroblasts and other mesenchymal cells. Cells exposed to $PDGF_1$ are rendered "competent", i.e., they are potentially able to leave G_0 and enter the cell cycle (12,24). Fibroblast growth factor from bovine brain or pituitary gland and a factor recently purified from bovine spinal cord can also recruit quiescent cells into the cell cycle (25).

Progression of cells through G_1 and S requires the continual presence of platelet-poor plasma (24,26). Cells exposed to only $PDGF_1$ will not synthesize new DNA. The concentration of plasma determines, in part, the rate of entry of cells into the S phase. Factors in plasma that can mediate the progression of cells through G_1 and S phases include insulin and Somatomedin C (27).

$PDGF_1$ also stimulates many activities in cells that occur much earlier than increased thymidine incorporation. These include: an increased rate of endocytosis of tracer molecules (i.e., ^{14}C-sucrose) within an hour of $PDGF_1$ exposure (28); increased cholesterol synthesis (17); increased turnover of phospholipids (29); and increased binding of low density lipoprotein (LDL) to specific high-affinity receptor for this lipoprotein (17). More recently, $PDGF_1$ has been shown to be a chemoattractant for smooth muscle cells and fibroblasts (30). A role for this factor in the development of the atherosclerotic plaque and in normal wound healing has been postulated. We have, however, been unable to show that preparations of $PDGF_1$ can accelerate normal wound healing in a hamster model system (31).

III. PLATELET-DERIVED GROWTH FACTOR FOR TRANSFORMED CELLS (PDGF$_2$)

The first evidence that there might be several growth factors present in platelet extracts came from attempts to characterize the platelet mitogen (32,33). As mentioned, growth promoting activity in crude platelet extracts for 3T3 cells (PDGF$_1$) was stable after heating to 100°C for 10 minutes. In contrast, growth promoting activity for SV40 virus transformed 3T3 (SV3T3) cells in crude platelet extracts (PDGF$_2$) was destroyed by heating at 100°C for 5 min (Figures 1A and 1B).

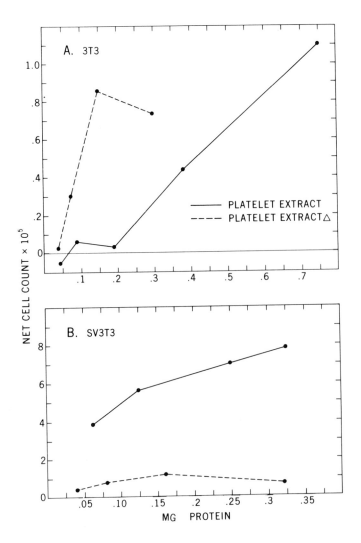

FIGURE 1. Heat Sensitivity of Mitogenic Activity for 3T3 and SV3T3 Cells from Human Platelets. Thirty to 80 units of outdated human platelet concentrates were pooled and spun at 163 x g for 10 min at room temperature to remove RBC. They were respun at 5875 x g for 10 min. The platelet button was washed and centrifuged 5 times at 5875 x g. Each wash was with 400 to 800 ml 0.85% (w/v) NaCl solution. The final platelet button was resuspended in 40 to 80 ml 0.85% NaCl solution. Washed platelets were either incubated at 37°C for 30 min or frozen and thawed 6 times and then centrifuged at 16,319 x g. The supernatant (platelet extract) was divided into 2 equal portions, and one portion was heated at 100°C for 5 min and then both portions were centrifigued at 500 x g. Both samples [heated (- -) and nonheated (—)] were sterilized using Millipore filters (0.22 μm) and tested in the standard assay for growth using the indicated amount of protein in 0.5 ml volume. In this assay, 3T3 and SV3T3 cells (10^5) were plated in 60 mm Falcon plastic dishes in 5 ml of Dulbecco's and Vogt's modification of Eagle's medium containing 0.4 and 0.15% (w/v) fetal calf serum (FCS), respectively, and cultures were incubated in 12% CO_2 at 37°C. This concentration of serum did not induce a significant increase in cell number per dish over a period of 4 days. The sample to be tested was added after 2-4 hours of incubation. Numbers of cells were determined in a Coulter counter 4 days after the start of the experiment. Net cell count was obtained by subtracting the number of cells in control plates (no additions) after 4 days of incubation. All cell counts were performed in duplicate; all experiments were repeated at least twice. [From Kepner and Lipton (33) with permission.]

These factors can be partially separated by gel filtration on a Sephadex G-100 gel column at pH 7.4 (Figure 2). The component that can selectively promote the growth of SV3T3 cells ($PDGF_2$) has a molecular weight of 72,000 daltons. Its effect appears to be quite specific in that the SV3T3-active fractions do not promote the growth of 3T3 cells (Figure 2). The platelet factor that promotes the growth of SV3T3 cells ($PDGF_2$) is stable on exposure to 4 M guandidine hydrochloride, but is destroyed by treatment with sodium metaperiodate (0.05 M at 4°C for 48 hr) and is partially inactivated by trypsin treatment.

$PDGF_2$ can be absorbed on to a Concanavalin A-Sepharose column and specifically eluted with methyl- β-D-glycopyranoside. Active fractions (Pool tubes #45-59) are 100-200 times more active than the platelet lysate in promoting SV3T3 growth. It would thus appear that the mitogenic activity for SV3T3 cells from human platelets ($PDGF_2$) is due to a glycoprotein with an isoelectric point of 7.8-8.3 (32,33). In this regard, $PDGF_2$ differs from $PDGF_1$ which focuses between 9.6 and 10.2 with a peak activity at 9.8. It should also be mentioned that partially purified fractions from Figures 2 and 3 that contain $PDGF_2$ activity do not induce competence in quiescent 3T3 cells.

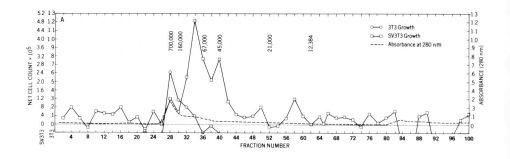

FIGURE 2. Sephadex G-100 Gel Filtration of Extract of Human Platelets. Platelet extracts were prepared as described in the legend to Figure 1. Six ml of extract were placed on a 3 x 80 cm Sephadex G-100 column containing 0.01 M Tris-HCl (pH 7.4) at 4°C. Five ml fractions were collected and sterilized using 0.22 µm Millipore filters. The growth assays for 3T3 and SV3T3 cells were performed as described in the legend to Figure 1 using 0.5 ml of each column fraction. Markers used were thyroglobulin (700,000), human γ-globulin (160,000), bovine albumin (67,000), ovalbumin (45,000), soybean trypsin inhibitor (21,000) and cytochrome c (12,000 daltons). [From Kepner and Lipton (33) with permission.]

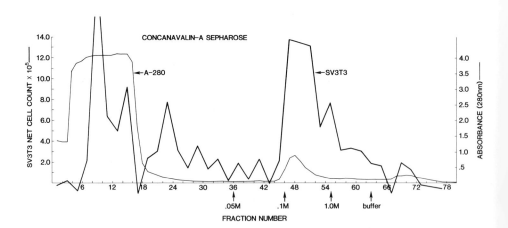

FIGURE 3. Con A-Sepharose Chromatography of PDGF$_2$ Activity. Platelet extracts were prepared as described in the legend to Figure 1. The platelet extract was then concentrated four-fold by lyophilization, dialyzed and 30 ml was placed on a 2 x 11.5 cm Con A-Sepharose column, 0.01 M Tris - 0.01 M NaCl (pH 8.0) at 4°C. After 100 ml were collected, a step wise gradient using 0.05, 0.1 and 1.0 M methyl- β -D-glucopyranoside as indicated was employed. Five ml fractions were collected and sterilized. From each column fraction, 0.25 ml was added to SV3T3 cells in a growth assay as described in the legend to Figure 1.

The preceding work was performed using cells transformed by the SV40 viral genome. Another means by which transformation can be induced is by incubation of cell cultures with chemical carcinogens. These cells, too, no longer grow in orderly fashion, have a decreased serum requirement and result in tumors when injected into animals. Treatment of an epithelial rat liver cell line, K-16, with N-acetoxy-2-acetylamino-fluorene produced a transformed cell line, W-8. This line is stimulated by fractions which contain PDGF$_2$ activity. Similarly, cell line NQ-T-1, derived from Balb/c 3T3 cells by treatment with 4-nitroquinoline 1-oxide, was stimulated to multiply by fractions containing both PDGF$_1$ and PDGF$_2$ activity while the parental Balb-3T3 line was stimulated only by fractions containing PDGF$_1$ activity.

Human platelet extract has also been shown to stimulate the multiplication of rat epithelial cell mammary tumor cells (34) and many cancer-derived cell lines (35,36). More recently platelet extracts have been shown to promote the growth of human cancer cells in the stem cell tumor assay system (37). Thus, the heat labile, non-dialyzable glycoprotein present in platelet extracts can promote the in vitro growth of a wide variety of transformed cells.

All the experiments described to this point were performed with cells grown in tissue culture. We next asked the question, can platelet extracts accelerate tumor growth in the whole animal? Oncogenic transformation of hamster embryo fibroblast (HEF) cells has been accomplished using ultraviolet (UV)-irradiated herpes simplex virus type 2 (HSV-2). Such virally transformed cells regularly produce tumors when injected into random-bred weanling Syrian hamsters (3-4 weeks old) (38,39). We chose this model because HSV-2 is a putative human tumor virus and consistently produces tumors.

One hundred HSV-2 transformed HEF cells were injected into the cheek pouch of fifty random-bred weanling female Syrian hamsters (3-4 weeks old) on day 1 only. The viability of injected cell suspensions was checked by trypan blue exclusion and was greater than 90 percent. This dose of cells was chosen for injection because in control experiments 85% of the animals receiving 10,000 cells developed tumors by week 4 after injection. In addition to tumor cells the initial injection contained either (a) 0.2 ml Krebs-Henseleit buffer (10 animals), (b) 0.2 ml Dulbecco's medium (10 animals) and (c) 0.2 ml crude platelet extract (15 animals). Repeat injections of 0.2 ml of

(a) to (c) were made into the appropriate animal's cheek pouch on days 2, 4 and 6 without cells.

Platelet extract for these experiments was prepared by pooling thirty to eighty units of outdated human platelet concentrates. This pool was spun at 163 x g for 10 min to remove RBC's. They were respun at 5875 x g for 10 min. The platelet button was washed and centrifuged 5 times at 5875 x g. Each wash was with 400-800 ml isotonic saline. The final platelet button was resuspended in 40-80 ml isotonic saline. The washed platelet button was incubated at 37°C for 30 min, then centrifuged at 16,319 x g. The supernatant (crude platelet extract) was concentrated four-fold by lyophilization and sterilized using a 0.22 μm Millipore filter.

Figures 4A and 4B summarize the results in hamsters injected in the cheek pouch with 100 HSV-2 transformed HEF cells. Each experiment was performed three times. Animals that received concomitant injections of either Krebs-Henseleit buffer or Dulbecco's medium did not develop tumors over the 15 week period of observation. Animals that were not injected with transformed cells and received only $PDGF_2$ also did not develop tumors. Thrirty-three percent of hamsters injected with platelet extract developed palpable tumors by week 7 (Figure 4A). At the termination of the experiment at week 14, sixty percent of hamsters injected with platelet extract developed readily visible tumors at the injection site (Figure 4B). Tumors were anaplastic spindle cell tumors with some epitheloid differentiation. These results were highly significant when compared to animals injected with Krebs buffer or Dulbecco's medium ($p < 0.001$). At the time they were sacrificed, all hamsters were free of disseminated tumors.

The mechanism of enhancement of tumor growth is speculative at present. We do feel that it is due to a direct stimulative effect resulting in enhanced multiplication of tumor cells and not due to immunosuppression of the host. The reason for this is that the hamster cheek pouch is an immunologically privileged sanctuary.

In conclusion, human platelets contain discrete macromolecules that promote the growth of 3T3 ($PDGF_1$) and SV3T3 cells ($PDGF_2$). Both appear to be proteins. The factor that promotes the growth of SV3T3 and a variety of other transformed cell lines is heat labile, non-dialyzable and has an isoelectric point of 7.8 - 8.3. Platelet extracts that contain $PDGF_2$ activity can promote the in vitro as well as in vivo growth of transformed cells. These observations would appear to offer several new strategies for cancer therapy such as (a) selective inhibition of the multiplication of cancer cells by removal or inhibition of the growth stimulatory glycoprotein $PDGF_2$, e.g., specific antibody to inhibit action or removal on appropriate ion exchange or adsorption resin and (b) use of the stimulatory features of $PDGF_2$ to promote tumor cells to enter a dividing state in which all the cells would be susceptible to cycle-active chemotherapy. At present many human tumors are refractory to chemotherapy because cells are in a dormant or non-dividing state.

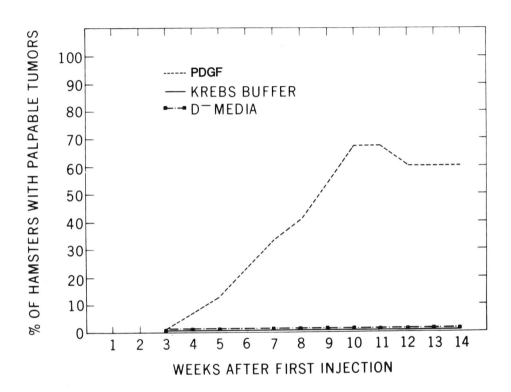

FIGURE 4. Effects of PDGF$_2$ on Hamster Tumors Formed by HSV-2 Transformed HEF Cells. [From Witkoski et al. (40) with permission.] 4A. Percentage of hamsters with palpable tumors after injection with the transformed cells and PDGF$_2$, Krebs–Henseleit buffer or Dulbecco's medium.

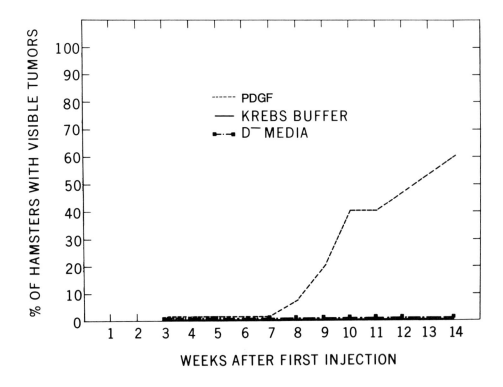

FIGURE 4B. Percentage of hamsters with visible tumors after injection with the transformed cells and PDGF$_2$, Krebs-Henseleit buffer and Dulbecco's medium.

IV. TRANSFORMING GROWTH FACTORS (TGF) FROM TUMOR CELLS

The transforming growth factors (TGFs) are a newly discovered class of cell growth agents. TGFs are low molecular weight polypeptides produced by rodent and human tumor cells and which are capable of reversibly stimulating nontransformed cells to grow as colonies in soft agar. Stimulation of anchorage-independent cell growth is the in vitro transformation parameter which most closely correlates with in vivo tumorigenicity (41). TGFs also have the capacity to stimulate the division of cell monolayers and to induce morphological cell changes.

TGF was first described in the culture medium of Moloney virus sarcoma transformed mouse cells and was called sarcoma growth factor (SGF) (42). Following this initial observation, several mammalian cells have been shown to contain or release related growth factors displaying several common biological and physiochemical characteristics (43). In vitro, the spontaneous release of TGFs has only been observed with transformed cell lines from different mammalian species: human tumor cells (44), spontaneously transformed rat cells and rat cells transformed by Kirsten murine sarcoma virus (45,46) or Simian virus 40 (SV40) (47) or Rous sarcoma virus (48) and chemically transformed mouse cells (49). But, in vivo, TGFs can be recovered by acid-ethanol extraction not only from grafted tumors in the rat and mouse (43) but also from normal mouse organs (50). More recently TGF activity has been identified in acid-ethanol extracts of human urine (51).

TGFs are acid and heat stable polypeptides which contain disulfide bonds (42,43). TGFs isolated from human sarcoma and carcinoma cell lines have molecular weights in the 7,000 and 20,000-23,000 size classes (44). The larger form has not been detected in the conditioned medium of tumor cells growing in culture. In contrast, a low molecular weight TGF activity (6,000-8,000 daltons) is found in human urine but a high molecular weight TGF activity (30,000-35,000 daltons) is found in the urine of many cancer patients (51). TGFs can compete with epidermal growth factor (EGF) for binding to the EGF cell membrane receptor and thus may be functionally related to this molecule (44,52). More recently, TGFs which do not compete with EGF for binding to its receptor have been identified in both normal and transformed rodent cells and have been shown to lack soft agar growth-promoting activity except in the presence of added EGF (50,53).

At present there is no answer as to what is the ultimate source of growth factor activity for cancer cells growing in humans. As outlined above such mitogenic activity may be produced by the cancer cells themselves or be released from circulating platelets. It would appear as if there are chemical differences between these two types of factors. It is possible that both factors may be involved in the growth of certain cancers. In other cancers one factor may play a dominant role in promoting growth. This information would be of utmost importance in learing to interrupt the influence of mitogenic factors on cancer cells and thus inhibit their growth.

V. CLINICAL TRIAL – ADJUVANT ASPIRIN THERAPY IN COLO-RECTAL CANCER

The intimate relationship between platelets and cancer cells appears to be an essential early step in tumor cells traversing the endothelial lining and establishing metastatic foci. It would thus appear logical to attempt to interrupt this contact using antiplatelet agents.

Antiplatelet agents have inhibited the spread of tumor cells in animal model systems. Gasic and coworkers (1,54) first reported on the antimetastatic effects of aspirin in two experimental animal model systems – MCA2 fibrosarcoma and T241 fibrosarcoma tumor cells. These same workers had previously reported that thrombocytopenia induced by either neuraminidase or antiplatelet serum significantly reduced metastasis formation upon injection of TA3 ascites tumor cells (55).

276

Kolenich et al. (56) also showed that aspirin administration resulted in a significant reduction in pulmonary metastases following injection of adenocarcinoma cells or KHT sarcoma cells in mice. However, negative results employing aspirin have been reported by Hilgard and coworkers using the V_2 carcinoma of rabbits (57) and Lewis lung carcinoma (58). The present study was designed to learn if aspirin could prevent the subsequent development of metastases in patients with Duke's "B_2" and "C" cancer of the colon.

A. Patient Selection and Treatment Protocol

Sixty-six patients with Duke's B_2 and C colon or rectal cancer (59) were selected for this study. All patients had undergone a "curative' resection for colo-rectal cancer (malignancy between the ileo-cecal valve and the anus). The surgery took place no more than 10 weeks before starting on this protocol. Patients were not receiving any medication known to affect platelet function.

Patients were stratified 1) as to whether they had a Duke's "B_2" or "C" lesion, 2) according to the site of the lesion in the colon (ascending, transverse, descending) or rectum and 3) whether they received radiation therapy or not. Patients were then randomized to receive either aspirin (ASA) 600 mg p.o. twice daily x 2 years or placebo (P). Compliance was checked in both groups by random measurement of blood salicylate levels.

B. Results

Sixty-six patients with Duke's "B_2" or "C" colon or rectal cancer were selected for study. Nine patients are inevaluable at this time (Table 1). Thus, there were 57 randomized, evaluable patients – 35 ASA (10 "B_2" + 25 "C") vs 22 P (3 "B_2 + 19 "C").

Table 1. Patients with Duke's B_2 or C Colo-Rectal Cancer.

66 Selected Patients

9 Inevaluable Patients

1 Lost to followup

2 Refused to take pills after randomization

1 Unsure patient took medication

5 On therapy less than one month

57 Evaluable Patients

The two groups of patients are comparable with respect to median number of positive lymph nodes at surgery (ASA 3 vs P 2) and number of patients who received radiation therapy (ASA 8 vs P 6). The median pre-operative carcinoembryonic antigen (CEA) was lower in the ASA group (median = 2.8) when compared to a median pre-op CEA of 6.7 in the placebo patients. The median duration of patients on study is 24 months for ASA and 28 months for P.

Life table analysis fails to demonstrate any difference in diseasefree (p = 0.66) (Figure 5) or overall survival (p = 0.90) (Figure 6) for these two groups of patients. In similar fashion, when only the Duke's "C" patients are analyzed there is no trend favoring the ASA treated patients. Sites of metastases are also similar for ASA and P patients. Most of the relapses occurred within the abdominal cavity. Only three patients had distant metastases without also having disease within the confines of the abdominal cavity.

We next looked to see if the time at which ASA therapy was started following surgery (within 2 or within 4 wk) affected disease-free or overall survival. Again no difference was found when compared with P patients (p = 0.48 and 0.91 at 2 and 4 wk, respectively).

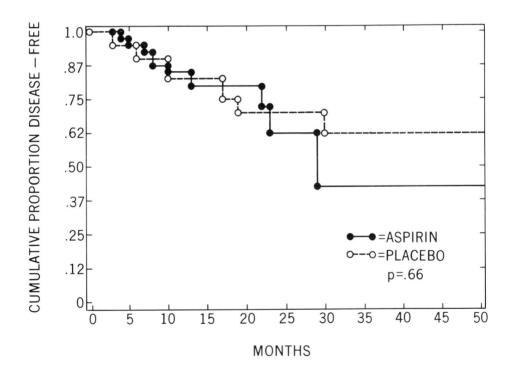

FIGURE 5. Life Table Analysis of Disease-Free Interval of Duke's B_2 and C Colo-Rectal Patients Treated with Aspirin or Placebo. [From Lipton et al. (60) with permission.]

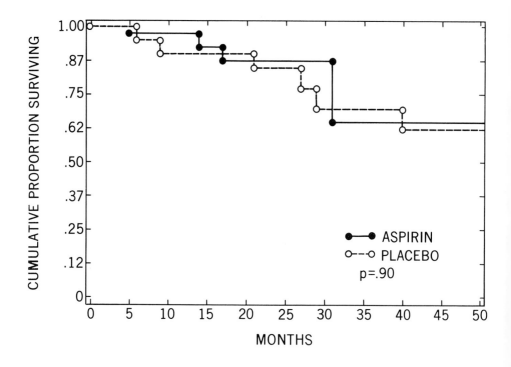

FIGURE 6. Life Table Analysis of Survival of Duke's B₂ and C Colo-Rectal Patients Treated with Aspirin or Placebo. [From Lipton et al. (60) with permission.]

Aspirin is a most commonly used medication in our society. As a result, compliance with any ASA study is always highly suspect. Random blood salicylate levels were obtained on selected patients. No P patient had a salicylate level greater than 3 mg/dl. By contrast, 10 of 12 ASA treated patients had a salicylate level of 4 mg/dl or greater (median = 6.4 mg/dl). The therapeutic range for salicylate level in our laboratory is 4-25 mg/dl. Toxicity in this study was minimal. No severe gastrointestinal or bleeding events were reported.

C. Future Directions

In this analysis of 57 evaluable patients with Duke's B₂ and C colo-rectal cancer we found no difference between patients treated with aspirin or placebo. Furthermore, there was no advantage in patients started on aspirin within 2 or 4 weeks of surgery when compared with placebo patients. No subgroup benefited from treatment with conventional dose aspirin.

Despite the lack of therapeutic efficacy reported in this trial with a conventional dose of aspirin we would still advocate further studies of antiplatelet therapy in man. Many variables must still be explored. Aspirin at the dose used above might be tried in other types of cancer. The dose of aspirin chosen was that used in many cardiovascular studies. This may well turn out to be too high. Platelet cyclooxygenase appears to be more sensitive to aspirin than the arterial endothelial cell cyclooxygenase (61) (See also Chapter 13). As a result "low dose" aspirin might have greater therapeutic efficacy. Finally, other antiplatelet agents also should be explored. These include phosphodiesterase inhibitors and agents that elevate prostacyclin levels (See Chapter 14). Current ongoing clinical studies will be outlined in a later chapter of this book.

ACKNOWLEDGEMENT

The authors wish to thank Mrs. Judy Weigel for her help in preparing this manuscript.

REFERENCES

1. Gasic GJ, Gasic TB, Galanti N, Johnson T and Murphy S. Int. J. Cancer 11:704-718, 1973.
2. Gasic GJ, Boettiger D, Catalfamo JL, Gasic TB and Stewart GJ. Cancer Res. 38:2950-2955, 1977.
3. Marcum JM, McGill M, Bastida E, Ordinas A and Jamieson GA. J. Lab. Clin. Med. 96:1046-1053, 1980.
4. Pearlstein E, Cooper LB and Karpatkin S. J. Lab. Clin. Med. 93:332-344, 1979.
5. Hilgard P and Gordon-Smith EC. Br. J. Haematol. 26:651-659, 1974.
6. Jones JD, Wallace AC and Fraser EF. J. Natl. Cancer Inst. 46:493-504, 1971.
7. Sindelar WF, Tralka TS and Ketcham AS. J. Surg. Res. 18:137-161, 1975.
8. Warren BA and Vales O. Br. J. Exp. Pathol. 53:301-313, 1972.
9. Hilgard P. Br. J. Cancer 28:429-435, 1973.
10. Balk SD. Proc. Natl. Acad. Sci. USA 68:271-276, 1971.
11. Kohler N and Lipton A. Exp. Cell Res. 87:297-301, 1974.
12. Ross R, Glomset B, Kariya B and Harker L. Proc. Natl. Acad. Sci. USA 71:1207-1210, 1974.
13. Rutherford RB and Ross R. J. Cell Biol. 69:196-203, 1976.
14. Heldin C-H, Westermark B and Wasteson A. Proc. Natl. Acad. Sci. USA 78:3664-3668, 1981.
15. Raines E and Ross R. J. Biol. Chem. 257:5154-5160, 1982.
16. Deuel TF, Huang JS, Profitt RT, Baenziger JR, Change D and Kennedy BB. J. Biol. Chem. 256:8896-8899, 1981.
17. Antoniades HN, Scher CD and Stiles CD. Proc. Natl. Acad. Sci. USA 76:1809-1813, 1979.
18. Heldin CH, Westermark B and Wasteson A. J. Biol. Chem. 257:4216-4221, 1982.
19. Bowen-Pope DF and Ross R. J. Biol. Chem. 257:5161-5171, 1982.
20. Glenn KC, Bowen-Pope DF and Ross R. J. Biol. Chem. 257:5172-5176, 1982.

280

21. Witte LD, Kaplan KL, Nossel HL, Lages BA, Weiss HJ and Goodman DS. Circ. Res. 42:402-406, 1978.
22. Kaplan KL, Broekman MJ, Chernoff A, Lesznik GR and Drillings M. Blood 53:604-609, 1979.
23. Chernoff A, Goodman DS and Levine RF. J. Clin. Invest. 65:926-929, 1980.
24. Pledger W, Stiles C, Antoniades H and Scher C. Proc. Natl. Acad. Sci. USA 74:2839-2845, 1978.
25. Jennings T, Jones R and Lipton A. J. Cell. Physiol. 100:273-277, 1979.
26. Vogel A, Raines E, Kariya B, Rivest M-J and Ross R. Proc. Natl. Acad. Sci. USA 75:2810-2814, 1978.
27. Clemmons DR and Van Wyk JJ. J. Cell. Physiol. 106:361-366, 1981.
28. Davies PF and Ross R. J. Cell Biol. 79:663-671, 1978.
29. Habenicht A, Glomset JA, King WC, Nist C, Mitchell DC and Ross R. J. Biol. Chem. 256:12329-12335, 1981.
30. Grotendorst GR, Chang T, Seppa HEJ, Kleinman HK and Martin GR. J. Cell. Physiol. 113:261-266, 1982.
31. Leitzel K, Cano C, Marks J and Lipton A. Manuscript submitted for publication.
32. Kepner N, Creasy G and Lipton A. In: Platelets: A Multidisciplinary Approach. (Eds. deGaetano G and Garattini S), Raven Press, New York, pp. 205-212, 1978.
33. Kepner N and Lipton A. Cancer Res. 41:430-432, 1981.
34. Eastment CT and Sirbasku DA. J. Cell. Physiol. 97:17-27, 1978.
35. Eastment CT and Sirbasku DA. In Vitro 16:694-699, 1980.
36. Hara Y, Steiner M and Baldini MG. Cancer Res. 40:1212-1216, 1980.
37. Cowan DH and Graham J. In: Interaction of Platelets and Tumor Cells (Eds. Jamieson GA and Scipio AR), Alan R. Liss, Inc., New York, pp. 249-268, 1982.
38. Duff R and Rapp F. Nature (London) 233:48-50, 1971.
39. Duff R and Rapp F. J. Virol. 8:469-477, 1971.
40. Witkoski E, Kempner N, Leitzel K, Rogers C, Jefferson LS and Lipton A. Cancer Res. 42:2350-2352, 1982.
41. Kahn P, Simon RS, Klein AS and Shin S. Cold Spring Harbor Symp. Quant. Biol. 44:695-702, 1980.
42. DeLarco JE and Todaro GJ. Proc. Natl. Acad. Sci. USA 75:4001-4005, 1978.
43. Roberts AB, Lamb LC, Newton DL, Sporn MB and DeLarco JE. Proc. Natl. Acad. Sci. USA 77:3494-3498, 1980.
44. Todaro GJ, Fryling C and DeLarco JE. Proc. Natl. Acad. Sci. USA 77:5258-5262, 1980.
45. Ozanne B, Fulton RJ and Kaplan PL. J. Cell. Physiol. 105:163-180, 1980.
46. DeLarco JE, Preston YA and Todaro GJ. J. Cell. Physiol. 109:143-152, 1981.
47. Kaplan PL, Topp WC and Ozanne B. Proc. Natl. Acad. Sci. USA 79:485-489, 1981.
48. Kryceve-Martinerie C, Lawrence DA, Crochet J, Jullien P and Vigier P. J. Cell. Physiol. 113:365-372, 1982.
49. Moses HL, Branum EL, Proper JA and Robinson RA. Cancer Res. 41:2842-2848, 1980.
50. Roberts AB, Anzano MA, Lamb LC, Smith JM and Sporn MB. Proc. Natl. Acad. Sci. USA 78:5339-5343, 1981.
51. Sherwin SA, Twardzik DR, Bohn WH, Cockley KD and Todaro GJ. Cancer Res. 43:403-407, 1983.
52. Marquardt H and Todaro GJ. J. Biol. Chem. 257:5220-5225, 1982.
53. Roberts AB, Anzano MA, Lamb LC, Smith JM, Frolik CA, Marquardt H, Todaro GJ and Sporn MB. Nature (London) 295:417-419, 1982.
54. Gasic GJ, Gasic TB and Murphy S. Lancet 2:932-933, 1977.
55. Gasic GJ, Gasic TB and Stewart CC. Proc. Natl. Acad. Sci. USA 61:46-52, 1968.
56. Kolenich JJ, Mansour EG and Flynn A. Lancet 2:932-933, 1977.
57. Wood S Jr. and Hilgard P. Lancet 2:1416-1417, 1972.
58. Hilgard P, Heller H and Schmidt CG. Z. Krebsforsch. 86:243-250, 1976.

59. Astler VB and Coller FA. Ann. Surg. 139:846–852, 1954.
60. Lipton A, Scialla S, Harvey H, Dixon R, Gordon R, Hamilton R, Ramsey H, Weltz M, Heckard R and White D. J. Med. 13:419–429, 1982.
61. Wu KK. J. Clin. Invest. 68:382–387, 1981.

CHAPTER 19.   ROLE OF THE VASCULAR ENDOTHELIUM IN HEMOSTASIS

BABETTE B. WEKSLER AND MARGARET LEWIN

I.   STRUCTURE OF ENDOTHELIUM

The vascular endothelium provides a thromboresistant, blood-compatible interface between the blood and the vessel wall. This monolayer of flattened, polygonal cells lines the entire vascular tree and thus comprises one of the largest surfaces of the body.

Considerable variation in structure and function exist in endothelium from different regions. The thickest endothelium is in the aorta (1 μm) and the thinnest in the capillaries (less than 0.1 μm) (1); the endothelium is continuous in arteries, veins and muscular capillaries but is fenestrated in the visceral capillaries (1). Arterial endothelium has complex tight intracellular junctions interpolated with gap junctions, whereas the junctions in veins are more loosely organized (2). Capillaries have only tight junctions; the endothelium of cerebral capillaries has particularly tight junctions which are important in constituting the blood-brain barrier (3,4). The luminal surface of aortic and large artery endothelium is relatively smooth, while that of the pulmonary vessels is covered with multiple microvilli, increasing the surface area markedly (1). Within the vascular tree, the capillaries comprise the greatest surface area, providing more than 1 m^2 surface (100,000,000 cells) per ml of blood volume (5).

Endothelial cells in arteries and veins are arranged in hemodynamically determined patterns aligned with their long axes in the direction of blood flow. However, near branch points and bifurcations where flow is not laminar, the cells assume a more polygonal shape without longitudinal orientation (1). The latter areas show more vaculated endothelial junctions, contain more lysosomes and endoplasmic reticulum, undergo greater cell turnover than do the flow-oriented areas (6) and display greater vascular permeability when tested with intravenous Evans blue dye.

Intact endothelium does not activate platelets or the coagulation mechanism, and thus is nonthrombogenic. This state involves both active and passive properties of the endothelium. Factors which contribute to endothelial thromboresistance include: 1) a negative surface charge, 2) binding of heparin-like substances on the luminal surface, 3) secretion by endothelium of antiplatelet and fibrinolytic substances, 4) the presence of proteinase inhibitors, 5) inactivation and/or regulation of coagulation factors on the surface and 6) clearance of coagulation factors, vasoactive mediators and autacoids.

II. ANTITHROMBOTIC FUNCTIONS OF ENDOTHELIUM

A. Surface Charge

First among the possible mechanisms by which endothelium maintains nonthrombogenicity is surface charge. Endothelial cells, like most cells, bear a net negative surface charge. Part of the negative charge results from the presence at the cell surface of sulfated glycosaminoglycans such as heparan sulfate and heparin-like substances which are synthesized by the endothelial cells and secreted to form a thick glycocalyx (7-9). Additional negative charge comes from sialic acid-containing surface glycoproteins. Distribution of the anionic cell surface sites in vessel segments and in cultured endothelial cells is uniform in undisturbed cells (10). However, after binding positively charged molecules such as cationized ferritin, anionic patches are rapidly formed on the luminal surface of the endothelial cells, followed by endocytosis of the bound cationic material and reappearance of new anionic sites on the cell surface (11,12). Neuraminidase treatment of the cells to eliminate sialic acid-dependent anionic sites removed about 50% of the binding sites for cationized ferritin (11). However, the negative charge of the luminal surface of endothelium does not appear to be the main factor in its thromboresistance, as the subendothelium, which is highly thrombogenic, is similarly negatively charged (1). Moreover, virus-transformed endothelium, which is thrombogenic for platelets, has a negative surface charge similar to that of normal endothelium (which does not produce platelet adherence) (13).

B. Heparin-like Substances

Another important factor in the nonthrombogenicity of the endothelial surface is the presence of heparan sulfate in the glycocalyx. This anticoagulant glycosaminoglycan is synthesized and secreted by endothelial cells. Heparan sulfate, although less highly charged than heparin and a less potent anticoagulant, can activate antithrombin III, and bind platelet factor 4 (PF4) and thrombin (14). The parts of the vasculature having the highest concentration of heparan and dermatan sulfates have the greatest thromboresistance (14).

In addition the endothelial surface coat efficiently binds heparin (15). Cultured endothelial cells bind up to 1,000,000 molecules heparin per cell in a time dependent, saturable process, and this heparin remains biologically active (15). Heparins of high and low anticoagulant potency bind equally well. Thus, the thromboresistant potential of endothelium can be enhanced in the presence of exogenous as well as endogenous heparin.

C. Proteinase Inhibitors

The plasma proteinase inhibitor, α_2-macroglobulin, is localized at the luminal surface of endothelial cells of arteries, veins and lymphatics. Since immunofluorescent staining techniques do not demonstrate α_2-macroglobulin in endothelial cytoplasm, this inhibitor probably originates elsewhere and then binds to the endothelial surface membrane. Another major plasma proteinase inhibitor, α_1-antitrypsin is not present on endothelial cells (16).

D.   Thrombin and the Endothelium

Thrombin is bound to vascular endothelium on its first pass through the circulation (5). Two populations of binding sites have been identified; these bind active thrombin and active site-inhibited thrombin (e.g., diisopropylfluorophosphate-treated thrombin) equally well (17). DIP-thrombin is 90% cleared (mainly in the lungs) within one min after intravenous or intraarterial infusion into rabbits. Active thrombin is less rapidly cleared, 55% remaining at 10 min, but is very rapidly bound to antithrombin III and circulates as a complex (18). Preconfluent endothelial cells, or cells proliferating after injury, bind 20 times more thrombin than do confluent endothelial cells (19). This increased thrombin-binding capacity of regenerating endothelium helps to inactivate excess proteinase activity locally generated after injury.

Thrombin has multiple effects upon endothelial function, some antithrombotic, others prothrombotic. It is of interest that thrombin can act as a cofactor which enhances the proliferative response of endothelial cells to other growth factors (20). Thrombin also stimulates the synthesis of the potent antiaggregant prostacyclin (PGI_2, see G below) in certain types of vascular endothelium, e.g., human (21,22) or ovine (23) umbilical venous endothelial cells, but does not stimulate PGI_2 synthesis in bovine or porcine aortic endothelium (21,24). Nevertheless, thrombin binding is a property of all types of endothelium. Prothrombotic functions of endothelial-bound thrombin include induction of endothelial cell contraction, the release of adenine nucleotides and von Willebrand factor (VWF) and the inhibition of plasminogen activator release (see E below).

E.   Endothelium and Fibrinolysis

Another important function of endothelium in hemostasis is its ability to potentiate the thrombin-catalyzed activation of Protein C (25,27). Protein C, a vitamin K dependent serine proteinase zymogen, is a potent anticoagulant and stimulator of fibrinolysis; it inactivates coagulation factors Va and VIIIa. The endothelium contains a cofactor for the activation of Protein C by thrombin (25). This cofactor, termed thrombomodulin, is a 75,000 dalton, calcium dependent protein which binds to thrombin on the endothelial cell surface and increases the rate of activation of Protein C by 20,000 fold (26,27). Activated Protein C also stimulates the release of plasminogen activator from endothelium (see below). Thus, by its role in the activation of Protein C, endothelium can modulate the inactivation of two coagulation factors (Va and VIIIa) and stimulate fibrinolysis. Activated Protein C can also inactivate the factor Xa receptor on platelets by cleaving its factor Va portion, and thus modulate platelet procoagulant activity as well (28).

The endothelium has an additional role in fibrinolysis: it synthesizes and secretes plasminogen activators and inhibitors. Tissue activator, a membrane bound protein, is produced and secreted by endothelial cells as a urokinase-like activator, a cytoplasmic protein (29,30). Confluent cells secrete more tissue activator than do proliferating endothelial cells, and tumor promoters such as phorbol ester enhance tissue activator secretion in vitro (30,31). The principal plasminogen activator of endothelial cells directly cleaves plasminogen to active plasmin; this process is catalyzed by fibrin (30). Fibrin binds the tissue activator in a complex which markedly enhances plasminogen cleavage. Since plasminogen also binds to fibrin the activity of the endothelial plasminogen activator is concentrated in areas of clot formation. The tissue activator has very little direct activity against fibrinogen and, therefore, preferentially stimulates fibrinolysis rather than fibrinogenolysis. Other agents, such as des-amino-D-arginine vasopressin, stimulate the release of endothelial plasminogen activator (32). Thrombin, in contrast, inhibits tissue activator secretion by endothelial cells (33). An acid labile inhibitor of plasminogen activation is present in the cytoplasm of endothelial cells and is released upon cell injury (30).

F. Other Surface Membrane Properties

Several surface enzymes of endothelial cells are important in modulating hemostasis. Angiotensin converting enzyme is localized to the luminal surface of endothelium particularly in the pulmonary vasculature but also in systemic vessels (34-36). This enzyme catalyzes the conversion of angiotensin I to angiotensin II, a potent vasoconstrictor which also induces PGI_2 synthesis by endothelium. Bradykinin, which can induce PGI_2 synthesis, is also inactivated by angiotensin converting enzyme (37). Pulmonary endothelium is also known to bind C3a, the anaphylatoxic peptide fragment of the third component of complement (38). Carboxypeptidase N (kininase II) which degrades C3a is also present on the surface of pulmonary endothelial cells (39).

Endothelium releases adenine nucleotides which are rapidly degraded by the ecto-ADPase present on the plasma membrane (40). The end product is adenosine which inhibits platelet aggregation. Thrombin induces adenine nucleotide release but factor Xa does not (41). The released nucleotide products may either promote platelet aggregation (ADP or ATP) or inhibit it (AMP or adenosine) depending on the relative rates of release and degradation.

Pulmonary endothelium in particular can inactivate many prostaglandins with vasoactive properties, such as PGE_1 and PGE_2, which are taken up by an active transport system and degraded intracellularly by prostaglandin dehydrogenases (42). PGI_2, however, is not taken up by this transport system and thus is not degraded by passage through the lung. Thus, many mechanisms exist by which endothelium can modulate the activity of vasoactive mediators.

G. Prostacyclin and Endothelium

In the early 1970's, a labile substance which inhibited platelet aggregation was extracted from endothelial cells although its nature was unknown (44). Since an ecto ADPase had been identified on vascular cells, adenosine was one possiblity (45). New findings that prostaglandins made by platelets could affect platelet function led Moncada et al. (46) to investigate whether vascular tissue produced similar platelet-aggregatory prostaglandins. Incubating platelets with extracts of vascular homogenates, they unexpectedly found a new prostaglandin produced by vascular tissue which inhibited platelet aggregation and produced vasodilation. This compound was identified as 9-deoxy-6,9 α-epoxy-delta-5-$PGF_{1\alpha}$, and given the trivial name prostacyclin (PGI_2). It was soon recognized as the major metabolite of arachidonate in vascular tissue. While PGI_2 was synthesized by the several layers of the vascular wall, the highest synthetic capacity was in the intima (47). Cultured endothelial cells from various sources, both arterial and venous, produce PGI_2 (24,48). Its synthesis is stimulated by mechanical trauma, hypotonicity, hypoxia, thrombin (in certain types of endothelium), trypsin, calcium ionophores, bradykinin, histamine and angiotensin II as well as the precursor substances arachidonate and prostaglandin endoperoxides (49). In several systems, endoperoxides derived from platelets can act as substrates for endothelial PGI_2 production (50), although the physiological relevance of such cell-cell transfer is not yet clear. (See also Chapter 13).

PGI_2 prevents the activation of platelets and may also reverse platelet activation returning platelets to a resting state. There is very little evidence that PGI_2 affects the coagulation process per se. Thus PGI_2 inhibits platelet shape change (51), prevents the development of PF3 or platelet procoagulant activity (51-52), prevents or reverses the induction of fibrinogen (53) and VWF (54) receptors on the platelet surface (49), inhibits aggregation by all aggregating stimuli including thrombin and prevents the release of platelet products such as beta thromboglobulin, PF4, ADP, serotonin and thromboxane A_2 (TXA_2) (49).

These activities of PGI_2 require nanomolar amounts, concentrations which can be achieved in the vicinity of the vessel wall. However, the importance of PGI_2 generation in the thromboresistance of normal endothelium is unclear. Prostacyclin does not seem to be the main factor preventing adherence of unstimulated platelets to the vascular wall since aspirin (which inhibits PGI_2 synthesis) does not affect platelet non-adherence to endothelium (55-56). However, platelets activated with thrombin show enhanced adherence to aspirin-treated endothelium probably reflecting the inability of PGI_2 to prevent platelet-platelet interaction (57). (Since this view is somewhat controversial, the reader may also wish to see Chapter 13). In animal models of thrombosis, pretreatment with very high doses of aspirin which are needed to inhibit vascular PGI_2 production leads only to a transient increase in the incidence and size of thrombi induced (58). Human vascular PGI_2 synthesis may, in contrast, be much more easily inhibited by small doses of aspirin (59,60). In general, platelet spreading after adhesion and platelet aggregation on the vascular subendothelium are inhibited by low nanomolar amounts of PGI_2 (61), whereas platelet adhesion to subendothelium is only prevented by supraphysiologic amounts (61,62). It therefore appears that PGI_2 produced by endothelium is important in limiting platelet reactivity – especially after vascular injury – but probably plays a minor role in maintaining the basal thromboresistance of the vascular surface.

III. PROTHROMBOTIC FUNCTIONS OF ENDOTHELIUM

While normal intact endothelium is nonthrombogenic it participates in the production of a highly thrombogenic subendothelium which is exposed to the blood upon endothelial injury. Moreover, injured endothelial cells release factors which activate the extrinsic (and perhaps also the intrinsic) pathway of coagulation; and virally or chemically transformed endothelial cells can themselves promote thrombosis.

A. Thrombogenic Glycoproteins

Endothelial cells synthesize and secrete factor VIII VWF (63), fibronectin (64) and thrombospondin (65) – adhesive glycoproteins which are highly thrombogenic, bind to thrombin-stimulated platelets and are found in the subendothelium, plasma and platelet alpha granules. Elucidating the complex interactions among these glycoproteins, platelets and the subendothelium is likely to reveal important factors governing thrombosis and the metastatic potential of malignant cells.

Coagulation factor VIII circulates as a complex composed of two separate components – VIII:C (coagulant) and VIII:Ag (antigen). Patients with von Willebrand's disease are deficient in VIII:VWR (von Willebrand factor) – the functional attribute of VIII:Ag multimers (66). VIII:Ag is synthesized by endothelial cells and is necessary for the first step in hemostatic plug formation: adhesion of platelets to (and their spreading on) the subendothelium (67). Thrombin mediates the release of VIII:Ag from human umbilical vein endothelial cells in culture without requiring cell lysis. This response is time and dose-dependent (68). The VIII:VWF found in platelet alpha granules is synthesized by the megakaryocyte (69). When released into the microenvironment by thrombin-stimulated platelets it probably participates in platelet-endothelial cell hemostatic interactions. There is no evidence that endothelial cells synthesize VIII:C which is responsible for the coagulation properties absent in severe hemophilia A; it source is unknown.

Fibronectin (cold-insoluble globulin) is a disulfide-linked dimer of 220,000 dalton subunits synthesized and secreted by endothelial cells _in_ _vitro_. It is incorporated into the subendothelial (extracellular) matrix (64) and at regions of cell-cell contact in sparse cultures but is not bound to the luminal surface of the endothelial cell (70).

Fibronectins are also synthesized by fibroblasts and, in lesser quantities, by a wide variety of other cells. The complex molecular structure of these large glycoproteins and their ability to stimulate cytoplasmic microfilament organization give them multiple biological functions. They play an important role in hemostasis and thrombosis, opsonization, phagocytosis, cytoskeletal microstructure, interactions of cells with extracellular matrices, embryonic cell migration and differentiation, and oncogenic transformation (71). They promote the adhesion and/or spreading of cells (including platelets) on such surfaces as collagen and fibrin (72) and bind to thrombin-stimulated platelets (73). In vitro studies suggest a physical connection between the fibronectin-containing extracellular matrix and the intracellular bundles of actin microfilaments (74).

In the third phase of coagulation, factor XIII transglutaminase cross-links fibronectin to fibrin (75). Fibroblasts avidly adhere to the cross-linked matrix. Fibronectin may serve as a structural template for the laying down of collagen fibers which can also be cross-linked to fibronectin by factor XIII transglutaminase (76,77).

Little fibronectin is found on the surface of transformed cells which are capable of producing extensive metastases. This suggests that fibronectin is needed to anchor cells and prevent metastatic spread (78,79). Indeed, transformed endothelial cells display thrombin on their luminal as well as basilar surfaces (80).

Thrombospondin is a disulfide-linked trimer which mediates the aggregation of thrombin-activated platelets by virtue of its lectin activity (81) and its ability to form complexes with fibrinogen (82). In vitro cross-linking experiments suggest an important interaction between platelet thrombospondin and fibronectin when platelets spread on solid, collagen-containing surfaces (72). Thrombospondin bound to thrombin-activated platelets might be the site of fibronectin attachment.

B. Changes in Endothelial Surface

The surface glycocalyx of endothelial cells can be altered by released platelet products which bind to heparan sulfate or which break down the sulfated glycosaminoglycans present at the luminal surface of the endothelium. Platelet factor 4, the cationic antiheparin protein from platelet alpha granules, binds to heparan sulfate or other heparin-like substances on endothelial cells (83). When released by platelet activation, a platelet endoglycosidase present in lysosomal granules can degrade cell-surface associated heparan sulfate in a specific manner (84). Endothelial cell heparins inhibit the growth of smooth muscle cells (85) by blocking the stimulatory effect of the platelet derived growth factor. Thus, release of heparinase by activated platelets can alter the regulation of vascular wall repair processes by its effect on endothelium.

When endothelial cells are disrupted the blood is exposed to the highly thrombogenic subendothelium. Such disruption can occur when the endothelial cells contract, creating gaps in the intracellular junctions. The endothelial cells lining the postcapillary venules are particularly sensitive to histamine, serotonin and bradykinin (products of platelet release and fluid phase coagulation) which cause endothelial cell contraction (86). In addition to exposing the subendothelium, injured endothelial cells release factors which activate the coagulation system directly.

Exposure of coagulation factor VII to tissue factor activates the extrinsic system of coagulation. Cultured endothelial cells contain sufficient tissue factor to accelerate coagulation markedly, and mechanical disruption of the cells leads to a several-fold increase in coagulation activity (87).

Injured endothelial cells may also activate the intrinsic system of coagulation. A serine proteinase – not yet characterized but associated with endothelial cell membranes and organelles and with subendothelial surfaces – can activate factor XII (88). Another factor associated with endothelial cells has been shown to enhance the activation of factors X and II and to induce cleavage of factor IX (89).

A major antithrombotic role for the endothelium is its production and secretion of PGI_2. Another arachidonate metabolite, PGE_2, inhibits the synthesis of PGI_2 in some types of vascular endothelium (90) and can interfere with PGI_2's inhibition of platelet aggregation (91). Exogenous agents such as aspirin (which acetylates cyclo-oxygenase) or lipid peroxides (which inactivate PGI_2 synthase) can interfere with PGI_2 production.

Certain blood vessels, in particular intrapulmonary arteries, have been found to synthesize significant amounts of TXA_2 as well as PGI_2 (92). Since TXA_2 is a potent platelet activator and a vasoconstrictor, its synthesis by vascular tissue is clearly prothrombotic.

Fibrinogen degradation products can injure human endothelial cells causing cell shrinkage, rounding up, bleb formation and detachment from the subendothelium; these products can also increase vascular permeability. In contrast, degradation products of fibronection, plasminogen or thrombin do not have these toxic effects (93). Fibrinogen fragment D infused in vivo into rabbits or exposed to cultured endothelial cells produced similar cell rounding, bleb formation and detachment without lethal injury; other fibrinogen fragments did not have this effect (94). These findings suggest that activation of the fibrinolytic system, for example, by tumor-induced mechanisms could produce local endothelial disruption permitting platelet or tumor cell aggregation at the subendothelium.

Whereas the normal intact endothelium is thromboresistant, viral transformation may interfere with its protective properties. SV40-treated endothelial cells, for example, interact with platelets, stimulating platelet adhesion and extensive interdigitation without platelet aggregation or release; these interactions are little affected by aspirin or PGI_2 (13).

IV. INTERACTION OF ENDOTHELIUM WITH BLOOD CELLS

As indicated above, normal vascular endothelium does not interact
with circulating platelets under normal flow conditions or with stasis
and the presence or absence of PGI_2 has little effect. Endothelium
which has been damaged, altered by mutagens (80) or virally
transformed (95) promotes platelet adhesion. The mechanism by which
this occurs is not well characterized but does not depend upon surface
charge, PGI_2 or glycosaminoglycans.

The interaction of endothelium with blood leukocytes presents a
very different picture. Normal leukocytes preferentially adhere to
normal vascular endothelium in comparison to fibroblasts, smooth
muscle cells or plastic surfaces (95,96). Arterial and venous
endothelium bind leukocytes equally well; in general, less adhesion
occurs under conditions of greater flow than in low flow settings or
stasis (95,97). Granulocytes and lymphocytes both adhere in similar
proportions. The adherence of leukocytes to the endothelium requires
divalent cations (Mg^{++} in particular) and is enhanced by the presence
of chemotactic agents such as the peptide formyl-methionyl-leucyl-
phenylalanine (96) or platelet activating factor (98), but is not
dependent on specific plasma proteins. The adherent leukocytes remain
rounded and can move freely over the surface of the endothelium or
penetrate via intercellular junctions to the subendothelium
(diapedesis). The process of adherence and migration can be affected
by PGI_2 (99), which can be inactivated by oxidatively active
leukocytes in contact with endothelium (100). Since activated
leukocytes can release tissue factor, leukocytes adhering to the
endothelium could promote local microthrombus formation.

While normal endothelium does not bear receptors for the Fc
portion of immunoglobulin or for C3b, the activated complement product
(101,102), receptors for Fc and C3b can be induced by viral infection
or trauma (103,104). Granulocyte adherence also increases after viral
infection of endothelial cells before the appearance of cytopathic
changes (105). Similarly, Ia determinants can be induced on normal
endothelium by exposure to lectins (which can be cleared by
endothelium) (106). Lectins have been found to stimulate lymphocyte
adherence (9). These alterations in the surface receptors of
endothelium may further promote leukocyte interaction. It is of
interest that blast cells are better able to adhere to, spread on and
penetrate through the endothelium than mature leukocytes (9).

When activated granulocytes bind to vascular endothelium,
secreted oxygen free radicals may inactivate PGI_2 synthase (107),
while the release of lysosomal enzymes can cause endothelial cell
detachment thus exposing the thrombogenic subendothelium (108).
Leukocyte elastase appears to be the enzyme responsible for
endothelial cell detachment while cathepsin G makes the cells
selectively unresponsive to thrombin stimulation of PGI_2 synthesis
(109). Changes induced in the vascular lining by exposure to
activated granulocytes would promote platelet activation and
initiation of thrombus formation.

Under certain conditions, erythrocytes also may adhere to the endothelium. Sickled erythrocytes will adhere to normal endothelial cells, possibly through increased fibrinogen on their surface (110) and erythrocytes infected with Falciparum malaria parasites specifically bind to normal endothelium both in vivo and in vitro via "knobs" which develop on the surface of the infected erythrocytes (111).

V. SUMMARY

The normal endothelium provides a thromboresistant surface which actively prevents platelet activation and platelet-initiated coagulation, regulates activated coagulation factors and promotes fibrinolysis. Multiple mechanisms contribute to endothelial thromboresistance, including the presence of anticoagulant and enzyme inhibitors on the endothelial surface, secretion of PGI_2, clearance of vasoactive substances and modulation of blood cell function. Injured endothelium, in contrast, exposes a highly thrombogenic surface to the flowing blood, releases procoagulant factors and develops increased vascular permeability. Endothelium thus represents a highly versatile tissue capable of a wide range of hemostatic responses to meet environmental challenges to normal hemostasis.

REFERENCES

1. Thorgeirsson G and Robertson AL. Am. J. Pathol. 93:803-848, 1978.
2. Simionescu M, Simionescu N and Palade GE. J. Cell Biol. 68:705-723, 1968.
3. Simionescu M, Simionescu N and Palade GE. J. Cell Biol. 67:863-885, 1975.
4. Hjelle JT, Baird-Lambert J, Cardinale G, Spector S and Udenfriend S. Proc. Natl. Acad. Sci. USA 75:4544-4548, 1978.
5. Owen WG. Arch. Pathol. Lab. Med. 106:209-213, 1982.
6. Gerrity RG, Richardson M, Somer JP, Bell FP and Schwartz CJ. Am. J. Pathol. 89:313-334, 1977.
7. Buonassisi V. Exp. Cell Res. 76:363-368, 1973.
8. Buonassisi V and Root M. Biochim. Biophys. Acta. 385:1-10, 1975.
9. DeBono DP. Adv. Microcirc. 7:68-95, 1977.
10. Pelikan P, Gimbrone MA and Corran RS. Atherosclerosis 32:69-80, 1979.
11. Skutelsky E and Danon D. J. Cell Biol. 71:232-241, 1976.
12. Simionescu M, Simionescu N, Silbert JE and Palade GE. J. Cell Biol. 90:614, 1981.
13. Curwen KD, Gimbrone MA, Jr. and Handin RI. Lab. Invest. 42:366-374, 1980.
14. Wight TN. Prog. Hemostasis Thromb. 5:1-40, 1981.
15. Glimelius B, Busch C and Hook M. Thromb. Res. 12:773-782, 1978.
16. Becker CG and Harpel PC. J. Exp. Med. 144:1-9, 1976.
17. Awbrey BJ, Hoak JC and Owen WG. J. Biol. Chem. 254:4092-4095, 1979.
18. Lollar P and Owen WG. J. Clin. Invest. 66:1222-1230, 1980.
19. Isaacs J, Savion N, Gospodarowicz D and Shuman MA. J. Cell Biol. 90:670-674, 1981.
20. Gospodarowicz D, Brown KD, Birdwell CR and Zetter BR. J. Cell Biol. 77:774-778, 1978.
21. Weksler BB, Ley CR and Jaffe EA. J. Clin. Invest. 62:923-930, 1978.
22. Czervionke RL, Smith JB and Hoak JC. Thromb. Res. 14:781-786, 1979.

23. Goldsmith J and Kisker CT. Thromb. Res. 25:131–136, 1982.
24. McIntyre EE, Pearson JD and Gordon JL. Nature (London) 271:549–551, 1978.
25. Esmon CT and Owen WG. Proc. Natl. Acad. Sci. USA 78:2249–2252, 1981.
26. Esmon NL, Owen WG and Esmon CT. J. Biol. Chem. 257:859–864, 1982.
27. Busch C and Owen WG. J. Clin. Invest. 69:726–729, 1982.
28. Dahlback B and Stenflo J. Eur. J. Biochem. 17:331–335, 1980.
29. Pugatch EMJ, Foster EA, MacFarlane E and Poole JCF. Br. J. Haematol. 18:669–681, 1970.
30. Loskutoff DJ and Edgington TS. Proc. Natl. Acad. Sci. USA 74:3903–3907, 1977.
31. Loskutoff DJ, Levin E and Mussoni L. In: Pathobiology of the Endothelial Cell (Eds. Nossel H and Vogel HJ) Acadademic Press, New York, pp. 167–182, 1982.
32. Shuman MA, Isaacs JD, Maerowitz T, Savion N, Gospodarowicz D, Glenn K, Cunningham D and Fenton JW II. Ann. N.Y. Acad. Sci. 370:57–66, 1981.
33. Cash J, Gader A and DaCosta J. Br. J. Haematol. 27:363–364, 1974.
34. Caldwell PRB, Seegal BC, Hsu KC, Das M and Soffer RL. Science 191:1050–1051, 1976.
35. Johnson AR and Erdos EG. J. Clin. Invest. 59:684–695, 1977.
36. Hayes LW, Goguen CA, Ching S and Slakey LL. Biochem. Biophys. Res. Commun. 82:1147–1153, 1978.
37. Hong SuChen L. Thromb. Res. 18:787–795, 1980.
38. Denny JB and Johnson AR. Immunology 36:169–177, 1979.
39. Ryan US, Ryan JW and Plummer TH. Circulation 66 (Suppl II) Abstract 667, 1982.
40. Pearson J and Gordon J. Nature (London) 281:384–386, 1979.
41. Lollar P and Owen W. Ann. N.Y. Acad. Sci. 371:51–56, 1981.
42. Ryan JW and Ryan US. Fed. Proc. Fed. Am. Soc. Exp. Biol. 36:2683–2691, 1977.
43. Saba SR and Mason RG. Thromb. Res. 5:747–757, 1974.
44. Lieberman G, Lewis G and Peters T. Lancet 2:330–332, 1977.
45. Moncada S, Gryglewski RJ and Bunting S. Nature (London) 263:663–665, 1976.
46. Moncada S, Herman AG, Higgs EA and Vane JR. Thromb. Res. 11:323–344, 1977.
47. Weksler BB, Marcus AJ and Jaffe EA. Proc. Natl. Acad. Sci. USA 74:3922–3926, 1977.
48. Baenziger NL, Becherer PR and Majerus PW. Cell 16:967–974, 1979.
49. Weksler BB. Prog. Hemostasis Thromb. 6:113–138, 1982.
50. Marcus AJ, Weksler BB, Jaffe EA and Broekman MJ. J. Clin. Invest. 66:979–986, 1980.
51. Ehrman ML and Jaffe EA. Prostaglandins 20:1103–1116, 1980.
52. Harsfalvi J, Muzbek L, Stadler I and Fesus L. Prostaglandins 20:935–945, 1980.
53. Hawiger J, Parkinson S and Timmons S. Nature (London) 283:195–197, 1980.
54. Fujimoto T, Ohara S and Hawiger J. J. Clin. Invest. 69:1212–1222, 1982.
55. Curwen KD, Kim H-Y, Vazquez M, Handin RI and Gimbrone MA, Jr. J. Lab. Clin. Med. 100:425–436, 1982.
56. Fry GL, Czervionke RL, Hoak JC, Smith JB and Haycraft DL. Blood 55:271–275, 1980.
57. Czervionke RL, Smith JB, Fry GL, Hoak JC and Haycroft DL. J. Clin. Invest. 63:1089–1092, 1979.
58. Kelton JG, Hirsh J, Carter J and Buchanan MR. J. Clin. Invest. 62:892–895, 1978.
59. Preston F, Greaves M, Jackson C, French A, Wyld P and Stoddard C. N. Engl. J. Med. 304:76–79, 1981.
60. Weksler B, Pett S, Tack-Goldman K, deRogue R, Subramanian V, Alonso D and Gay D. Clin. Res. 30:509A, 1982.
61. Weiss HJ and Turitto VT. Blood 53:244–250, 1979.
62. Adelman B, Stemerman MB, Mennell D and Handin RI. Blood 58:198–205, 1981.
63. Jaffe E, Hoyer L and Nachman R. Proc. Natl. Acad. Sci. USA 71:1906–1909, 1974.
64. Jaffe E and Mosher D. J. Exp. Med. 147:1779–1791, 1978.

65. Mosher D, Doyle M and Jaffe E. J. Cell Biol. 93:343-348, 1982.
66. Weiss H, Hoyer L, Rickles F, Varma A and Rogers J. J. Clin. Invest. 52:2708-2716, 1973.
67. Sakariassen K, Bolhuis P and Sixma J. Nature (London) 279:636-638, 1979.
68. Levine J, Harlan J, Harker L, Joseph M and Counts R. Blood 60:531-534, 1982.
69. Nachman R, Levine R and Jaffe E. J. Clin. Invest. 60:914-921, 1977.
70. Birdwell C, Gospodarowicz D and Nicholson G. Proc. Natl. Acad. Sci. USA 75:3273-3277, 1978.
71. Hynes R and Yamada K. J. Cell Biol. 95:369-377, 1982.
72. Lahav J, Schwartz M and Hynes R. Cell 31:253-262, 1982.
73. Singer I. Cell 16:675-685, 1979.
74. Plow E and Ginsberg M. J. Biol. Chem. 256:9477-9482, 1981.
75. Mosher D. Biochim. Biophys. Acta 491:205-210, 1977.
76. Mosher D, Schad P and Kleinman H. J. Clin. Invest. 64:781-787, 1979.
77. Engvall E and Ruoslahti E. Int. J. Cancer 20:1-5, 1977.
78. Chen L, Burridge K, Murray A, Walsh M, Copple C, Bushnell A, McDougall J and Gallemore P. Ann. N.Y. Acad. Sci. 312:366-381, 1978.
79. Chen L, Murray A, Segal R, Bushnell A and Walsh M. Cell 14:377-391, 1978.
80. Zetter B, Johnson L, Shuman M and Gospodarowicz D. Cell 14:501-509, 1978.
81. Jaffe E, Leung L, Nachman R, Levin R and Mosher D. Nature (London) 295:246-248, 1982.
82. Leung L and Nachman R. J. Clin. Invest. 70:542-549, 1982.
83. Busch C, Dawes J, Pepper D and Wasteson A. Thromb. Res. 19:129-137, 1980.
84. Wasteson A, Glimelius B, Busch C, Westermark B, Heldin C and Norling B. Thromb. Res. 11:309-321, 1977.
85. Castellot J, Favreau L, Karnovsky M and Rosenberg R. J. Biol. Chem. 257:11256-11260, 1982.
86. Majno G, Shea S and Leaventhal M. J. Cell Biol. 42:647-672, 1969.
87. Maynard J, Dreyer B, Pitlick F and Nemerson Y. Blood 50:387-396, 1977.
88. Wiggins R, Loskutoff D, Cochrane C, Griffin J and Edgington T. J. Clin. Invest. 65:197-206, 1980.
89. Osterud B. Haemostasis 8:324-331, 1979.
90. Tomasi V, Meringolo C, Bartolini G and Orlandi M. Nature (London) 273:670-671, 1978.
91. Gordon J, Pearson J and MacIntyre D. Nature (London) 278:480, 1979.
92. Salzman P, Salmon J and Moncada S. J. Pharmacol. Exp. Therap. 215:240-247, 1980.
93. Busch C and Gerdin B. Thromb. Res. 22:33-39, 1981.
94. Dang C, Bell W, Kaiser D and Wong A. Blood 60:209a, 1982.
95. Beesley J, Pearson J, Carleton J, Hutchings A and Gordon J. J. Cell Sci. 33:85-101, 1978.
96. Hoover R, Folger R, Haering W, Ware P and Karnovsky M. J. Cell Sci. 45:73-86, 1980.
97. Taylor R, Price T, Schwartz S and Dale D. J. Clin. Invest. 67:584-587, 1981.
98. Ingraham L, Coates T, Allen J, Higgins C, Baehner R and Boxer L. Blood 59:1259-1266, 1982.
99. Boxer L, Allen J, Schmidt M, Yoder M and Baehner R. J. Lab. Clin. Med. 95:672-678, 1980.
100. Weksler B, Knapp J and Tack-Goldman K. Clin. Res. 27:466A, ???.
101. Ryan U, Schultz D, DelVecchio P and Ryan J. Science 208:748-479, 1980.
102. Shingu M, Hashimoto Y, Johnson A and Hurd E. Proc. Soc. Exp. Biol. Med. 167:147-155, 1981.
103. Cines D, Lyss A, Bina M, Corkery R, Kefalides N and Friedman H. J. Clin. Invest. 69:123-128, 1982.

104. Ryan U, Schultz D and Ryan J. Science 214:557-558, 1981.
105. MacGregor R, Friedman H, Macarak E and Kefalides N. J. Clin. Invest. 65:1469-1477, 1980.
106. Pober and Gimbrone M, Jr. Proc. Natl. Acad. Sci. USA 79:6641-6645, 1982.
107. Weiss S, Turk J and Needleman P. Blood 53:1191-1196, 1979.
108. Harlan J, Kille P, Harker L, Striker G and Wright D. J. Clin. Invest. 68:1394-1403, 1981.
109. Weksler B, Brower M, deRoque R, Jaffe E and Tack-Goldman K. Blood 60 (Suppl. 1):225A, 1982.
110. Hebbel R, Yamada O, Moldow C, Jacob H, White J and Eaton J. J. Clin. Invest. 65:154-160, 1980.
111. Udeinya I, Schmidt J, Aikawa M, Miller L and Green I. Science 213:555-557, 1981.

CHAPTER 20. THE CELLULAR INTERACTIONS OF METASTATIC TUMOR CELLS WITH
SPECIAL REFERENCE TO ENDOTHELIAL CELLS AND THEIR BASAL LAMINA-LIKE
MATRIX

GARTH L. NICOLSON, TATSURO IRIMURA, MOTOWO NAKAJIMA, TIMOTHY V. UPDYKE
AND GEORGE POSTE

I. INTRODUCTION

Major goals in the prevention of cancer deaths are understanding
how malignant tumor cells spread from primary sites to establish near
or distant metastases and preventing this process from occurring.
Metastasis involves a complex sequence of events in which malignant
cells invade the surrounding host tissues, penetrate into lymphatics
and blood vessels, detach from the primary tumor mass and spread to
other sites where they must implant, invade and finally proliferate to
form new metastatic colonies (for reviews see 1-8). This sequence is
discussed in the reviews cited above; the present article will be
limited to a discussion of the final events involved in the formation
of hematogenous metastases (8).

Distant hematogenous metastasis often occurs to particular
secondary sites where tumor colonies grow and eventually kill their
host (4,9). Although the locations of most regional metastases can be
explained strictly on anatomical or mechanical grounds, such as the
efferent venous and lymphatic drainage (9), distant blood-borne organ
colonization by malignant cells often does not follow this pattern
(4). The formation of hematogenous metastases requires that
blood-borne tumor cells must arrest within the microcirculation by
adhesion to the wall of a blood vessel, usually a capillary or
post-capillary venule, and subsequently penetrate the vessel wall to
reach the extravascular tissues where they proliferate to generate
metastatic colonies. This suggests that hematogenous metastasis
formation requires recognition of target organ cells or stroma by the
circulating metastatic cells, selective survival and/or growth at
specific distant sites or a combination of these processes (4,10).
Thus, the blood vasculature is not merely a mechanical conduit for the
transport of malignant cells from primary tumors; it is most likely
involved in determining the anatomic locations of secondary tumors.

There are several properties of malignant cells that appear to be
important for the successful completion of each step of the metastatic
process (3-8). The fact that malignant cells can enter the
circulation does not mean that implantation, invasion and metastatic
colonization will follow. There are numerous examples where the
presence of malignant cells or their emboli in the blood does not
correlate with metastatic disease (11). It appears that most
malignant cells die rapidly in the circulation and only a very small
fraction of the circulating tumor cells survive to form hematogenous

metastatic colonies (1,3,8,12). Kinetic studies of tumor cell distribution after injection of radiolabeled malignant cells by intravenous or intracardiac routes have shown that tumor cells can recirculate to microvascular organ sites other than those first encountered by the blood-borne cells (13,14).

Evidence for the ability of metastatic cells to "home" to and grow in particular organs such as the lung has been obtained by implanting murine lung tissue into the thighs of syngeneic mice and examining whether lung-colonizing tumor cells can recirculate to and form metastatic colonies at these ectopic sites (15-17). Hart and Fidler (17) noted that there is no difference in the immediate distribution patterns of lung-colonizing tumor cells in ectopically implanted lung or kidney tissues suggesting that events subsequent to implantation (invasion, survival, vascularization, etc.) are important in determining tumor colonization of the ectopic organ. However, there are some problems with this interpretation (6). The first of these is that a substantial portion of the vascular system in the ectopic implants may be from the surrounding tissues. In addition, the mere localization of tumor cells in the ectopic implant in no way determines their exact location within the tissue. Many of these cells would not be expected to extravasate and survive to form tumor colonies.

During their transport in the blood, malignant cells are known to be involved in several types of cellular and noncellular interactions. For example, blood-borne tumor cells can undergo interactions with other tumor cells, circulating host cells and soluble blood components as well as with the cells of the vascular endothelium. This last type of interaction will be the focus of the present article. However, it should be understood that the abilities of malignant cells to escape from the vascular compartment, establish a proper microenvironment and avoid host defense mechanisms are also essential characteristics for successful metastasis formation (3-8).

It is now well established that malignant tumors are populated by cells with differing phenotypic properties and that only certain subpopulations of tumor cells within primary tumors are endowed with metastatic properties (for reviews see 4,5,18). It is thought that as malignant tumors grow, variant cell subpopulations progressively arise which are subject to host selection pressures, creating tumors composed of various subpopulations possessing differing properties. This has been described by Foulds (19,20) as the phenomenon of tumor or neoplastic evolution or progression where each tumor gradually changes, acquiring or losing certain characteristics in the face of host selection pressures. As a result of neoplastic progression, malignant tumors become more heterogenous. A variety of experiments utilizing _in_ _vivo_ or _in_ _vitro_ selection techniques or tumor cell cloning procedures have provided strong evidence for the phenotypic variability of tumor cell subpopulations in malignant neoplasms (for review see 2-6).

Using selection and/or cloning techniques subpopulations of malignant cells have been obtained which are particularly useful in studies of the role of tumor and/or host properties in metastasis.

However, the success in obtaining such subpopulations does not guarantee that their phenotypes will remain stable during propagation in vivo or in vitro. Several studies have shown that great care must be taken with potentially unstable tumor cell subpopulations in order to avoid changes in metastatic properties and/or other phenotypes (3-6,18). However, by comparing known low and high metastatic phenotype cells from the same tumor, tumor cell properties essential in certain steps of the metastatic process can begin to be identified and eventually studied in detail (3-6,21,22).

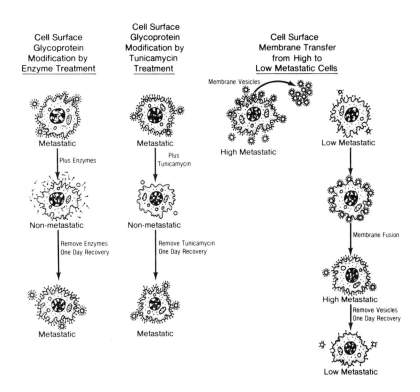

FIGURE 1. Three Major Lines of Evidence Supporting a Role for Cell Surfaces in Blood-Borne Tumor Cell Arrest. Left panel demonstrates that enzymatic modification of cell surface components can change malignant cell implantation properties. Center panel indicates that selective biosynthetic modification(s) of surface glycoproteins can inhibit metastatic processes. Right panel illustrates that the transfer of portion of the plasma membrane from highly metastatic tumor cells to cells of low metastatic potential can temporarily render the latter more metastatic in blood-borne implantation experiments. [From Nicolson and Poste (6) with permission.]

Many of the interactions of malignant cells with their environment, including host cells, are mediated by cell surface constituents (4,8,21,23). Three major lines of evidence have been used to demonstrate the involvement of cell surface components in certain aspects of metastasis, particularly blood-borne tumor cell implantation (Figure 1). The first of these is that enzymatic modifications of cell surface components can alter tumor cell implantation in the microcirculation and subsequent metastasis formation without modifying tumor cell viability (24,25). Second, specific biosynthetic modifications of cell surface glycoproteins have been shown to inhibit blood-borne implantation and experimental metastasis (26,27). Finally, the role of the cell surface in metastasis has been demonstrated by the transfer of portions of plasma membrane from highly metastatic B16 melanoma cells to B16 cells of low metastatic potential (28). In addition, there are numerous examples in which differences in the display, dynamics, amount or structure of cell surface proteins and glycoproteins may be involved in determining metastatic properties (4,5,21,22).

II. THE CELLULAR INTERACTIONS OF METASTATIC TUMOR CELLS DURING DISSEMINATION IN THE BLOOD

During tumor cell transport in the lymph or blood, several different types of cellular interactions can occur including homotypic adhesion of malignant cells to form multicellular tumor emboli. It has been established that such tumor emboli can implant with greater efficiency than single tumor cells (29,30). This suggests that mechanical factors, such as the size and deformability of the circulating tumor cells or their emboli as well as host capillary deformability, can modify the lodgment properties of metastatic cells in the first capillary bed encountered (31-33). However, tumor cell emboli often pass through capillaries after initial arrest and recirculate to other organ sites (13,14,34,35).

Using the B16 melanoma system we have examined the possible relationship between homotypic adhesive properties and blood-borne implantation. This has been possible because of the availability of B16 melanoma sublines that have been selected for increased abilities to colonize lung (B16-F10) (36), ovary (B16-O13) (37) or brain (B16-B15b) (38). In addition, in vitro selection procedures have also been used to obtain B16 sublines with increased potential for tissue invasion (B16-BL6) (39), increased resistance to lymphocyte-mediated cytolysis (B16-F10^{Lr6}) (40), decreased sensitivity to toxic doses of lectins (41), increased ability to invade veins (42) or increased detachment from growth substrata (43). Winkelhake and Nicolson (44) utilizing lung-colonizing variants of B16 found that B16 sublines with higher lung colonization potentials showed greater tendencies to form homotypic aggregates in vitro. Expansion of these data by examining several other selected B16 sublines indicates that highly metastatic B16 sublines have high rates of homotypic adhesion, while B16 sublines with low potential for forming experimental metastases generally have lower rates of homotypic adhesion (Figure 2). Similar results have been obtained using other metastatic tumor systems (45). These data

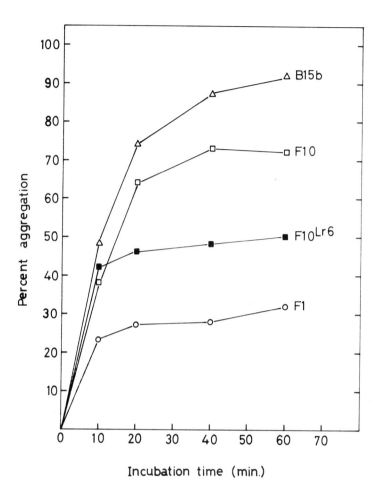

FIGURE 2. Time Course of Homotypic Aggregation of Metastatic Variants of the B16 Melanoma. Subconfluent cells were removed with buffered 2 mM EDTA (26). The cells were washed once in aggregation medium (AM) consisting of Dulbecco's minimal essential medium (1 mg/ml D-glucose, 1 mM pyruvate, no bicarbonate), 50 mM HEPES, 1% bovine serum albumin (crystallized; Sigma), 300 mOsmolar, pH 7.45 at 25°C, and counted using an electronic particle counter. Single cells (200,000) in 0.2 ml AM were placed in 1 dram opti-clear vials (Fisher) and rotated in a lab-line shaker (3/4 inch orbit) at 165 rpm (RCF = 0.295) at 37°C . Aggregation kinetics were determined by computing the percentage of single cells lost from the zero time half-maximal single cell channel settings for each cell line versus time. Results are expressed as percent aggregation versus incubation time in min. Each symbol represents the average of duplicate samples (S.D. < 10% of Data).

are pertinent to the findings that multicellular aggregates are more effective in implanting in the microcirculation, resulting in more efficient metastasis formation (29,30). Although the actual mechanisms of these tumor cell interactions have not been determined, a recent report by Raz and Lotan (46) that several human and rodent tumor cells possess cell surface lectins that appear to be specific for galactosyl- or asialogalactosyl-containing components could point the way to isolation and characterization of tumor cell surface adhesive molecules.

Blood-borne malignant cells also interact with other circulating host cells, such as platelets and lymphocytes. The interaction of malignant cells with platelets is thought to be important in facilitating blood-borne implantation by the formation of platelet-tumor cell emboli. Circumstantial support for this concept is provided by data showing that experimental metastasis in certain systems can be inhibited by inducing thrombocytopenia via administration of antiplatelet agents (47-50). Using the B16 melanoma system Gasic et al. (51) demonstrated that sublines of high lung implantation and experimental metastasis abilities aggregated at faster rates with platelets in vitro than sublines of low metastatic potential. Platelet aggregation activities have been demonstrated in a wide variety of tumor cell lines (for review see 4) and these activities have been localized to the tumor cell surface membrane (51,52). Hara et al. (53) have partially characterized a tumor cell-platelet aggregating activity, which they have found is a cell surface glycoprotein. Recently Honn et al. (54) have determined that tumor cell platelet aggregating activity is related to a cathepsin B-like proteinase in experiments where cysteine proteinase inhibitors blocked platelet aggregation.

Determining the mechanism of platelet-tumor cell interactions in the circulation may eventually be important in the development of new antimetastatic treatments (55). However, not all tumor cells appear to be associated with platelets during blood-borne transport and implantation (56). In some metastatic systems there is no correlation between platelet aggregation abilities and the incidence of spontaneous or experimental metastasis (J. Estrada and G.L. Nicolson, unpublished data).

Metastatic tumor cells can also undergo heterotypic adhesion with host lymphocytes. Fidler (57) found that B16 melanoma sublines with high lung colonization potential adhered to host lymphocytes at higher rates than B16 sublines of low lung colonization potential. Using sequential selection procedures based on lymphocyte-mediated cytolysis of B16 cells, Fidler et al. (40) selected B16 sublines that were more resistant to lymophocyte-mediated cytolysis than the parental B16 line. These lymphocyte-resistant B16 sublines were much less heterotypically adhesive in vitro and they also formed fewer experimental lung metastases in vivo (40,58).

Another important aspect of tumor cell-lymphocyte interactions involves host natural defense mechanisms against circulating tumor cells. The natural killer (NK) cell system is believed to be particularly important in killing blood-borne malignant cells (for review see 59). However, NK cell—mediated destruction of malignant cells in the blood cannot explain the rapid death of tumor cells in the circulation within approximately one day after their entry into the blood. Passive processes such as the inabilities of tumor cells to withstand the excessive shear forces and deformation in the microcirculation are thought to be responsible for the demise of most blood—borne tumor cells. Nonetheless, NK-mediated killing mechanisms have been show to be important in some metastatic systems. Gorelik et al. (60) found that mixing spleen cells with metastatic 3LL carcinoma cells before subcutaneous implantation reduced the incidence of spontaneous metastasis. These authors then selected NK-resistant sublines from the 3LL tumor (61). After eight selections for NK resistance, there was a dramatic decrease in NK-mediated cell lysis in the selected 3LL cells and the selected cells showed an increase in their abilities to metastasize spontaneously to lung. Hanna and Fidler (62) obtained similar results when they sequentially selected B16 melanoma cells in vitro for NK resistant cells using mature nude mice as the NK effector cell source. They found that the NK-resistant B16 sublines had enhanced metastatic potentials and had gained the capacity to metastasize in adult nude mice in contrast to the parental tumor lines which failed to form experimental metastases in adult nude mice.

Many tumor cells are thromboplastic and elicit fibrin formation during blood-borne transport or soon after their implantation in capillary beds (56,63,64). During blood-borne arrest fibrin clots can form at the site of tumor cell implantation (64) and under certain conditions this can result in vessel wall damage and accumulation of neutrophils (65) or platelets (66). However, Fidler et al. (1) have questioned whether fibrin formation is essential to the survival of blood-borne malignant cells. Warren (56) has reviewed the evidence for and against the role of fibrin in blood-borne metastasis and has concluded that in many cases fibrin formation is not essential for implantation or metastatic spread of tumor cells because in some experimental systems there is no relationship between tumor thromboplastin levels, fibrin formation and metastatic potential (67), nor is there evidence for fibrin deposition at the implantation site in many experimental metastasis systems (67 and Chapter 8).

Once malignant cells have implanted in the microcirculation, they usually escape from the vascular compartment by invasion through the blood vessel wall rather than by expansive growth and rupture of the endothelial vessels (68,69). Malignant cells can escape through defects in the endothelial wall (70) but the more usual route of extravasation involves tumor cell invasion between adjacent endothelial cells (71-74) or penetration of the endothelial cell cytoplasm by tumor cell pseudopodia (68,75). This is followed by adhesion to and subsequent destruction of the underlying endothelial basal lamina or basement membrane (see Section III).

After extravasation out of the circulatory compartment, metastatic cells interact with parenchymal cells and the tissue stroma at secondary sites. These interactions have been modeled in vitro using several experimental approaches. We have measured the abilities of B16 melanoma cells to heterotypically adhere to suspended organ cells in vitro and found that lung-colonizing B16 cells adhered at faster rates to lung cells than to other organ cells (76). More recently, using small pieces of organ tissue we noted that organ-selected melanoma sublines possess differing abilities to attach to and invade tissues such as lung, ovary and heart (4). Similar organ cell-tumor cell interactions have been reported by Phondke et al. (77). Using leukemia cells that preferentially colonize spleen, these authors found that the tumor cells adhered to spleen but not to isolated lung cells (77). Similarly, Schirrmacher et al. (78) have found that liver-colonizing mouse lymphoma cells adhere to mouse hepatocytes in relation to their metastatic potentials. The mechanisms involved in these intercellular interactions have not been determined; however, there is some evidence that they probably involve cell surface glycoproteins. In the studies of Schlepper-Schafer et al. (79), Walker carcinoma, BD10 lymphoma and Yoshida hepatoma cells, but not rat 5222 leukemia cells, were found to bind to normal rat hepatocytes while they all bound to normal liver Kupffer cells. Inhibition studies indicated that N-acetylgalactosaminyl- or galactosyl-specific lectins on the normal cells were probably involved in these interactions. In the studies of Schirrmacher et al. (78) liver-colonizing metastatic ESb cells, but not nonmetastatic Eb cells, formed multicellular rosettes with hepatocytes. Neuraminidase treatment abolished ESb cell adhesion to hepatocytes, suggesting that the cellular interactions may be mediated by lectin receptors on the normal cells that can bind to tumor cell sialoglycoproteins.

Experiments on the interactions of metastatic tumor cells with artificial culture substrata in vitro have shown that in some tumor systems there is a relationship between these interactions and metastatic potential. However, the relationship of these interactions to the important adhesive events that occur in vivo during the metastatic sequence is unclear. For example, adhesion of MCB-31 carcinoma cells to glass surfaces correlates inversely with metastatic potential (80), and B16 melanoma (43) and fibrosarcoma cells (81,82) resistant to removal from culture substratum by EDTA or trypsin treatment have higher experimental metastatic properties in vivo. Although Varani et al. (82) have found a correlation between attachment to plastic surfaces or detachment from endothelial cell monolayers and metastasis, extrapolation of such experiments to events that occur in vivo may be unrealistic.

Efforts to relate specific tumor cell properties to blood-borne implantation and extravasation in the circulation have been hindered until recently by the lack of suitable experimental systems. Studies on the kinetics of arrest and clearance of radiolabeled tumor cells introduced into the circulation have been useful in monitoring differences in average tumor cell distributions in different organs, in screening potential therapeutic agents for inhibition of tumor cell implantation and in determining differences in tumor cell survival at different sites (6,8,22,55). However, such methods have provided little insight into the cellular and molecular mechanisms underlying these phenomena. Progress in identifying the mechanisms involved in tumor cell implantation has depended upon the development of in vitro models that permit study of the interactions of tumor cells with vascular endothelium and endothelial basal lamina using techniques that would be difficult or impossible to employ <u>in vivo</u>. This approach involves interacting tumor cells with vascular endothelial cells grown on cellular (83) or noncellular (72,73,84) substrata or, alternatively, using excised intact blood vessels maintained in perfusion chambers (42).

III. THE INTERACTIONS OF METASTATIC TUMOR CELLS WITH VASCULAR
     ENDOTHELIAL CELLS AND THEIR BASAL LAMINA-LIKE MATRIX

The first cell type encountered by malignant cells at sites where they initiate distant blood-borne organ colonization are the endothelial cells lining the microcirculation. The interactions of circulating tumor cells with endothelial cells may in certain

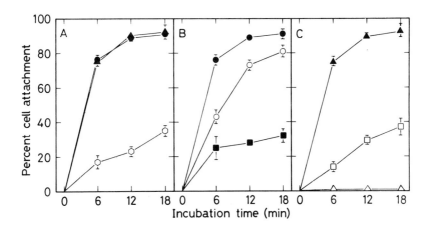

FIGURE 3. Rates of Attachment of Radiolabeled Murine B16-F10 Melanoma Cells to Endothelial Cell Monolayers, Basal Lamina-Like Extracellular Matrix Produced by Endothelial Cells or Immobilized Fibronectin <u>In Vitro</u>. A, Adhesion of untreated B16-F10 cells to untreated endothelial cell monolayers (○), endothelial matrix (●) or immobilized-fibronectin (▲). B, Adhesion of untreated (○, ●) or tunicamycin-treated (0.5 μg/ml for 24 hr) (■) B16-F10 cells to endothelial extracellular matrix or matrix pretreated with 400 μg/ml purified antifibronectin antibody (○). C, Adhesion of of untreated (△, ▲) or tunicamycin-treated (0.5 μg/ml for 24 hr) (□) B16-F10 cells to immobilized-fibronectin or immobilized-fibronectin pretreated with 400 μg/ml antifibronectin (△). [From Irimura <u>et al</u>. (100) with permission.]

circumstances be specific, because endothelial cells from different locations possess unique characteristics that reflect their tissue origin. This has been shown in experiments where antigenic differences have been found between endothelial cells established from different organs (85) and in our own experiments where brain-colonizing B16 cells attached at higher rates to brain endothelial cells than to lung endothelial cells (74). Each organ may thus have its own "recognition" system based on unique determinants expressed on vascular endothelial cells or on their underlying basal lamina.

Blood-borne tumor cells are commonly found to adhere to the junctional region between adjacent endothelial cells and especially to regions of exposed subendothelial basal lamina (65,71,86). Similar results have been obtained in _in vitro_ experiments utilizing monolayers of vascular endothelial cells (72-74). For example, we have shown that metastatic tumor cells exhibit greater adhesive affinities to the basal lamina-like matrix synthesized by endothelial cells than to the apical surfaces of the endothelial cells (Figure 3) (87,88). This may explain why metastatic tumor cells move from the lumen of a blood vessel to an extravascular position.

After initial attachment of tumor cells to the apical endothelial cell surface, they appear to induce local endothelial cell retraction, after which they then migrate to and spread on the underlying basal lamina-like matrix (Figure 4) (72-74). A wide range of neoplastic and non-neoplastic cells have been examined for their abilities to adhere to monolayer cultures of endothelial cells and to stimulate endothelial cell retraction. Apart from lymphocytes and platelets which do not adhere to undamaged endothelium, no significant differences were found in the adhesive behaviors of metastatic cells and several non-metastatic or non-neoplastic cell lines. Examination of the cells attached to vascular endothelial cell monolayers has revealed that of the cells that adhere to a model endothelium few undergo spreading and most remain rounded in shape. In addition, the predominant adhesion of tumor cells occurs at the junctional region between adjacent endothelial cells, suggesting that this region represents a specialized domain of the endothelial cell surface or that exposure of the underlying matrix has occurred in this area.

The distinguishing characteristic of metastatic cells appears to be in their abilities to underlap adjacent endothelial cells, solubilize regions of basal lamina-like matrix and migrate through this structure (Figure 4). Similar events have been found to occur _in vivo_ (65,71,89) and infiltration of malignant cells through the endothelial cell layer does not result in loss of endothelial cell viability. Following invasion, endothelial cells quickly reconstruct disrupted junctions to reform an intact monolayer (Figure 4). Consistent with the extensive tumor cell heterogeneity that exists in most if not all tumor systems, considerable variation exists in the times required for individual tumor cells to attach to and invade through endothelial monolayers (72-74). This is also consistent with the differences reported in the speed with which different tumor cells extravasate from blood vessels _in vivo_ (89,90).

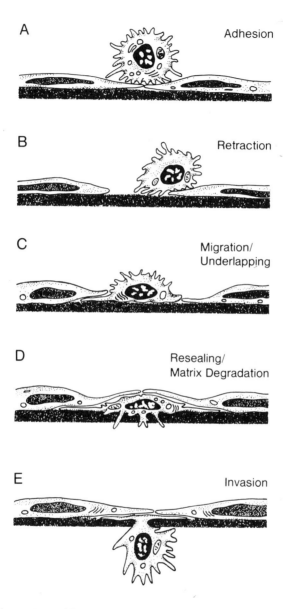

FIGURE 4. Schematic Illustration of the Sequence of Events During Blood–Borne Metastatic Cell Attachment and Invasion of Vascular Endothelium and Underlying Basal Lamina-Like Matrix. A, Malignant cell attachment to endothelial cells; B, endothelial cell retraction; C, tumor cell migration and attachment to the underlying matrix; D, local destruction of the endothelial basal lamina-like matrix and E, invasion of the malignant cell into surrounding tissue. [From Nicolson (4) with permission.]

Components in the basal lamina-like matrix synthesized by endothelial cells differ from components on the apical endothelial cell surface and these differences are probably important in the preferential adhesion of metastatic cells to the basal lamina-like matrix. The matrix synthesized by endothelial cells contains glycoproteins such as fibronectin (87,88,91) and laminin (92-94), collagens, particularly type IV (95-97), and sulfated proteoglycans (98-100). These basal lamina components are likely to be involved in adhesive interactions with metastatic tumor cells. In fact, this has been shown in assays in which the binding of tumor cells to specific matrix components is blocked by antibodies (Figure 3) (88) or where purified, immobilized matrix components are tested for tumor cell adhesive capacities (Figure 3) (95-97). For example, metastatic B16 melanoma cells adhere with similar rapid kinetics to immobilized-fibronectin and subendothelial basal lamina-like matrix synthesized by vascular endothelial cells. However, while adhesion to immobilized-fibronectin is completely blocked by an affinity-purified antibody to fibronectin, adhesion to basal lamina-like matrix is only partially inhibited by such antibodies (Figure 3) (100 see also Chapter 21). These results suggest that metastatic tumor cells probably use a variety of adhesive mechanisms in concert to attach to endothelial cell basal lamina and each class of adhesive interactions may act independently and play only a partial role in cell-matrix adhesion (4,88).

In support of the view that metastatic tumor cells use a variety of adhesive mechanisms to attach to basal lamina, Murray et al. (95) found that metastatic cells attached in relation to their metastatic potentials to type IV collagen, but not to other collagen types. In addition, Terranova et al. (101) utilized laminin complexes to demonstrate that this glycoprotein was important in adhesion of tumor cells to collagen. In these experiments laminin-dependent adhesion correlated with the metastatic capacities of various tumor sublines.

Tumor cell surface glycoproteins have been implicated in metastatic cell attachment to basal lamina-like matrix as well as to immobilized matrix components. Tunicamycin, an inhibitor of glycoprotein biosynthesis, effectively blocks tumor cell-endothelial cell adhesion as well as tumor cell-fibronectin adhesion (Figure 3) (26,27,100). This drug appears to modify cell surface glycoproteins, such as those on B16 melanoma cells, without modifying the major surface proteins detected by lactoperoxidase-catalyzed iodination (26). The effects of tunicamycin are reversible within one day after drug removal from cultures of melanoma cells. By examining the loss of metastatic properties during tunicamycin treatment of B16 melanoma cells, we were able to relate the biologic properties in this system to the disappearance of a specific class of cell surface components, in this case the sialogalactoproteins on B16 cells. Treatment of B16 melanoma cells with tunicamycin also blocked blood-borne implantation and experimental metastasis (26,27). Modification of B16 melanoma cell surface glycoconjugates by enzymes can also result in loss of cell recognition and metastatic properties (24). We have attempted to purify B16 melanoma cell surface sialogalactoproteins and to examine their affinity to endothelial basal lamina-like matrix (102). In contrast to B16 melanoma cells, isolated B16 sialogalactoproteins possess low affinities for endothelial matrix (102), again suggesting that B16 cell adhesion to matrix results from multiple adhesive interactions (4,88).

IV. DEGRADATION OF ENDOTHELIAL BASAL LAMINA-LIKE MATRIX BY METASTATIC TUMOR CELLS

Components of the basal lamina-like matrix synthesized by endothelial cells in vitro can be used to study mechanisms of basal lamina destruction by metastatic tumor cells. Although mechanical disruption and enzymatic degradation have both been postulated as important in the penetration of basal lamina by metastatic cells, we and other investigators have concentrated on the role of tumor cell degradative enzymes in this process. Mechanical disruption of basal lamina by metastatic tumor cells is postulated strictly on morphological observations, whereas proposals for enzymatic mechanisms are based on direct measurements of various tumor cell enzymes. As candidate enzymes, collagenase specific for type IV collagen and proteineases capable of degrading matrix glycoproteins, such as fibronectin and laminin, have been proposed as important in extravasation (for review see 4, 103; see also Chapter 21). In addition, it is unlikely that simple mechanical disruption can explain mechanisms of extravasation, because metastatic tumor cells can easily penetrate endothelial basal lamina-like matrix (72-74,83,84) and intact blood vessel walls (39,42) in vitro under conditions of minimal mechanical pressure.

Mechanisms of extravasation which do not require special circumstances, such as excessive tumor pressure due to cell proliferation, are more likely to be involved in basal lamina penetration. In support of enzymatic mechanisms Liotta et al. (104) have shown that highly metastatic B16 cells possess higher collagenase activities than B16 cells of low metastatic potential, but only against type IV collagen, the major collagen component of basal lamina. When several B16 sublines were measured for collagenase activities against type I or type II collagen, they were similar, indicating that highly metastatic cells possess enzymes that can degrade major collagen components of the basal lamina. Lysosomal proteinases and glycosidases may also be important in basal lamina digestion. Sloane et al. (105,106) have reported that B16 melanoma cells of high metastatic potential possess high levels of lysosomal enzymes such as cathepsin B. The presence of cathepsin B in metastatic cells is interesting, because this cysteine proteinase may be involved in the activation of latent collagenase to active collagenase (see Chapter 12).

It is now known that metastatic tumor cells have the capacities to degrade all of the major components of the endothelial basal lamina-like matrix. To show this, the components of the basal lamina-like matrix synthesized by endothelial cells in vitro can be radiolabeled with appropriate precursors, and by monitoring the release of radiolabel on exposure to tumor cells it is possible to determine the susceptibility of different matrix components to enzymatic degradation by tumor cells and to eventually identify the tumor cell enzymes involved. For example, when metastatic B16 cells are seeded onto [^{3}H]leucine-labeled, cell-free endothelial matrix, radiolabel is released into the media in the form of solubilized macromolecules that are 90–95% precipitable with 10% trichloroacetic acid. Highly metastatic B16 melanoma sublines release [^{3}H]leucine-labeled molecules from endothelial matrix at higher rates than B16 cells of lower metastatic potential (74,99). Using endothelial cell matrix we have found that the predominant glycoproteins solubilized by B16 melanoma cells are fibronectin and laminin. Fibronectin is released into the media in a new form of slightly lower ($M_r \sim 10,000$) molecular weight. Analysis of endothelial matrix fibronectin by SDS-polyacrylamide gel electrophoresis indicates that the matrix fibronectin subunits are $M_r \sim 230,000$ suggesting that the tumor cell solubilized fibronectin is modified by tumor cell proteinases or glycosidases (98).

Metastatic tumor cells also have enzymes capable of solubilizing basal lamina proteoglycans. This can be measured by examining the solubilization of [^{35}S]sulfated proteoglycans from endothelial matrix. The major glycosaminoglycan side chains of the endothelial matrix proteoglycans are molecules of $M_r \sim 25,000 - 30,000$. Addition of metastatic tumor cells to endothelial matrix results in the release of glycosaminoglycan fragments which are approximately one-third their original size and > 95% heparan sulfate (98). The composition of the glycosaminoglycan fragments solubilized by metastatic cells indicates that these cells possess an endoglycosidase capable of cleaving heparan sulfate molecules at intrachain sites. The release of these solubilized heparan sulfate fragments from endothelial matrix occurs at higher rates when B16 melanoma sublines of high metastatic and invasive potentials are compared with similar sublines of low metastatic and invasive potentials (74,99).

We have examined the abilities of metastatic B16 cells to degrade purified lung heparan sulfate glycosaminoglycans in vitro. In this assay we measure the appearance of heparan sulfate degradation products using polyacrylamide gel electrophoresis in 1,3-diamino-propane-acetate buffer according to Nakajima et al. (99). The rates of total heparan sulfate degradation by various B16 melanoma sublines and the rates of appearance of degradation products of decreased molecular weights (Figure 5) indicate that high molecular weight heparan sulfate is degraded to large fragments rather than monosaccharides. These data are consistent with our previous data suggesting that B16 melanoma cells have an endoglycosidase capable of cleaving heparan sulfate (98). When various B16 sublines are compared for their heparan sulfate-degrading activities using either intact cells (Figure 6) or their cell-free homogenates (Figure 7), we find that the B16 melanoma sublines with the highest lung colonization potentials have the highest heparan sulfate degradation activities.

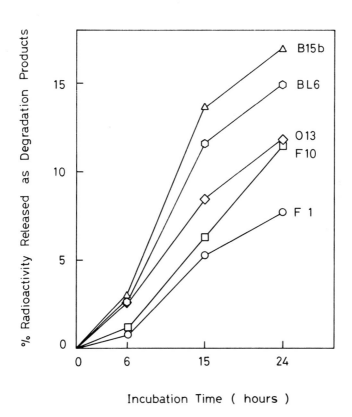

FIGURE 5. Solubilization of Sulfate Glycosaminoglycans from Subendothelial Matrix by Metastatic Variants of the Murine B16 Melanoma. Endothelial cell cultures were labeled metabolically with sodium [^{35}S]sulfate (25 µ Ci/ml) in sulfate-depleted medium plus 10 percent fetal bovine serum for one week, and subendothelial matrix was prepared according to Kramer et al. (98). B16 melanoma cells were grown, harvested and 2 ml of cell suspension plated on matrix in 35 mm culture dishes at a concentration of 150,000 cells/ml. At various times during the incubation at 37°C aliquots of the media were removed and centrifuged at 40,000 x g for 30 min. The radioactivity in the supernatants was determined by liquid scintillation counting. Spontaneous release of radioactivity by a nonenzymatic process (98) has been subtracted from the raw data. Each symbol represents the average of triplicate samples (S.D. < 1%). [From Nakajima et al. (99) with permission.]

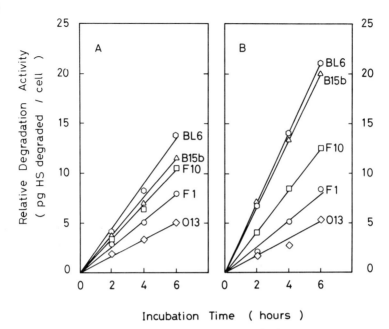

FIGURE 6. Time Course of Heparan Sulfate (HS) Degradation by Intact, Viable B16 Melanoma Cells. B16 cells (100,000) were indubated with 50 μg purified bovine lung HS for various times in 200 μl medium containing 20 mM Tricine (pH 7.3) at 37°C. Upon incubation with B16 cells the relative degradation activities were calculated from the decrease in total area of the HS peak (A) or the decrease in area of the high molecular weight half of the HS peak (B). Results are expressed as pg HS degraded/cell. Each symbol represents the average of quadriplicate samples (S.D. < 10% of data). [From Irimura et al. (100) with permission.]

In order to rapidly determine the size distributions of a variety of glycosaminoglycans and their fragments we have recently developed an analytical system using high performance liquid chromatography (107). With this system we have found that lung heparan sulfate, and also heparan sulfate from various other sources, is degraded into large molecular weight fragments by glycosidases derived from metastatic cells. For example, heparan sulfate synthesized by PYS-2 embryonic carcinoma cells ($M_r \sim 11,000$) is fragmented into molecules of average $M_r \sim 6,000$ (Figure 8) in the presence of D-saccharic acid 1,4-lactone, an inhibitor of exo-β-glucuronidase. The result indicates that metastatic cells have an endoglycosidase which recognizes a sequence in the heparan sulfate chain.

We have now more precisely determined the heparan sulfate cleavage points produced by incubation with B16 melanoma glycosidases. Bovine lung heparan sulfate fragments previously reduced with $NaBH_4$ at their reducing termini have been isolated and labeled at their newly formed reducing terminal ends with $NaB[^3H]_4$. The labeled reducing

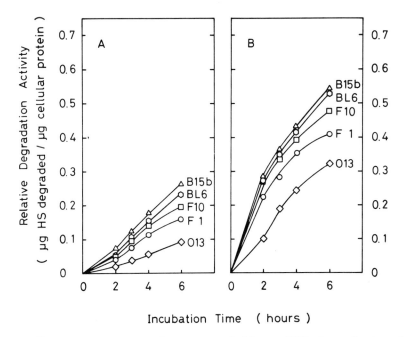

FIGURE 7. Time Course of Heparan Sulfate (HS) Degradation by Cell Homogenates of B16 Melanoma Cells. Fifty μg of purified bovine lung HS was incubated with each B16 cell homogenate (40 μg protein) or boiled cell homogenate in 70 μl of 0.1 M sodium phosphate, 0.2% (v/v) Triton X-100 and 0.15 M sodium chloride (pH 6.0) at 37°C for various times. After incubation, the mixtures were centrifuged to remove debris and 2 μl of the supernatants was applied to 6% polyacrylamide gels in 50 mM 1,3-diaminopropane-acetate buffer, pH 9.0. Electrophoresis was performed at 120 V for 60 min at 4°C. Electrophoresed gels were fixed and then stained with 0.1% toluidine blue in 1% acetic acid, destained and scanned at 525 nm to quantitate the glycosaminoglycans. The relative degradation activities were calculated from the decrease in total area of the HS peak (A) or the decrease in area of the high molecular weight half of the HS peak (B). Results are expressed as μg HS degraded/μg cellular protein. Each symbol represents the average of quadriplicate samples (S.D. < 10% of data). [From Irimura et al. (100) with permission.]

terminal sugars have been analyzed after acid hydrolysis or nitrous acid deamination followed by mild acid hydrolysis using descending paper chromatography and high voltage paper electrophoresis. Greater than 90% of the reducing terminal sugars of the heparan sulfate fragments are glucuronic acid, indicating the heparan sulfate degrading enzymes from B16 melanoma are endoglucuronidases.

312

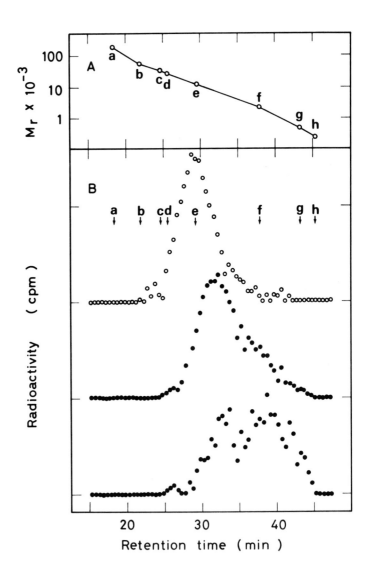

FIGURE 8. High Performance Liquid Chromatographic Analysis of [^{35}S]-Labeled HS from PYS-2 Embryonic Carcinoma Cells and of Fragments Produced by B16 Melanoma Cell Heparanases.

A. Logarithmic plot of the molecular weights versus the retention times of standard glycans separated on two sequential 0.7 x 75 cm columns of Fractogel-TSK (Toyopearl) HW-55(S). Elution was performed with 0.2 M sodium chloride at a flow rate of 1.0 ml/min at 55°C. Standard glycans used are: a, HA from human umbilical cord (M_r ∿ 230,000); b, C6S from shark cartilage (M_r ∿ 60,000); c, HS from bovine lung (M_r ∿ 34,000); d, DS from hog mucosal tissue (M_r ∿ 27,000); e, heparin from hog mucosal tissue (M_r ∿ 11,000); f, monosyalosyl-biantenary complex-type glycopeptide from porcine thyroglobulin (M_r ∿ 2,165); g, tri-N-acetylchitotriose (M_r ∿ 627); h, N-acetyl-glucosamine (M_r ∿ 221).

B. Elution profiles of cellular heparan sulfate produced by PYS-2 embryonic carcinoma (upper) and its fragments after incubation with B16 melanoma cell extract in the presence (middle) or absence (lower) of D-saccharic acid 1,4-lactone. 2,500 cpm of [^{35}S]HS (4 μ g glucuronolactone) was incubated at 37°C for 1.5 hr with B16 melanoma cell extract (30 μg cellular protein) in 100 μl of 0.1 M sodium phosphate buffer, pH 6.0, containing 0.2% Triton X-100, 0.15 M sodium chloride and 0.05% sodium azide. D-saccharic acid 1,4-lactone was added at a final concentration of 20 mM (middle). The reaction was stopped by chilling and the addition of one tenth volume of cold 50% trichloroacetic acid. After centrifugation at 9,000 x g the supernatant was delivered directly into the injection port. Fractions corresponding to 30s were collected and counted; a-f indicate the eluting positions of the standard glycans.

Heparan sulfate endoglycosidases have been described in various tissues, such as skin fibroblasts (108), rat liver cells (109), human platelets (110) and placenta (111). Ogren and Lindahl (112) have noted that murine mastocytoma cells contain a heparin-specific endoglucuronidase that is capable of cleaving macromolecular heparin into physiologically active, intermediate molecular weight fragments. A heparan sulfate endoglycosidase has been purified recently from normal human platelets (113). Heparan sulfate endoglycosidases in normal cells may be important in restructuring the basal lamina during angiogenesis and during blood leukocyte extravasation. However, it is not known whether there are regulatory or structural differences between the heparan sulfate endoglycosidases of tumor and nontumor cells.

V. INTERACTIONS OF METASTATIC TUMOR CELLS WITH INTACT BLOOD VESSELS

A new system which has been devised to quantitate tumor invasion through an endothelial tissue matrix and achieve simultaneous recovery of the invasive cells is the blood vessel perfusion-invasion chamber system developed by Poste et al. (42) (Figure 8). In this system tumor cells interact with segments of vein maintained in a perfusion

314

apparatus. This allows tumor cells to interact with either the outer elements of the vessel or the luminal endothelial cell surface, in the latter case by inverting the blood vessels before their insertion into the chamber. Using this arrangement is is possible to study intravasation and extravasation with the same apparatus. Another feature of this apparatus is that malignant cells that can successfully invade and cross the wall of the vein can be recovered in the internal perfusion circuit and can later be compared with noninvasive cells harvested from the outer injection chamber. Thus, the blood vessel perfusion-invasion system (Figure 9) offers excellent opportunities for studying the events in initial penetration of the tumor cells into blood vessels, as well as the invasion of malignant cells into extravascular tissues after implantation. The perfusion-invasion apparatus can also be utilized with mixtures of host cells, such as lymphocytes, platelets and so on, along with metastatic or nonmetastatic tumor cells to determine the roles of these normal host cells in implantation and extravasation (42).

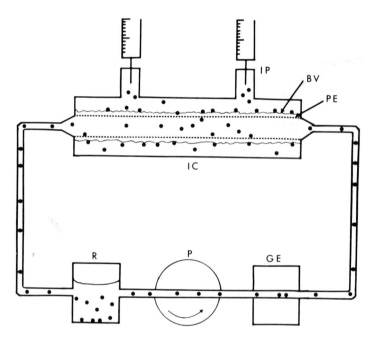

FIGURE 9. Schematic Illustration of a Perfusion Chamber System to Study the Ability of Tumor Cells to Invade Segments of Vein. A segment of vein (BV) is fitted over a central tube of porous ultrahigh molecular weight polyethylene (PE) containing 20 μm diameter pores. Tumor cells are introduced into the invasion chamber (IC) via injection ports (IP). Any cells that invade and cross the vessel then pass through pores in the PE tube to enter the internal perfusion circuit where they can be harvested from a reservoir (R). A peristaltic pump (P) and a gas exchanger (GE) are used to ensure flow of culture medium through the chamber at the correct CO_2 content and pH. The various components of the unit are not drawn to scale. [From Poste et al. (42) with permission.]

Although the perfusion-invasion apparatus in its current design offers new opportunity to study cellular interactions during blood-borne implantation and extravasation, it has one major drawback. Only large diameter vessels or veins can be used, because the small size and delicate structure of capillary networks precludes their use in this apparatus. Since the normal mode of blood-borne implantation and invasion takes place in the microcirculation and rarely in the large diameter veins or vessels similar to those used in the perfusion-invasion apparatus, studies using this system may not accurately reflect the events that occur during implantation and invasion in the microcirculation. Miniaturization of the perfusion system may be one possible solution to eliminate this deficiency, though this will not be a simple task.

VI. SUMMARY

Blood-borne metastasis often occurs to specific organ sites in vivo suggesting that recognition of target organ endothelial cells or their stroma by circulating metastatic tumor cells may be important in the metastatic process. In addition, cellular interactions during blood-borne transport, such as the interactions between tumor cells and between tumor cells and platelets and tumor cells and lymphocytes can affect the outcome of metastatic colonization. By using vascular endothelial cells as an in vitro model for blood vessel endothelium, we have examined the important steps in blood-borne tumor cell attachment and secondary invasion. These studies have revealed that metastatic cells attach more strongly and rapidly to the endothelial basal lamina-like matrix than to the apical surface of endothelial cells and this difference may be due, in part, to the exclusive presence of adhesive molecules such as fibronectin, laminin and possibly proteoglycans in the matrix. Tumor cell surface glycoproteins are also important in endothelial cell and matrix interactions, because preventing their appearance on tumor cell surfaces with specific biosynthetic inhibitors blocks malignant cell binding to endothelial cells or their matrix and abolishes blood-borne implantation properties. During invasion of the vascular endothelum metastatic cells must degrade and then penetrate the basal lamina. Metastatic cells possess proteinases and glycosidases capable of solubilizing the major endothelial basal lamina-like components. We have examined the solubilization of endothelial matrix glycosamino-glycans utilizing radiolabeled matrix and purified heparan sulfate substrates. Metastatic melanoma cells possess enzymes capable of cleaving heparan sulfate at intrachain glucuronide linkages resulting in the production of intermediate molecular weight heparan sulfate fragments.

ACKNOWLEDGEMENTS

Our studies are supported by USPHS grants RO1-CA28844, CA28867 and CA29571 from the National Cancer Institute to G.L. Nicolson, institutional grant IN-121B to T. Irimura and IN-34 to M. Nakajima, from the American Cancer Society, and USPHS grants RO1-CA18260 and CA30192 from the National Cancer Institute to G. Poste.

316

REFERENCES

1. Fidler IJ, Gersten DM and Hart IR. Adv. Cancer Res. 28:149–250, 1978.
2. Poste G and Fidler IJ. Nature (London) 283:139–146, 1980.
3. Fidler IJ and Nicolson GL. Cancer Biol. Rev. 2:171–234, 1981.
4. Nicolson GL. Biochim. Biophys. Acta 695:113–176, 1982.
5. Poste G. Cancer Metastasis Rev. 1:141–199, 1982.
6. Nicolson GL and Poste G. Curr. Probl. Cancer 7(6):1–83, 1982.
7. Nicolson GL and Poste G. Curr. Probl. Cancer 7(7):1–43, 1983.
8. Nicolson GL and Poste G. Int. Rev. Exp. Pathol., in press, 1983.
9. Sugarbaker EV. Cancer Biol. Rev. 2:235–278, 1981.
10. Hart IR. Cancer Metastasis Rev. 1:5–16, 1982.
11. Salsbury AJ. Cancer Treatment Rev. 2:55–72, 1975.
12. Fidler IJ. In: Fundamental Aspects of Metastasis (Ed. Weiss L), North-Holland, Amsterdam, pp. 257–289, 1976.
13. Fidler IJ and Nicolson GL. J. Natl. Cancer Inst. 57:1199–1202, 1976.
14. Fidler IJ and Nicolson GL. J. Natl. Cancer Inst. 58:1867–1872, 1977.
15. Kinsey DL. Cancer (Philadelphia) 13:674–676, 1960.
16. Sugarbaker EV, Cohen AM and Ketcham AS. Ann. Surg. 174:161–166, 1971.
17. Hart IR and Fidler IJ. Cancer Res. 40:2281–2287, 1980.
18. Hart IR and Fidler IJ. Biochim. Biophys. Acta 651:37–50, 1981.
19. Foulds L. J. Natl. Cancer Inst. 17:701–712, 1956.
20. Foulds L. J. Natl. Cancer Inst. 17:713–754, 1956.
21. Nicolson GL. In: Tumor Invasion and Metastasis (Eds. Liotta L and Hart IR), Martinus Nijhoff Publishers, The Hague, pp. 57–59, 1982.
22. Poste G. In: Cancer Invasion and Metastasis (Eds. Hart IR and Liotta L), Marcel Dekker, New York, pp. 148–177, 1982.
23. Nicolson GL. Biochim. Biophys. Acta 458:1–72, 1976.
24. Hagmar B and Norrby K. Int. J. Cancer 11:663–675, 1973.
25. Fidler IJ. Methods Cancer Res. 15:399–439, 1978.
26. Irimura T, Gonzalez R and Nicolson GL. Cancer Res. 41:3411–3418, 1981.
27. Irimura T and Nicolson GL. J. Supramol. Struct. Cell. Biochem. 17:325–336, 1981.
28. Poste G and Nicolson GL. Proc. Natl. Acad. Sci. USA 77:399–403, 1980.
29. Fidler IJ. Eur. J. Cancer 9:223–227, 1973.
30. Liotta LA, Kleinerman J and Saidel GM. Cancer Res. 36:889–894, 1976.
31. Sato H, Khato J, Sato T and Suzuki M. Gann Monogr. Cancer Res. 20:3, 1977.
32. Zeidman I and Buss JM. Cancer Res. 12:731–733, 1952.
33. Sato H and Suzuki M. In: Fundamental Aspects of Metastasis (Ed. Weiss L), North-Holland, Amsterdam, pp. 311–317, 1976.
34. Zeidman I. Cancer Res. 21:38–39, 1961.
35. Fisher B and Fisher ER. Cancer Res. 27:421–425, 1967.
36. Fidler IJ. Nature (London) New Biol. 242:148–149, 1973.
37. Brunson KW and Nicolson GL. J. Supramol. Struct. 11:517–528, 1979.
38. Miner KM, Kawaguchi T, Uba GW and Nicolson GL. Cancer Res. 42:4631–4638, 1982.
39. Hart IR. Am. J. Pathol. 97:587–600, 1979.
40. Fidler IJ, Gersten DM and Budmen MB. Cancer Res. 36:3160–3165, 1976.
41. Tao T-W and Burger MM. Nature (London) 270:437–438, 1977.
42. Poste G, Doll J, Hart IR and Fidler IJ. Cancer Res. 40:1636–1644, 1980.
43. Briles EB and Kornfeld S. J. Natl. Cancer Inst. 60:1217–1222, 1978.
44. Winkelhake JL and Nicolson GL. J. Natl. Cancer Inst. 56:285–291, 1976.
45. Nicolson GL. Am. Zool. 18:77–86, 1978.
46. Raz A and Lotan R. Cancer Res. 41:3642–3647, 1981.
47. Gasic GJ, Gasic TB and Murphy S. Lancet 2:932–933, 1972.
48. Fisher B and Fisher ER. Surgery 50:240–247, 1961.

49. Gastpar H. J. Med. 8:103-121, 1977.
50. Brown JM. Cancer Res. 33:1217-1224, 1973.
51. Pearlstein E, Salk PL, Yogeeswaran G and Karpatkin S. Proc. Natl. Acad. Sci. USA 77:4336-4339, 1980.
52. Gasic GJ, Boettiger D, Catalfamo JL, Gasic TB and Stewart GJ. Cancer Res. 38:2950-2955, 1978.
53. Hara Y, Steiner M and Baldini MG. Cancer Res. 40:1217-1221, 1980.
54. Honn KV, Cavanaugh P, Evens C, Taylor JD and Sloane BF. Science 217:540-542, 1982.
55. Giraldi T and Sava G. Anticancer Res. 1:163-174, 1981.
56. Warren BA. Cancer Biol. Rev. 2:95-169, 1981.
57. Fidler IJ. Cancer Res. 35:218-224, 1975.
58. Fidler IJ and Bucana C. Cancer Res. 37:3945-3956, 1977.
59. Hanna N. Cancer Metastasis Rev. 1:45-64, 1982.
60. Gorelik E, Fogel M, Feldman M and Segal S. J. Natl. Cancer Inst. 63:1397-1404, 1979.
61. Gorelik E, Fogel M, DeBaetselier P, Katsav S, Feldman M and Segal S. In: Tumor Invasion and Metastasis (Eds. Liotta L and Hart IR), Martinus Nijhoff, The Hague, pp. 133-146, 1982.
62. Hanna N and Fidler IJ. J. Natl. Cancer Inst. 66:1183-1190, 1981.
63. Chew E-C and Wallace AC. Cancer Res. 36:1904-1909, 1976.
64. Chew E-C, Josephson RK and Wallace AC. In: Fundamental Aspects of Metastasis (Ed. Weiss L), North-Holland, Amsterdam, pp. 121-150, 1976.
65. Warren BA. In: Thrombosis: Pathogenesis and Clinical Trials (Eds. Deutsch E, Brinkhous KM, Lechner K and Hinnom S), F.K. Schattauer Verlag, Stuttgart-New York, pp. 139-156, 1973.
66. Hilgard P. Br. J. Cancer 28:429-435, 1973.
67. Kenjo M, Oka K, Kohga S, Tanaka K, Oboshi S, Hayata Y and Yasumoto K. Br. J. Cancer 39:15-23, 1979.
68. Dingemans KP. J. Natl. Cancer Inst. 53:1813-1819, 1974.
69. Nakamura K, Kawaguchi T, Asahina S, Sakurai T, Ebina Y, Yokoya S and Morita M. Gann Monogr. Cancer Res. 20:57-71, 1977.
70. Wood S Jr. Arch. Pathol. 66:550-568, 1958.
71. Sindelar WF, Tralka TS and Ketcham AS. J. Surg. Res. 18:137-161, 1975.
72. Kramer RH and Nicolson GL. Proc. Natl. Acad. Sci. USA 76:5704-5708, 1979.
73. Kramer RH and Nicolson GL. In: International Cell Biology 1980-1981 (Ed. Schweiger S), Springer-Verlag, Heidelberg, pp. 794-799, 1981.
74. Nicolson GL. J. Histochem. Cytochem. 30:214-220, 1982.
75. Roos E and Dingemans KP. Biochim. Biophys. Acta 560:135-166, 1979.
76. Nicolson GL and Winkelhake JL. Nature (London) 255:230-232, 1975.
77. Phondke GP, Madyastha KR, Madyastha PR and Barth RF. J. Natl. Cancer Inst. 66:643-647, 1981.
78. Schirrmacher V, Cheinsong-Popov R and Arnheiter H. J. Exp. Med. 151:984-989, 1980.
79. Schlepper-Schaffer J, Friedrich E and Kolb H. Eur. J. Cell Biol. 25:95-102, 1981.
80. Cottler-Fox M, Ryd W, Hagmar B and Fox CH. Int. J. Cancer 26:689-694, 1980.
81. Varani J, Orr W and Ward PA. J. Natl. Cancer Inst. 64:1173-1178, 1980.
82. Varani J, Lovett EJ, Elgebaly S, Lundy J and Ward PA. Am. J. Pathol. 101:345-352, 1982.
83. Jones PA. Proc. Natl. Acad. Sci. USA 76:1882-1886, 1979.
84. Zamora PO, Danielson KG and Hosick HL. Cancer Res. 40:4631-4639, 1980.
85. Joseph J, Miao T, Alby L, Grieves J, Houser B, Kubai L, Morrissey L, Sidky YA, Watt SL and Auerbach G. In: Endothelial Cell Identification and Culture Methods (Ed. Thilo D), Karger, Basel, in press, 1983.

86. Carr I, McGinty F and Norris P. J. Pathol. 118:91-99, 1976.
87. Kramer RH, Gonzalez R and Nicolson GL. Int. J. Cancer 26:639-645, 1980.
88. Nicolson GL, Irimura T, Gonzalez R and Rouslahti E. Exp. Cell Res. 135:461-465, 1981.
89. Ludatsher RM, Luse SA and Suntzeff V. Cancer Res. 27:1939-1952, 1967.
90. Wood S Jr. Bull. Schweitz. Akad. Med. Wiss. 20:92-121, 1964.
91. Birdwell CC, Gospodarowicz D and Nicolson GL. Proc. Natl. Acad. Sci. USA 75:3273-3277, 1978.
92. Terranova VP, Rohrbach DH and Martin GR. Cell 22:719-726, 1980.
93. Gospodarowicz D, Greenberg G, Foidart JM and Savion N. J. Cell. Physiol. 107:171-183, 1981.
94. Vlodavsky I and Gospodarowicz D. Nature (London) 289:303-306, 1981.
95. Murray CJ, Liotta LA, Rennard SE and Martin GL. Cancer Res. 40:347-351, 1980.
96. Liotta LA, Tryggvason K, Garbisa S, Robey PG and Marray JC. In: Metastatic Tumor Growth (Ed. Grundmann C), Verlag, New York, pp. 21-30, 1980.
97. Howard BV, Macarak EJ, Gunson D and Kefalides NA. Proc. Natl. Acad. Sci. USA 73:2361-2364, 1976.
98. Kramer RH, Vogel KG and Nicolson GL. J. Biol. Chem. 257:2678-2686, 1982.
99. Nakajima M, Irimura T, DiFerrante DT, DiFerrante N and Nicolson GL. Science in press, 1983.
100. Irimura T, Nakajima M and Nicolson GL. Gann Monogr. Cancer Res. in press, 1983.
101. Terranova VP, Liotta LA, Russo RG and Martin GR. Cancer Res. 42:2265-2269, 1982.
102. Irimura T and Nicolson GL. J. Cell Biol. 91:118a, 1981.
103. Liotta LA, Thorgeirsson UP and Garbisa S. Cancer Metastasis Rev. 1:227-288, 1982.
104. Liotta LA, Tryggvason S, Garbisa S, Hart IR, Foltz CM and Shafie S. Nature (London) 284:67-68, 1980.
105. Sloane BF, Dunn JR and Honn KV. Science 212:1151-1153, 1981.
106. Sloane BF, Honn KV, Sadler JG, Turner WA, Kimpson JJ and Taylor JD. Cancer Res. 42:980-986, 1982.
107. Irimura T, Nakajima M, DiFerrante N and Nicolson GL. Anal. Biochem., in press, 1983.
108. Klein U, Kresse H and von Figura K. Biochem. Biophys. Res. Commun. 69:158-166, 1976.
109. Hook M, Wasteson A and Oldberg A. Biochem. Biophys. Res. Commun. 67:1422-1428, 1975.
110. Wasteson A, Glimelius B, Bush D, Westermark D, Heldin C-H and Norling B. Thromb. Res. 11:309-311, 1977.
111. Klein U and von Figura K. Biochem. Biophys. Res. Commun. 73:569-576, 1976.
112. Ogren S and Lindahl U. J. Biol. Chem. 250:2690-2697, 1975.
113. Oosta GM, Favreau LV, Beeler DL and Rosenberg RD. J. Biol. Chem. 257:11249-12255, 1982.

CHAPTER 21.   INTERACTION OF TUMOR CELLS WITH THE BASEMENT MEMBRANE OF ENDOTHELIUM

LANCE A. LIOTTA AND RONALD H. GOLDFARB

I.   INTRODUCTION

Intense clinical and experimental interest continues to be placed on cancer invasion and metastasis since these pathologic processes are widely considered to be the major cause of death resulting from malignant disease (1-3).   In addition, the properties of invasion and metastasis define the malignant phenotype of tumor cells (1-3).   Tumor cells with metastatic potential, which comprise only a subpopulation of the heterogenous cells within the primary neoplasm, can only give rise to secondary metastatic colonization following numerous and complex tumor cell-host interactions (4); for example, invasive, metastatic cells penetrate a number of host extracellular matrices and barriers.   This chapter will review recent findings dealing with the interaction of malignant cells with one particular type of extracellular matrix that is encountered by invasive tumor cells at several steps of the metastatic process: the basement membrane. Following an overview dealing with the structure and function of basement membranes, including vascular basement membranes, emphasis will be placed on the discrete steps involved in tumor cell-basement membrane interaction: tumor cell attachment, basement membrane dissolution mediated by tumor cell-derived proteolytic enzymes and subsequent tumor cell locomotion through localized domains of degraded basement membrane in the proximity of invading tumor cells.   The potential significance of knowledge gained from the exploration of biochemical mechanisms involved in tumor cell-mediated degradation of the basement membrane will be discussed relative to the possible diagnosis and therapy of human metastatic disease.

II.   STRUCTURE AND FUNCTION OF BASEMENT MEMBRANES

Metastasizing tumor cells interact with the basement membrane (BM) at more than one step during their dissemination from the primary tumor and eventual growth as a metastatic colony (5).   The BM, which delineates boundaries between tissue compartments and forms a scaffolding support for organ parenchymal cells, is usually a resilient and stable structural barrier with a slow turn-over rate (5,6).   However, in several pathologic conditions, including tumor invasion and mammary involution, the BM undergoes a rapid and localized degradation.   The intact BM does not normally contain pores large enough for tumor cells to passively migrate through; even the passage of colloidal carbon is excluded by undegraded BM (5).   The structure and biochemical composition of this complex extracellular matrix, which serves as both a selective permeability and supporting element, is described below.

The BM is composed of collagenous, glycoprotein and proteoglycan components and is organized into three predominant units (5-8). The lamina lucida externa is a 20-40 nm wide electron-lucent region localized on the BM side facing organ parenchymal cells. The lamina densa, also known as the basal lamina, is a 20-100 nm wide middle layer which is both amorphous and electron dense. The lamina lucida interna, found at the interface of the BM and connective tissue stroma, is an electron-lucent region of variable width. Anchoring filaments of 2-8 nm form bridges between the tonofilament-desmosome complex and the laminia densa within the epithelial BM (5). Anchoring fibers with a periodic banding pattern, smaller in size than anchoring fibrils, as well as tubular microfilaments, span between the lamina densa and the interstitial collagen of connective tissue stroma (8). Attachment glycoproteins such as laminin (9) and fibronectin (10-11) as well as proteoglycans (12-14) are contained within the lamina lucida externa (5). Proteoglycans may play some role in regulation of BM permeability (13). It is widely held that the lamina densa zone is the structural component of the BM that contains type IV collagen (15-18). Type V collagen is an additional type of BM-associated collagen located adjacent to the lamina densa on the stromal side (14,19,20). Whereas type IV collagen is uniquely localized to the BM, type V collagen is also found in structural elements other than the BM (e.g., interstitial connective tissue, stromal elastic fibers). Various structural components of the BM will be described relative to their function in tumor cell-BM interaction at the levels of attachment, degradation and locomotion.

III. ATTACHMENT OF TUMOR CELLS TO BASEMENT MEMBRANES

It has generally been found that both malignant and normal cells demonstrate optimal cell attachment to the subendothelial matrix rather than to intact vascular endothelial cell monolayers (5,21-24). Indeed, it has been demonstrated that tumor cell attachment and invasion takes place under conditions where the endothelial cell lining is modified or injured to expose the subendothelium of the basal lamina (5,21). In large blood vessels, tumor cells bind preferentially to regions of exposed basement membrane in vivo (25,26). It has been suggested that malignant cells induce endothelial cell retraction upon adhering to vascular endothelial cells and expose the underlying basal lamina which in turn leads to facilitation of tumor cell binding to the endothelial basal lamina (27).

Evidence to date suggests that BM penetration during tumor invasion takes place in three steps, the first of which appears to be preferential tumor cell binding to the exposed BM as compared to the surface of the endothelium resting on the BM or to the surface of the endothelium (1,5). Recent studies have indicated that during attachment many cell types utilize various attachment proteins such as fibronectin or laminin and do not bind directly to various collagenous matrices (28). Attachment of metastatic cells to the BM may be mediated by laminin and fibronectin, as discussed below (29-31).

A number of studies have shown that interaction of various cell types with extracellular collagenous matrices demonstrate substantial specificity in binding (28). For example, many cells of mesenchymal origin, including fibroblasts, myoblasts and smooth muscle cells, employ fibronectin for binding to collagen (28,32). Chondrocytes utilize the glycoprotein chondronectin to bind to cartilage-specific type II collagen in cartilage (33). Cells which interact with basement membrane-associated type IV collagen appear to utilize laminin as an attachment protein (29). A number of studies have examined the role of fibronectin and laminin in the attachment of metastatic and nonmetastatic tumor cells to extracellular matrices and their subcomponents.

It has been reported that certain metastatic cells attach more rapidly to type IV collagen than to type I collagen whereas nonmetastatic cells preferentially bind to type I collagen (34). Additional studies have shown that metastatic and nonmetastatic cells utilize different attachment proteins in their interactions with various collagens (30). Laminin has been found to enhance the attachment of metastatic cells to type IV collagen whereas fibronectin increased the attachment of nonmetastatic tumor cells to both type I and type IV collagen (30). Serum, which contains fibronectin but lacks laminin, stimulated the attachment of nonmetastatic cells but not metastatic cells (30). In the absence of attachment factors tumor cells attached slowly to type IV collagen and attachment was dependent upon biosynthesis of endogenous attachment factors (30). Although it was demonstrated that antibody to laminin blocked the attachment of metastatic cells to type IV collagen, it was found that antibody to fibronectin blocked the attachment of nonmetastatic cells. In the case of metastatic PM2 sarcoma and B16 BL6 melanoma cells it has been found that metastatic cells preferentially utilize laminin over fibronectin in binding to type IV collagen; in contrast, in the case of nonmetastatic C3H cells, fibronectin showed greater reactivity than laminin in mediating such attachment (3). Attachment studies by other investigators have shown contrasting results. It has been reported, for example, that melanoma cells use fibronectin to attach to the subendothelial matrix synthesized by cultured endothelial cells (24). It has also been reported that sarcoma cells, of fibroblastic origin, utilize fibronectin for attachment whereas carcinomas, of epithelial origin, employ laminin (35). These disparate findings may be related to the use of different substrates in binding studies, i.e., purified basement membrane type IV collagen (30) versus subendothelial matrix from cultured cells (35).

A. Selection for Metastatic Cells by Binding to Laminin or
    Fibronectin

The metastatic activity of cells separated on the basis of attachment to type IV collagen mediated by laminin or fibronectin has been reported (30). The number of pulmonary metastases that developed following i.v. injection of equal numbers of viable cells into mice was employed as an index of the metastatic potential of cells; it was found that PM2 cells showed a ten-fold increase in the number of pulmonary metastases if selected in vitro by attachment to type IV collagen in the presence of laminin, when compared to cells that did not attach to type IV collagen under these conditions (30). In the case of BL6 cells, a five-fold difference in the number of metastases was observed between the laminin attached and unattached cells. It has also been observed that cells which attach to type IV collagen with laminin show a three-fold increase with PM2 cells and an eight-fold enhancement with the BL6 cells in metastatic activity when compared to the metastatic potential of the same cells selected by fibronectin-mediated attachment to type IV collagen (30). Nonmetastatic C3H sarcoma cells could not be selected for metastatic activity on the basis of attachment to type IV collagen mediated by either laminin or fibronectin. A decrease in metastatic ability was noted when metastatic cells were preincubated with anti-laminin antibody prior to i.v. injection (30). It has also been found that metastatic sarcoma and melanoma cells that utilize laminin for attachment to type IV collagen are retained in the lungs and form more metastases than either parental cells or cells that do not bind by laminin to type IV collagen (30). It, therefore, appears that laminin binding affinity may be a correlate of metastatic activity. It has recently been demonstrated that high metastatic cells, but not low metastatic cells express laminin or a laminin-like moiety (36). It was suggested that the laminin-like substance could facilitate cell attachment and play a role in selecting for the differential phenotype of metastatic potential. A number of studies dealing with the role of laminin in various aspects of adhesion have recently been described (37-43). Additional interest in laminin has been generated as a consequence of studies dealing with laminin receptors as well as laminin fragments, as described below.

B. Tumor Cell Surface Receptors for Laminin

It has recently been reported that human MCF-7 breast carcinoma cells possess a receptor on their surface that has a high binding affinity (Kd = 2nM) for laminin (44; Figure 1). It was found that exogenous laminin can stimulate up to 80% of MCF-7 cells to bind to type IV collagen whereas fibronectin stimulated only 20% to bind to the same substrate (44). It is of interest that ZR-75-1 and T47-D breast carcinoma cell lines can use either laminin or fibronectin for attachment to type IV collagen, and show decreased laminin binding capacity in comparison to MCF-7 cells (44). The specific high affinity receptors for laminin, present on attached as well as suspended MCF-7 cells, are reminiscent of those for various hormones and growth factors associated with breast tumor metabolism and growth and indeed the Kd of the MCF-7 laminin receptor is similar to affinity constants noted for other growth factors such as epidermal growth factor (44). It, therefore, appears that laminin may act, at least in part, as a growth factor in the promotion of cell attachment and spreading and subsequently in the stimulation of cell division.

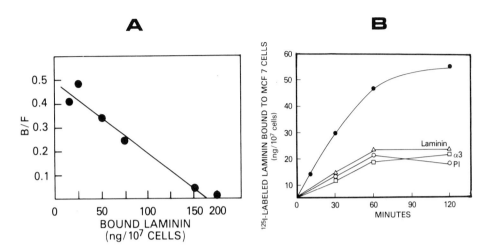

FIGURE 1. Binding of ^{125}I-Laminin to MCF-7 Breast Carcinoma Cells.
A. Scatchard plot of the ^{125}I-laminin binding to MCF-7 cells. Least
squares analysis demonstrates an r value of 0.98 for a linear fit
(44). B. Time course of binding with or without 100x competition by
unlabeled, intact laminin or purified, unlabeled proteinase-derived
laminin fragments (31,44,55). Pl and α3; see Figure 2.

It has been suggested that free laminin binding sites on the cell
surface of tumor cells may facilitate interaction of metastatic cells
with the vascular basement membrane and contribute to extravasation
and metastasis formation. The isolation of a tumor cell laminin
receptor, from detergent extracts of B16 BL6 melanoma cell plasma
membranes, has recently been described (45). BL6 melanoma cells
contain approximately 110,000 binding sites on the cell surface for
laminin (45). A single class of laminin receptors can be observed
upon detergent treatment of isolated melanoma cell plasma membranes.
The receptor has been purified 900-fold by laminin affinity
chromatography and has a Mr of 67,000 (45); the receptor binds to
laminin with high affinity (Kd = 2 nM) and is similar to binding noted
with whole cells. A laminin receptor has also been isolated from
murine fibrosarcoma cells (46); this high affinity laminin receptor,
which under reducing conditions has a Mr of 69,000, appears to be a
subunit or component part of a larger cell surface receptor protein.

C. Molecular Structure and Function of Laminin and Proteinase-
Derived Fragments of Laminin

Recent electron microscopic studies have shown that the
configuration of the laminin molecule is an asymmetric "cross" with

one long arm (77 nm) and three short arms (36-37 nm) with a diameter
of 2 nm (47,48; Figure 2). Since intact laminin binds to heparin and
heparin sulfate (49,50), in addition to mediating the attachment of
metastatic cells to type IV collagen, it has been of interest to
determine which molecular domains of the laminin molecule participate
in these diverse biologic functions (48). In order to study which
molecular domains participate in which biologic functions it is
necessary to produce specific molecular fragments of laminin and
correlate their structures with their biologic activities. For
example, although the whole laminin molecule appears as a cross-shaped
structure (Figure 2), it had previously been impossible to
experimentally determine which arms contributed to either the alpha or
beta subunits noted on gel electrophoresis, or which arms contributed
to various binding phenomena. Early studies had examined the effect
of pepsin-mediated hydrolysis of laminin (51). Treatment of laminin
with pepsin has led to the identification of P1 (Mr = 290,000) and P2
(Mr = 45,000) fragments (51). P1 and P2 peptides were shown to differ
in amino acid composition as well as immunochemical properties (51).
The P1 fragment, upon reduction, migrates on gel electrophoresis as a
series of low molecular weight components suggesting that pepsin
produces nicks in laminin which are evident upon removal of disulfide
bonds.

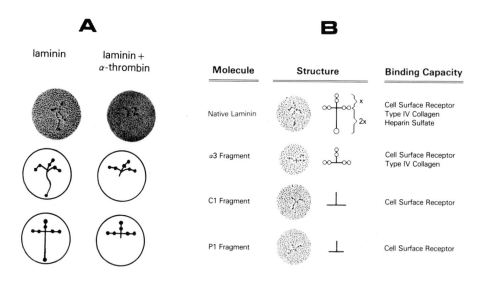

FIGURE 2. Structural and Functional Properties of Laminin and its
Proteinase-Derived Fragments. A. Alpha thrombin removes the 400 kDa
beta chain within the long arm of laminin. The remaining three 200
kDa short arms are embodied within the alpha subunit (31,44,55). B.
Structural and functional properties of laminin and its proteinase-
derived fragments. Representative electron micrographs of laminin or
purified laminin-derived fragments are depicted (31,44,55).

We have recently employed a number of additional proteolytic enzymes and utilized rotary shadowing electron microscopy to further probe the role of characteristic rod-like and globular domains of laminin (Figure 2). Alpha thrombin and plasmin are among the enzymes we have employed for this purpose. During our studies dealing with laminin degradation we had noted that homogeneously purified alpha thrombin selectively degraded the beta subunit of laminin (52-54). In contrast plasmin degraded both alpha and beta chains yielding fragments of 180,000 and 140,000 Mr (54). We have recently extended this observation to isolate the native alpha subunit of laminin and to study its structure by electron microscopy and its function as an attachment factor (31). Upon selective proteolysis of laminin with alpha thrombin, the beta subunit was removed with no change in the size or quantity of alpha subunit (31); the total mass of the laminin molecule was reduced by approximately 40% upon removal of the beta subunit. Upon electron microscopy it was found that the alpha subunit was missing the long arm and had no changes in the length of the short arms (Figure 2; 31). It was also noted that this subunit of laminin mediated the attachment of human squamous carcinoma cells to type IV collagen whereas such attachment properties were lost upon treatment of intact laminin with pepsin (31). It is known from electron microscopy experiments that P1 pepsin fragments lack both the long arm and the globular end regions of the three short laminin arms (31,48). It, therefore, appears that the beta subunit of laminin is apparently not required for adhesion to type IV collagen; it has indeed been noted that the P1 fragment of laminin inhibits tumor cell attachment to type IV collagen (31). Our studies have also shown that the P1 fragment of intact laminin is identical with the pepsin-derived fragment of the isolated alpha subunit (31); it, therefore, appears that the P1 fragment is within the central region of the alpha subunit. Since the alpha subunit, but not the P1 fragment, mediates tumor cell attachment to type IV collagen, it appears that the globular end regions of the short arms are required for attachment to take place. Since both the alpha subunit and the P1 fragment bind to the tumor cell surface, but only the alpha subunit mediates attachment to type IV collagen, it is likely that the globular end regions of the short arms of laminin bind to type IV collagen. Our results, therefore, indicate that the beta subunit of laminin is found within the long arm of the laminin molecule and that the alpha subunit is comprised of three similar chains of 200 kDa.

We have also further evaluated the relative proteolytic susceptibility of the alpha and beta subunits by using a variety of additional serine proteinases (55). It was found that chymotrypsin, plasmin and cathepsin G all degraded both the beta and alpha subunits resulting in limited digestion products. Cathepsin G and chymotrypsin both produced two major fragments of 130,000 and 160,000 Mr. Studies of digestion with time indicated that the 400 kDa beta subunit was digested far more rapidly than the alpha subunit thereby suggesting that the major fragments (greater than 100,000 Mr) produced by chymotrypsin, plasmin and cathepsin G were derived from the alpha subunit (55). Alpha subunit derivation was confirmed by first digesting laminin with alpha thrombin to completely remove the beta subunit, followed by digestion with cathepsin G, chymotrypsin or plasmin. We have, therefore, concluded that the beta subunit of laminin is highly proteinase-labile while the alpha subunit contains a large domain resistant to serine proteinases (55). Electron microscopy of the purified laminin fragments derived from digestion with cathepsin G has revealed that the proteinase resistant region of the alpha subunit contains three arms of similar morphological appearance (32 nm) and contains the intersection of the three short arms of the intact laminin molecule (55). This finding is consistent with the finding that the intersection of the short arms is resistant to proteolytic activity of pepsin (48). The proteinase resistance of the alpha subunit may be related to its high cysteine content (31). The length of the arms of the cathepsin G-derived fragment is shorter by 5-6 nm than the short arms of the intact molecule and it is possible that the end region-globular domains are modified in size. The T-shaped proteinase-resistant region of the laminin molecule has an apparent Mr of 350,000 but in the presence of reducing reagents migrates in electrophoresis as two major components of 130,000 and 160,000 daltons. Since two different major components are observed after reduction, the three short arms may be different in chemical composition or there may be a heterogenous distribution of interchain disulfide bonds (55).

We have also recently probed the domains of laminin that participate functionally in cell attachment to type IV collagen. Whereas native laminin binds to both cell surfaces as well as to type IV collagen, proteinase-derived fragments of laminin retain some but not all of the binding properties of the intact molecule (44). Digestion of laminin with alpha thrombin does not affect the cell binding or type IV attachment properties (Figure 2). The alpha-3 600,000 Mr fragment derived from thrombin digestion is, as noted above, missing the long arm of the laminin molecule but retains the three short arms plus their globular domains. The Pl and cathepsin G (Cl) fragments, in which the long arm of the molecule is removed and the globular regions of the short arms are modified, bind to the cell surface and block cell attachment to type IV collagen (Figure 2). We have concluded from these studies that the major cell receptor binding site on the laminin molecule exists within the midregion or intersection point of the three short arms of the laminin molecule (44). It also appears that the type IV collagen binding domain is on or near the globular regions of the short arms since pepsin or cathepsin G treatment abrogates their attachment to type IV collagen (Figure 2). Since the Pl or Cl fragment inhibits cell attachment it appears that these fragments saturate cell surface receptors for laminin. These fragments, however, lack the type IV collagen binding domain and fail to mediate the attachment of cells to type IV collagen.

We have recently examined the location and nature of carbohydrate moieties on the laminin molecule by employing a series of lectins and examining their binding affinity for proteinase-derived, purified fragments of laminin (manuscript submitted for publication). We have found that alpha-D-galactosyl end groups are markedly enriched in the globular end regions of the short arms when compared to the rod-shaped portions of laminin. Alpha-D-mannopyranosyl residues are present on both the globular end regions and the rod shaped portions of intact laminin, whereas exposed N-acetyl-D-galactosaminyl end groups are absent or present in low amounts in laminin. We have also noted that specific terminated oligosaccharide units are enriched on the rod-shaped regions of the short arms when compared to globular end regions of laminin. The significance of these findings relative to the attachment of metastatic cells to type IV collagen mediated by laminin has not yet been fully established.

Recent studies with elastase-dervied fragments of laminin have also indicated the existence of proteinase-resistant domains of laminin similar to those described above (56). In contrast to our findings, however, it was observed that plasmin cleaved primarily the heavy chain and the long arm but only upon destruction of the alpha helix content by prolonged heat treatment (56). Other investigators have confirmed our findings with plasmin (A. Vaheri, personal communication). It is of interest that an elastase-generated laminin fragment of 50,000 Mr, termed fragment 3, was able to bind to heparin-Sepharose (56). Under conditions of limited proteolysis of laminin with elastase or pepsin seven laminin fragments have recently been described (57). Proteinase fragments derived in this manner have also been employed to delineate the relationship between biologic function and molecular domains of laminin. Fragments 5, 6 and 7 had Mr of 30,000 to 50,000. It was observed that fragments 1, 5 and 6 promoted the attachment of rat hepatocytes to plastic (57). It is of interest that elastase generated fragments E5 and E6 were found to be small globules when examined by rotary shadowing electron microscopy (57). Fragments 5 and 6 appeared to play a role in promoting cell spreading of hepatocytes and therefore may play some role in the initiation of DNA synthesis and cell proliferation (57). Although it has not yet been shown whether elastase-derived fragments play a role in binding phenomena associated with metastatic cells, it is of interest that the E1-4 fragment appears to share some similarity with the thrombin-derived fragment described above (55,57). Studies with elastase and pepsin-derived fragments have to date been unable to define a type IV collagen binding site (57). It is also of interest that fragments 1, 5 and 6 appear to be separate domains with hepatocyte-binding ability. Since attachment of hepatocytes to fragments, but not to intact laminin, could be inhibited with specific antibodies, it has been suggested that the intact protein may contain an additional hepatocyte-binding site (57).

In summary, it is clear that laminin and its molecular domains play important roles in attachment properties of metastatic cells which have profound implications for the mechanism of tumor invasion and metastasis. Purified proteinase-derived fragments of laminin have been used to map the binding domains of the cross-shaped laminin molecule. The receptor for metastatic cells binds to a proteinase-resistant disulfide-bonded intersection region of the three short arms and the globular end regions of the three short arms bind to type IV BM collagen. In contrast, the long arm binds to heparin sulfate proteoglycan. A proteinase-derived fragment of laminin, C1, binds to the receptor and blocks tumor cell attachment in vitro and intravenous metastasis formation in vivo.

Recent studies with laminin have indicated that this attachment glycoprotein may have significance to phenomena beyond those described above. Studies with mononuclear phagocytes have suggested that laminin may play a role in the regulation of movement of cells across the BM during inflammation, whereas studies with E. coli and Streptococci suggest that laminin may play a role in certain bacterial infections (58,59).

D. Adhesive Behavior of Metastatic Cells

Recent attention has focused on the role of cell surface glyco-sphingolipids and glycoproteins in malignant transformation and metastasis (60-62). It has been reported that the ability of murine tumor cells to metastasize from a subcutaneous site is well correlated with cell surface sialic acid content and particularly with the degree of sialylation of galactosyl and N-acetylgalactosaminyl residues within cell surface glycoconjugates (63). A positive correlation was noted between the degree of sialylation, neuraminidase-releasable sialic acid and metastatic potential; in contrast the total cell sialic acid content of tumor cells showed only a rough correlation with metastatic potential (60,63). Recent studies have employed non-metastatic wheat germ agglutinin-resistant (WGA[R]) mutants of the highly metastatic MDAY-D2 tumor to further examine the role of cell surface carbohydrate composition and metastasis (64). It has been found that WGA[R] cells have a 3-4 fold reduction in neuraminidase-accessible cell surface sialic acid and show enhanced attachment to BM type IV collagen and fibronectin but not to laminin (61,64). It has been suggested that cell attachment to fibronectin and type IV collagen may require carbohydrate chains which are potential acceptors of terminal sialic acid residues (64). A plastic adherent line of a highly invasive and metastatic murine T cell lymphoma has recently been found to have lost its metastatic potential, and to have modified binding sites for terminal N-acetylgalactosamine residues (65). Sialic acid masked such sites on metastatic cells whereas they appeared to be unmasked on the low metastatic plastic adherent cells; metastatic revertants did not express the lectin receptor sites due to sialic acid masking (65). It has been suggested that the masking of specific lectin receptor sites on the cell surface of tumor cells may play a key role in adherence characteristics of metastastic cells (61,65).

It has also been reported that treatment of malignant cells with neuraminidase can shift the distribution of metastatic colonization from the lungs to the liver (66). Incubation of tumor cells with tunicamycin, an inhibitor of cell glycosylation, leads to morphologic and adhesive changes, as well as to inhibition of the metastatic potential of intravenously injected B16 melanoma cells; this modification of metastatic reactivity was reversed upon removal of the drug from cells in culture and upon recovery in tunicamycin-free media (67,68). For a comprehensive review dealing with the role of the cell surface of malignant cells relative to metastatic spread and colonization the reader is directed to recent reviews (27,62,69 and Chapter 20).

Although tumor cells adhere preferentially to the subendothelial matrix as compared to intact vascular endothelial cells, considerable interest has also been focused on tumor cell–endothelial cell interactions (27,62). It has been argued that stable adhesion or attachment to the capillary endothelium is required to prevent detachment and recirculation and thereby allow secondary and more stable tumor cell attachment to the subendothelial matrix to take place. Specific adhesive interactions between tumor cells and cells of host organs may play a key role in determining the organ distribution of metastatic cell subpopulations through site-specific adherence in the capillary beds of specific organs (62). A precedent for selectivity in organ binding as a consequence of cell-endothelium interaction exists in the case of lymphocyte recognition of lymph node endothelium during lymphocyte recirculation (70,71). It has also been recently reported that metastatic cells binding to cultured endothelial cells exhibit organ specificity (27,62). B16 sublines selected for enhanced lung metastasis attached to lung cells at a faster rate than to cells of other organs not involved in metastatic colonization (62). Leukemic cells that form splenic metastases but fail to colonize the lung adhered to isolated spleen cells but not to isolated lung cells and liver-colonizing lymphoma cell lines bound to hepatocytes in proportion to their metastatic potential (for review see 62). In addition, brain-selected B16 melanoma cells adhered at faster rates to endothelial cell monolayers derived from brain when compared to lung-selected B16 melanoma variants (62). Both in vivo and in vitro selection techniques have been employed to identify variant cell lines with enhanced abilities to colonize liver, lung, ovary or brain (72). For example, B16F1 variants have been described which metastasize to the rhinal fissure between the cerebral cortex and the olfactory bulb of the mouse brain (73). It is interesting to note that this brain-colonizing subline did not give an advantage in giving rise to brain tumors if directly injected into the brain by intracerebral implantation, when compared to non-selected B16F1 cells (72,73). The results suggest that the ability of brain-homing cells to give rise to metastases in the brain is linked to their ability to home, become arrested and then colonize the brain (72,73).

It has been suggested that malignant cells adhere to vascular endothelial cells and upon stimulation of endothelial cell retraction expose the underlying basal lamina with subsequent migration and adherence of metastatic cells to the basal lamina (63). It is of interest that brain-selected B16 melanoma cells adhere at faster rates to exposed endothelial cell basal lamina, or extracellular matrix, at faster rates compared to endothelial cell surfaces (62); it has therefore been argued that this cell type would be expected to preferentially bind to regions of injured endothelium (21,62). Recent studies with a Dba/2 T lymphoma system have indicated that non-metastatic cells retain a spheroid shape upon interaction with the subendothelial extracellular matrix whereas metastatic variants showed both flatter morphology and the formation of long pseudopods; it has been suggested that pseudopod formation may play a role in endothelial cell penetration (21). As for other systems, Dba/2 T lymphoma cells attached to the subendothelial matrix faster and more firmly than to an intact monolayer of vascular endothelial cells (21).

Aspects of tumor cell interaction with the endothelium have also been examined relative to the role of platelet adherence to tumor cells. It has been suggested that platelets might contribute to metastasis by stabilizing initial tumor cell interaction with the vascular endothelium and by protecting tumor cells prior to tumor invasion (74,75). It has recently been proposed that tumor cells or tumor cell shed vesicles can favor platelet aggregation by shifting the intravascular balance between prostacyclin and thromboxane A_2 (75); the significance of prostacyclin and thromboxane in platelet- tumor cell interaction and platelet-tumor cell-vessel wall interactions relative to tumor metastasis has been extensively reviewed (75 and Chapter 14). It has been proposed that arachidonic acid metabolism in the tumor cell, the platelet and the vessel wall plays a role in tumor cell arrest in the microvasculature and in attachment prior to growth into a metastatic foci (75). It has also been proposed that prostacyclin functions as an antimetastatic agent by inhibition of tumor cell-platelet association, platelet-vessel wall interaction or tumor cell-vessel wall interaction (75).

IV. BM DEGRADATION MEDIATED BY TUMOR CELL-DERIVED PROTEOLYTIC ENZYMES

Following binding of malignant cells to the exposed BM, the second step involved in tumor cell penetration of the BM is local degradation of the BM (5). Local dissolution of the BM takes place at the point of tumor cell contact and can result in protrusion of tumor cell pseudopodia through the BM (5). Histological studies have demonstrated local and rapid BM breakdown during tumor invasion (5). A substantial body of evidence has indicated that penetration of the BM involves proteolytic enzymes directly or indirectly associated with tumor cells (1,3). Multiple enzymes may be responsible for BM dissolution and separate enzymes may degrade the collagenous and non-collagenous constitutents of the BM (76). The reader is directed to a number of recent reviews that have summarized the role of proteolytic enzymes in various aspects of metastatic tumor cell invasion (5,11,21,62,77-81). A number of approaches have been used to characterize the proteolytic enzymes responsible for BM degradation (5,76). In one approach, known purified enzymes have been employed to determine their effect on preparations of intact BM in vitro or on isolated purified components of the BM. Another approach has been the identification, purification and characterization of proteolytic enzymes secreted by metastatic tumor cells which have the capacity to degrade BM components. To date a large number of enzymes have been identified which have the potential to degrade at least some BM proteins (5,76-81).

A. Role of Type IV Collagenase and Type V Collagenase in BM Degradation, Tumor Invasion and Metastasis

Recent studies have indicated that collagenases are an important family of metallo proteinases that play a role in facilitating tumor cell invasion of the extracellular matrix (5). Distinct collagenolytic metallo proteinases have been identified which degrade specific types of collagen. A collagenase which recognizes type IV collagen in the BM and is distinct from classic collagenases has been shown to be elevated in a number of metastatic cells, as described below.

Type IV collagenolytic activity of cultured metastatic cells has been found in both an active form and a latent form (5,77,82-86). The latent form, secreted into the culture medium, can be activated with plasmin or trypsin. The enzyme is a metallo proteinase which is inhibited by alpha 2 macroglobulin, EDTA and cartilage-derived natural collagenase inhibitors but not by DFP, PMSF or N-ethylmaleimide (5). Type IV collagenase purified from human tumor cells migrates as a doublet on gel electrophoresis with a Mr of 70 kDa (5). The enzymatic activity of type IV collagenase is assayed on biosynthetically labeled and acid extracted type IV collagen purified from organ cultures of EHS sarcoma (5). At 37°C the enzyme cleaves the substrate into several fragments (5). Below 35°C, however, specific large cleavage products are obtained (83). It appears that type IV collagenase produces a specific cleavage within a pepsin-resistant domain of type IV collagen (5). Degradation of type IV collagen by type IV collagenase at 25°C produces a major cleavage product at a region approximately one third of the way from one end of the intact substrate (5). The exact sequence of the cleavage site remains unknown. Although type IV collagen does not degrade collagens I, II, III or V or native elastin, it is still unknown whether type IV collagen is the enzyme's only substrate.

At least one group of metastatic murine tumors shows a correlation between production of type IV collagenase and capacity to yield spontaneous metastases (85). To date, all highly metastatic tumors that we have tested, including carcinomas, fibrosarcomas, hepatomas, reticulum cell sarcomas and melanomas, consistently displayed elevated type IV collagenase activity when compared to benign control cells (5). In cases of tumor cells derived from the same parent, a quantitative relationship has been found between the amount of type IV collagenolytic activity and metastasis formation (5,77); in some cases tumor cells with type IV collagenolytic activity were poorly metastatic. This is not surprising since it is unlikely that a quantitative difference in this proteinase would correlate with metastatic propensity in all types of tumors. It would seem necessary that some minimal ability to degrade BM collagen would be required for hematogenous metastasis.

A separate tumor metallo proteinase produced by metastatic cells has been identified which preferentially degraded type V collagen (87). This enzyme, which fails to degrade type IV collagen, produces specific large molecular weight cleavage products of type V collagen.

It should also be kept in mind that separate metallo proteinases which degrade collagens type IV and V are not unique to tumor cells. For example a type V collagen-degrading enzyme has also been identified in normal alveolar macrophages (88) and a type IV collagen-degrading elastase has been identified and isolated from human polymorphonuclear leukocytes (89). Enzymes that degrade both type IV and type V collagens have been found in normal involuting epithelial ducts (90). These enzymes, which can contribute to BM degradation during metastatic tumor invasion, probably also play some role in the selective physiologic turnover of BM during normal tissue remodeling (77).

B. Role of Plasminogen Activator and Plasmin in BM Degradation, Tumor Invasion and Metastasis

Plasminogen activators (PA) are neutral serine proteinases that proteolytically convert the serum proenzyme plasminogen to the active neutral serine proteinase plasmin. PA has been found to play a role in the degradative functions and migration of a number of normal cell types in various normal and pathologic aspects of tissue remodeling (for review see 91). The role of PA in cellular migration, tissue remodeling and invasive processes is evident in various aspects of malignant transformation (78,92). The production of PA and the proteolytic activation of plasminogen to plasmin has been correlated with many processes that characterize the malignant phenotype (for review see 92). The PA/plasmin system plays a role in anchorage independent growth in agar, tumorigenesis of viral transformants in nude mice, tumorigenesis of hormone dependent murine mammary carcinoma cells and bromodeoxyuridine-regulated murine melanoma cells, tumor promoter treatment of normal and transformed cells and the temperature-sensitive expression of the Rous sarcoma virus src gene product (92); the PA/plasmin system has also been correlated with the induction of cellular proliferation and loss of intracellular actin cables. Although normal cells involved in invasive activity produce PA activity, it appears that normal cell PA synthesis is under regulation of a temporal, hormonal or developmental nature which does not regulate tumor cell PA production (92). For example, extensive degradation of the Graafian follicle at the time of ovulation and invasive embryonic implantation of trophoblasts show only transient production of PA coincident with the invasive phase of these processes (91,92). Since the phenomena of malignant transformation, cell migration and tissue remodeling may be associated with BM changes, PA and plasmin have recently been examined for their effects in degradation of the BM, tumor invasion and metastasis.

It has been found that matrix glycoproteins are sensitive to hydrolysis by plasmin and that the generation of plasmin plays an important role in glycoprotein degradation by macrophages as well as by tumor cells (79,93-96). PA and plasmin have been extensively examined for their effects on both glycoprotein and collagenous components of the BM (5,53,76). Homogeneously pure human PA (urokinase) was incubated with isolated components of the BM as well as with whole, intact human BM (53,76). The BM components investigated were acid extracted type IV collagen, pepsin fragments of collagen type IV and laminin (76); in addition, type V collagen associated with the peri-BM zone was studied. Fibronectin or any of the other BM components that were examined by SDS polyacrylamide gel electrophoresis following incubation with pure human PA were not significantly degraded (53,76). Under the same conditions, pure human plasmin, as well as pure human alpha thrombin, cleaved fibronectin and laminin but not type IV collagen or type V collagen (76). These findings were in agreement with those noted for degradation of the extracellular matrix (96). Additional studies have indicated that solubilization of BM glycoproteins, in a hamster lung BM, is also primarily due to PA-mediated degradation (97). Whereas PA was unable to cleave either fibronectin or laminin, plasmin was found to cleave both fibronectin as well as both the alpha and beta chains of laminin (76). In addition, it was noted that plasmin alone could not degrade the intact BM as judged by immunofluorescent localization studies with anti-type IV collagen antibodies and anti-laminin antibodies. Plasmin treatment cannot completely destroy the BM lamina densa (76). Plasmin treatment of the BM leads to a loss of immunoreactivity for anti-laminin antisera but not of immunoreactivity for anti-type IV collagen antisera, which is preserved within the BM following plasmin treatment (76). It, therefore, appears that the BM components studied are poor substrates for PA (urokinase) and that plasmin alone is not capable of complete degradation of the BM. It should be noted that the potential role of tissue type PA, rather than urokinase, has not yet been explored relative to degradation of BM components and the possible existence of additional BM substrates for PA remains an open question (92).

A number of studies have examined whether a quantitative relationship exists between PA production by malignant cells and metastatic potential in vivo (92). Studies with melanoma variant sublines of differing metastasizing capabilities have given conflicting results. Whereas one report has indicated that low metastatic B16F1 and variants of increasing metastatic potential, B16F5, B16F10 and B16F13, showed similar and high levels of PA activity, a quantitative difference in PA production between B16F1 and B16F10 sublines has also been described (98,99). Although studies with metastatic variants from a cloned epitheloid cell line of hepatic origin have shown no correlation between metastatic ability and fibrinolytic activity, quantitative models of metastasis employing HEp-3 human epidermoid carcinoma cells in the chick embryo have utiilized PA as a marker for HEp-3 metastasis in both chick embryos and in newly hatched chicks (100,101). Studies with human colon tumors have shown that tumor samples produced high PA levels in comparison to normal mucosal samples and a correlation was found between high PA levels in tumors and an invasive and metastatic phenotype (102). In contrast, primary and metastatic human breast cancers did not show significant differences in their PA content (103). However, PA levels have been correlated with the metastatic spread of rat prostatic adenocarcinoma cells (104). Studies with UV2237 fibrosarcoma cells have shown that some cloned tumor cell lines with high in vivo metastatic potential produce low levels of PA when compared to cells with a lower metastatic capability (105); nevertheless, clones with low PA activity are highly metastatic in immunosuppressed hosts (105). We have recently observed that homogenously purified PAs (high and low Mr urokinase) are angiogenic in the rabbit cornea whereas DFP-inhibited preparations are not angiogenic (R.H. Goldfarb, G. Murano and L.A. Liotta, unpublished observations). Our results suggest that PA may function, in part, by contributing to the process of tumor neovascularization and thereby contribute to this aspect of metastatic tumor invasion. For more detailed accounts of the role of PA in metastasis the reader is directed to a number of recent reviews (62,78,92,106-108).

C. Enzymatic Cascade for BM Degradation

A number of studies have examined the interactions among different proteolytic enzymes in degradation of the BM. Emphasis has been placed on the interaction of PA and type IV collagenase in mediating dissolution of the BM by acting in concert (5,76,78). Plasmin, in addition to being capable of degrading BM laminin and fibronectin, also has the capacity to activate latent type IV and latent type V collagenases (5,109). Plasmin may, therefore, aid in the enzymatic destruction of the BM through the activation of latent metallo proteinases which degrade collagen, glycosaminoglycan or glycoprotein components of the BM (76). In addition, plasmin may play some role in removal of the glycoprotein component of the BM and in exposing type IV collagen for degradation by additional enzymes. It has been suggested that PA may play an important role in the regulation of a cascade of enzyme activation relative to BM degradation and that this function may indeed be the major role of PA in tumor invasion (5,76,96). Recent reports have suggested that the activation of latent BM collagenase in vivo may be facilitated by PA by the activation of plasminogen to plasmin, and that the secretion of BM collagenase concomitantly with PA is a prerequisite for metastasis (110). Studies with the subendothelial matrix of cloned bovine endothelial cells have also indicated that the PA/plasmin system plays a key role in matrix degradation (111). Four human tumor cell lines, that produce high PA levels, digested matrix glycoproteins under conditions that allowed for the generation of active plasmin (111). It was reported that HT1080 cells, in the absence of plasminogen, showed reduced but significant degradation of the subendothelial matrix indicating that such matrix digestion was either due to the direct enzymatic activity of PA (112,113) or due to an uncharacterized enzyme produced by this cell type (111). In contrast, in the case of one human rhabdomyosarcoma line, no plasminogen-independent matrix degradation was noted (111). HT1080 clones which secrete either small or large amounts of PA, but have similar cell-associated PA activity, were found to digest the subendothelial matrix at similar rates (111). It has, therefore, been suggested that the cell-associated form of PA, known to be associated with the plasma membrane (113,114), may be mainly responsible for glycoprotein degradation (111); alternatively an additional plasminogen-independent enzyme may be involved. In this regard, it is interesting to note that leukocytes, macrophages and highly metastatic cells were found to secrete laminin-degrading proteinases which showed significant enhancement of laminin degradation in the presence of plasminogen (76). Although this finding supports a role for plasmin-mediated degradation of laminin, it also appears that additional neutral proteinases other than plasmin may be involved in the degradation of laminin since degradation also took place in the absence of plasminogen (76). An additional study has determined that metastatic tumor cell contact with the subendothelial matrix induces enhanced solubilization of the matrix in a plasminogen-independent process (115). It was, therefore, concluded that plasmin is not required for matrix solubilization; however, it was noted that plasminogen could enhance matrix solubilization when serum inhibitors are inactivated (115). Since acid-treated serum stimulated matrix solubilization even in the absence of plasminogen, it was suggested that B16 melanoma cells may secrete, or have on their cell surface, proteinase-inhibitor sensitive proteinases which may be PA or some additional neutral proteinase (115).

The degradation of proteoglycans by metastatic cells has also been examined (115). Solubilization of sulfated proteoglycans, which was not dependent upon plasminogen, appeared to require tumor cell-subendothelial matrix interaction (115). Sulfated glycosaminoglycan chains released by the metastatic cells were shorter than chains found following treatment with alkaline borohydride (115). The results, therefore, suggested that the metastatic cells produce a glycosidase. In a study directed at the relationship of heparan sulfate degradation to the invasive and metastatic behavior of B16 melanoma sublines, evidence was provided for the production of a heparan sulfate endoglycosidase (116). It was noted that invasive and metastatic B16F10 sublines degraded matrix glycosaminoglycans at faster rates than sublines of lower metastatic capacity (23,116). It was, therefore, suggested that this enzymatic activity may play a role in extravasation and lung colonization of B16 cells. It has also been noted that highly metastatic ESb T cell lymphoma cells solubilize subendothelial glycosaminoglycans with greater ability than low metastatic Eb cells, and it has been suggested that enhanced degradation of sulfated proteoglycans may facilitate hematogenous metastasis (117).

Recent studies have demonstrated that a cathepsin B-like activity in B16F10 cells was elevated when compared to the B16F1 variant (118). It has been suggested that a cathepsin B-like cysteine proteinase may play a direct or regulatory role in tumor metastasis (118,119 and Chapter 12). We have recently examined the role of a purified tumor cathepsin B-like proteinase on degradation of various BM components. Our preliminary results suggest that this proteinase has the capacity to cleave both the long arm of laminin as well as fibronectin (L.A. Liotta, B.F. Sloane, K.V. Honn and R.H. Goldfarb, unpublished observations); additional studies are in progress to determine whether cascading zymogen activation reactions and regulatory interactions exist among cathepsin B, PA, plasmin and type IV collagenase.

V. TUMOR CELL LOCOMOTION INTO VACANCY CREATED BY PROTEOLYTIC DEGRADATION OF THE BM

The third step in penetration of the BM by metastatic tumor cells is locomotion through the BM defect generated by localized proteolysis of the BM (5). It appears that the direction of locomotion may be influenced by chemotactic factors derived from serum, connective tissue or host cells (120-122). It has been reported that a number of chemotactic stimuli including the C5a-derived tumor cell chemotactic peptide, N-formyl-methionyl-leucyl-phenylalanine (FMLP) and 12-0-tetradecanoyl phorbol ester induce a rapid, transient adherence response (123). It has been speculated that this phenomenon, which may be mediated by lipoxygenase metabolites of arachidonic acid, may influence tumor cell localization in vivo (123). We have recently shown that FMLP significantly stimulated the migration of invasive, metastatic M5076 cells through amnion connective tissue at a concentration similar to that found optimal for stimulating migration of phagocytes and tumor cells across artificial porous filters (124,125).

Metastatic cell locomotion has also been examined from the viewpoint of cell detachment (126); it has been argued that detachment of malignant cells from the substrata through which they migrate is a key step in the locomotion of metastatic cells. Recent studies have indicated that considerable metabolism of and changing intermolecular associations of proteoglycans take place during the movement of fibroblasts over the extracellular matrix (127).

Considerable attention has also been directed towards the possible role in tumor cell locomotion of proteinases with degradative potential for BM components (127). In this regard it is interesting to note that cellular serine proteinases have been shown to induce chemotaxis (128,129) and that alpha thrombin has recently been shown to be a chemoattractant for human monocytes (130). In addition, the PA/plasmin system has also been linked to enhanced cell migration, including enhanced tumor cell migration (131-133).

VI. POTENTIAL SIGNIFICANCE OF METASTATIC CELL DEGRADATION OF THE BM TO DIAGNOSIS AND THERAPY OF HUMAN CANCER

A thorough understanding of the mechanisms of BM degradation by invasive metastatic tumor cells may provide important insights into the diagnosis and therapy of human malignant disease. For example, it has been shown that micrometastases of breast carcinoma can be detected by the presence of BM collagen (134). It has also been suggested that immunoperoxidase staining with antibodies to specific components of the BM may be of diagnostic use in the delineation of intraductal carcinoma from true microinvasive breast carcinoma and the identification of micrometastases in distal sites (135). In intraductal carcinoma it has been found that intact BM surrounds the ducts and lobules when examined by antibodies to type IV collagen and laminin, these antibodies yield extracellular linear staining patterns. In intraductal carcinoma with microinvasion, fragmentation and absence of the BM at areas of microinvasion have been observed (135). It was also observed that metastatic breast carcinoma and infiltrating carcinoma were usually devoid of surrounding extracellular BM containing type IV collagen and laminin. Immunoreactivity directed at type IV collagenase has also been utilized in studies dealing with invasive breast carcinoma. In contrast to benign epithelium, invasive carcinoma cells which show a loss of BM components also show specific cytoplasmic reactivity to type IV collagenase (136). We have reported that the demonstration of type IV collagenase immunoreactivity in human breast carcinoma is useful in both identification of the invasive process in tissue sections, as well as gaining insight into the pathophysiology of tumor spread (136). Additional studies have examined changes in BM in breast cancer by immunohistochemical staining for laminin, and it has been suggested that staining for laminin may be a useful test for the detection of micrometastases in lymph nodes (137).

Studies dealing with the submolecular domains of laminin, and studies dealing with invasive proteolytic degradation of the BM suggest novel mechanisms for the treatment of human metastatic disease. Characterization of the specific domain of laminin that modifies tumor cell attachment suggests the synthesis of a cell binding analogue, or type IV collagen-binding analogue, that might be used therapeutically to reduce hematogenous metastasis (31,44,55). Studies described in this review suggest that a number of proteolytic enzymes, perhaps working in a cascade-like manner, play a role in degradation of BM collagenous, glycoprotein and proteoglycan components. The actual cascade of BM degradation in vivo probably takes place adjacent to the tumor cell surface where the local concentration of degradative enzymes is sufficiently high to negate natural proteolytic inhibitors that are ubiquitious throughout the extracellular matrix and are present in serum. Although it is unlikely that a quantitative difference will be noted for each degradative enzyme which may be involved in the metastatic capability of all tumor types, it would seem to be necessary that a minimal ability for BM degradation is required for hematogenous metastasis. If proteinases are indeed playing an in vivo role their action is probably restricted to a local pericellular locus under the control or balance of enzyme and tissue proteinase inhibitors (5). Whether this balance can be therapeutically altered in favor of the host is unknown and remains to be determined. It is likely that critical analysis of this question will be dependent upon the development of specific, efficient, non-toxic, potent, bioavailable inhibitors, as previously suggested (138). In summary, a thorough understanding of the mechanism of tumor cell attachment, dissolution and locomotion with respect to the BM may yield critical insights into the early diagnosis of micrometastatic disease, and lead to the identification of mechanisms for the treatment and/or prevention of hematogenous metastatic dissemination.

REFERENCES

1. Liotta LA and Hart IR. Tumor Invasion and Metastasis. Martinus Nijhoff, The Hague, 1982.
2. Grundmann E. Metastatic Tumor Growth. Gustav Fischer Verlag, Stuttgart, 1980.
3. Strauli P, Barrett AJ and Baici A. Proteinases and Tumor Invasion. Raven Press, New York, 1980.
4. Fidler IJ, Gersten DM and Hart IR. Adv. Cancer Res. 28:149-250, 1978.
5. Liotta LA, Garbisa S and Tryggvason K. In: Tumor Invasion and Metastasis (Eds. Liotta LA and Hart IR), Martinus Nijhoff, The Hague, pp. 319-333, 1982.
6. Liotta LA, Tryggvason K, Garbisa S, Gehron-Robey P and Murray JC. In: Metastatic Tumor Growth (Ed. Grundmann E), Gustav Fischer Verlag, Stuttgart, pp. 21-30, 1980.
7. Vracko R. Am. J. Pathol. 77:314-320, 1974.
8. Daroczy J, Feldmann J and Kiraly K. Front. Matrix Biol. 7:208-234, 1979.
9. Timpl R, Rohde H, Gehron-Robey P, Rennard S, Foidart JM and Martin GR. J. Biol. Chem. 254:9933-9937, 1979.

338

10. Mosesson MW and Amrani DL.   Blood 56:145–148, 1980.
11. Alitalo K and Vaheri A.   Adv. Cancer Res. 37 111–158, 1982.
12. Bernfield MR, Cohn RH and Banerjee SD.   Am. Zool. 13:1067–1083, 1973.
13. Caulfield JP and Farquhar MG.   J. Cell Biol. 63:883–903, 1974.
14. Hassell J, Gehron-Robey R, Barrach H, Wilczek J, Rennard S and Martin GR.   Proc. Natl. Acad. Sci. USA 77:4494–4498, 1981.
15. Kefalides NA.   Biology and Chemistry of Basement Membranes.   Academic Press, New York, 1978.
16. Miller EJ.   Mol. Cell. Biochem. 13:165–192, 1976.
17. Bornstein P and Sage H.   Annu. Rev. Biochem. 49:957–1003, 1980.
18. Timpl R, Martin GR, Bruckner P, Wick G and Wiedemann H.   Eur. J. Biochem. 84:43–50, 1978.
19. Burgeson RE, EL Adli FA, Kaitila II and Hollister DW.   Proc. Natl. Acad. Sci. USA 73:2579–2580, 1976.
20. Madri JA and Furthmayr H.   Am. J. Pathol. 94:323–331, 1980.
21. Vlodavsky I, Schirrmacher V, Ariav Y and Fuks Z.   Invasion Metastasis 3:81–97, 1983.
22. Kramer RH, Gonzalez R and Nicolson GL.   Int. J. Cancer 26 639–644, 1980.
23. Vlodavsky I, Ariav Y, Atzmon R and Fuks Z.   Exp. Cell Res. 140:149–159, 1982.
24. Nicolson GL, Irimura T, Gonzalez RS and Rusohlahti E.   Exp. Cell Res. 135:461–465, 1981.
25. Warren BA and Vales O.   Br. J. Exp. Pathol. 53 301–311, 1972.
26. Poste G and Fidler IJ.   Nature (London) 283 139–146, 1980.
27. Nicolson GL.   In: Tumor Invasion and Metastasis (Eds. Liotta LA and Hart IR), Martinus Nijhoff, The Hague, pp. 319–333, 1982.
28. Kleinman HK, Klebe RJ and Martin GR.   J. Cell Biol. 88:473–485, 1981.
29. Terranova VP, Rohrbach DH and Martin GR.   Cell 22:719–726, 1980.
30. Terranova VP, Liotta LA, Russo RG and Martin GR.   Cancer Res. 42:2265–2269, 1982.
31. Rao CN, Margulies IMK, Tralka TS, Terranova VP, Madri JA and Liotta LA.   J. Biol. Chem. 257:9740–9744, 1982.
32. Grinnell F and Field MK.   Cell 18 117–128, 1979.
33. Miller EJ and Matukas VJ.   Proc. Natl. Acad. Sci. USA 64:1264–1268, 1969.
34. Murray JC, Liotta LA, Rennard SI and Martin GR.   Cancer Res. 40:347–351, 1980.
35. Vlodavsky I and Gospodarowicz D.   Nature (London) 289:304–306, 1981.
36. Varani J, Lovett EJ, McCoy JP, Shibata S, Maddox DE, Goldstein IJ and Wicha M.   Am. J. Pathol. 111:27–34, 1983.
37. Hogan B.   Nature (London) 290 737–738, 1981.
38. Johansson S, Kjellen L, Hook M and Timpl R.   J. Cell Biol. 90:260–264, 1981.
39. Damnon MY.   In Vitro 18:997–1003, 1982.
40. Crouchman JR, Hook M, Rees DA and Timpl R.   J. Cell Biol. 96:177–183, 1983.
41. Leivo I.   J. Histochem. Cytochem. 31:35–45, 1983.
42. Macarak EJ and Howard PS.   J. Cell. Physiol. 116 76–86, 1983.
43. Kennedy DW, Rohrbach DH, Martin GR, Momoi T and Yamada KM.   J. Cell. Physiol. 114:257–262, 1983.
44. Terranova VP, Rao CN, Kalebic T, Margulies IM and Liotta LA.   Proc. Natl. Acad. Sci. USA 80:444–448, 1983.
45. Rao CN, Barsky SH, Terranova VP and Liotta LA.   Biochem. Biophys. Res. Commun. 111:804–808, 1983.
46. Malinoff HL and Wicha MS.   J. Cell Biol. 96:1475–1479, 1983.
47. Engel J, Odermatt E, Engel A, Madri JA, Furthmayr H, Rohde H and Timpl R.   J. Mol. Biol. 150 97–120, 1981.
48. Timpl R, Engel J and Martin GR.   Trends Biochem. Sci. 8:207–209, 1983.
49. Sakashita S, Engvall E and Ruoslahti E.   FEBS Lett. 116:243–246, 1980.

0. Delrosso M, Cappelletti R, Viti M, Vanucchi S and Chiarngi V. Biochem. J. 199:699-704, 1981.
1. Rohde H. Bachinger HP and Timpl R. Hoppe-Seyler's Z. Physiol. Chem. 361:1651-1660, 1980.
2. Liotta LA, Goldfarb RH and Terranova VP. Thromb. Res. 21:663-673, 1981.
3. Goldfarb RH, Liotta LA and Garbisa S. Proc. Am. Assoc. Cancer Res. 22:59, 1981.
4. Liotta LA, Goldfarb RH, Brundage R, Siegal GP, Terranova VP and Garbisa S. Cancer Res. 41:4629-4636, 1981.
5. Rao CN, Margulies IMK, Goldfarb RH, Madri JA, Woodley DT and Liotta LA. Arch. Biochem. Biophys. 219:65-70, 1982.
6. Ott U, Odermatt E, Engel J, Furthmayr H and Timpl R. Eur. J. Biochem. 123:63-72, 1982.
7. Timpl R, Johansson S, vad Delden V, Oberbaumer I and Hook M. J. Biol. Chem. 258:8922-8927, 1983.
8. Giavazzi R and Hart IR. Exp. Cell. Res. 146:391-399, 1983.
9. Speziale P, Hook M, Wadstrom T and Timpl R. FEBS Lett. 146:55-58, 1982.
10. Yogeeswaran G. Adv. Cancer Res. 38:289-350, 1983.
11. Schirrmacher V, Altevogt P, Fogel M, Dennis J, Waller CA, Barz D, Schwartz R, Cheingsong-Popov R, Springer G, Robinson PJ, Nebe T, Brossmer W, Vlodavsky I, Pawletz N, Zimmerman H-P and Uhlenbruck G. Invasion Metastasis 2:313-360, 1982.
12. Nicolson GL. Biochim. Biophys. Acta. 695 113-176, 1982.
13. Yogeeswaran G and Salk PL. Science 212 1514-1516, 1981.
14. Dennis J, Waller C, Timpl R and Schirrmacher V. Nature (London) 300:274-275, 1982.
15. Fogel M, Altevogt P and Schirrmacher V. J. Exp. Med. 157:371-376, 1983.
16. Sinha BK and Goldenberg GJ. Cancer (Philadelphia) 34:1956-1961, 1974.
17. Irimura T, Gonzalez R and Nicolson GL. Cancer Res. 41 3411-3418, 1981.
18. Irimura T and Nicolson GL. J. Supramol. Struct. Cell. Biochem. 17 325-336, 1981.
19. Turner GA. Invasion Metastasis 2:197-216, 1982.
20. Stamper HB and Woodruff JJ. J. Exp. Med. 144:828-833, 1976.
21. Chin Y, Carey GD and Woodruff JJ. J. Immunol. 129:1911-1915, 1982.
22. Nicolson GL. In: Cancer Achievements, Challenges and Prospects for the 1980's (Eds. Burchenal JH and Oettgen HF), Grune and Stratton, New York, pp. 477-490, 1980.
23. Brunson KW, Beattie G and Nicolson GL. Nature (London) 272 543-545, 1978.
24. Karpatkin S and Pearlstein E. Ann. Intern. Med. 95:636-641, 1981.
25. Honn KV, Busse WD and Sloane BF. Biochem. Pharmacol. 32:1-11, 1983.
26. Liotta LA, Goldfarb RH, Brundage R, Siegal GP, Terranova V and Garbisa S. Cancer Res. 41:4629-4636, 1981.
27. Liotta LA, Thorgeirsson UP and Garbisa S. Cancer Metastasis Rev. 1 277-288, 1982.
28. Goldfarb RH. In: Tumor Invasion and Metastasis (Eds. Liotta LA and Hart IR), Martinus Nijhoff, The Hague, pp. 375-390, 1982.
29. Jones PA and De Clerck YA. Cancer Metastasis Rev. 1:289-317, 1982.
30. Pauli BU, Schwartz DE, Thonar EJ-M and Kuettner KE. Cancer Metastasis Rev. 2:129-152, 1983.
31. Mareel M. Cancer Metastasis Rev. 2:201-218, 1983.
32. Liotta LA, Abe S, Gehron-Robey P and Martin GR. Proc. Natl. Acad. Sci. USA 76 2268-2272, 1979.
33. Liotta LA, Tryggvason K, Garbisa S, Gehron-Robey P and Abe S. Biochemistry 20:100-104, 1981.
34. Salo T, Liotta LA and Tryggvason K. J. Biol. Chem. 258:3058-3063, 1983.

85. Liotta LA, Tryggvason K, Garbisa S, Hart I, Foltz CM and Shafie S. Nature (London) 284:67-68, 1980.
86. Garbisa S, Kniska K, Tryggvason K, Foltz C and Liotta LA. Cancer Lett. 9:359-366, 1980.
87. Liotta LA, Lanzer WL and Garbisa S. Biochem. Biophys. Res. Commun. 98 184-190, 1981.
88. Mainardi CL, Seyer JM and Kang AH. Biochem. Biophys. Res. Commun. 97:1108-1115, 1980.
89. Mainardi CL, Dixit SN and Kang AH. J. Biol. Chem. 255:5435-5441, 1980.
90. Liotta LA, Wicha MS, Foidart JM, Rennard SI, Garbisa S and Kidwell WR. Lab. Invest. 41:511-518, 1979.
91. Reich E. In: Molecular Basis of Degradative Processes (Eds. Berlin RD, Herrman H, Lepow IR and Tanzer JM), Academic Press, New York, pp. 155-169. 1978.
92. Goldfarb RH. Annu. Rep. Med. Chem. 18:257-264, 1983.
93. Werb Z, Banda MJ and Jones PA. J. Exp. Med. 152:1340-1357, 1980.
94. Jones PA and Scott-Burden T. Biochem. Biophys. Res. Commun. 86:71-77, 1979.
95. Jones PA and Werb Z. J. Exp. Med. 152:1527-1536, 1980.
96. Jones PA and DeClerck Y. Cancer Res. 40:3222-3227, 1980.
97. Sheela S and Barrett JC. Carcinogenesis 3:363-369, 1982.
98. Nicolson GL, Winkelhake JL and Nussey AC. In: Fundamental Aspects of Metastasis (Ed. Weiss L), North Holland, Amsterdam, pp. 291-303, 1976.
99. Wang BS, McLoughlin GA, Richie JP and Mannick JA. Cancer Res. 40:288-292, 1980.
100. Talmadge JE, Starkey JR and Stanford DR. J. Supramol. Struct. Cell. Biochem. 15:139-151, 1981.
101. Ossowski L and Reich E. Cancer Res. 40:2300-2309, 1980.
102. Corasanti JG, Celik C, Camiolo SM, Mittelman A, Evers AJC, Barbasch A, Hobika GH and Markus G. J. Natl. Cancer Inst. 65:345-351, 1980.
103. Evers JL, Patel J, Madeja JM, Schneider SL, Hobika GH, Camiolo S and Markus G. Cancer Res. 42:219-226, 1982.
104. Pollard M, Luckert PH and Ruckner-Kardoss E. Fed. Proc. Fed. Am. Soc. Exp. Biol. 42 773, 1983.
105. Roblin R. Cancer Biol. Rev. 2:59-94, 1981.
106. Cederholm-Williams SA. Invasion Metastasis 1:85-97, 1981.
107. Barrett JC and Sheela S. In: Tumor Invasion and Metastasis (Eds. Liotta LA and Hart IR), Martinus Nijhoff, The Hague, pp. 359-374, 1982.
108. Markus G. In: Progress in Fibrinolysis, Vol 6 (Eds. Davidson JF, Nilsson IM, Astedt B), Churchill-Livingstone, Edinburgh, pp. 587-604, 1981.
109. Paranjpe M, Engel L, Young N and Liotta LA. Life Sci. 26:1223-1231, 1980.
110. Salo T, Liotta LA, Keski-Oja J, Turpeenniemi-Hujanen T and Tryggvason K. Int. J. Cancer 30:669-673, 1982.
111. Laug WE, DeClerck YA and Jones PA. Cancer Res. 43:1827-1834, 1983.
112. Quigley JP and Goldfarb RH. J. Cell Biol. 79:73a, 1978.
113. Quigley JP, Goldfarb RH, Scheiner CJ, O'Donnell-Tormey J and Yeo TK. Prog. Clin. Biol. Res. 41:773-796, 1980.
114. Quigley JP. J. Cell Biol. 71 472-486, 1976.
115. Kramer RH, Vogel KG and Nicolson GL. J. Biol. Chem. 257 2678-2686, 1982.
116. Nakajima M, Irimura T, DiFerrante D, DiFerrante N and Nicolson GL. Science 220:611-613, 1983.
117. Vlodavsky I, Fuks Z, Bar-Ner M, Ariav Y and Schirrmacher V. Cancer Res. 43:2704-2711, 1983.
118. Sloane BF, Honn KV, Sadler JG. Turner WA, Kimpson JJ and Taylor JD. Cancer Res. 42:980-986, 1982.
119. Sloane BF, Dunn JR and Honn KV. Science 212:1151-1153, 1981.

120. Orr W, Varani J and Ward PA. Am. J. Pathol. 93:405–422, 1978.
121. Orr W, Varani J, Gondek MD, Ward PA and Mudny GR. Science 203 176–179, 1979.
122. Varani J and Ward PA. In: Tumor Invasion and Metastasis (Eds. Liotta LA and Hart IR), Martinus Nijhoff, The Hague, pp. 98–112, 1982.
123. Varani J. Cancer Metastasis Rev. 1:17–28, 1982.
124. Thorgeirsson UP, Liotta LA, Kalebic T, Margulies IM, Thomas K, Rios–Candelore M and Russo RG. J. Natl. Cancer Inst. 69:1049–1054, 1982.
125. Russo RG, Thorgeirsson U and Liotta LA. In: Tumor Invasion and Metstasis (Eds. Liotta LA and Hart IR), Martinus Nijhoff, The Hague, pp. 173–187, 1982.
126. Weiss L and Ward PM. Cancer Metastasis Rev. 2:111–127, 1983.
127. Lark MW and Culp LA. Biochemistry 22:2289–2296, 1983.
128. Thomas CA Yost FJ, Snyderman R, Hatcher BB and Lazarus G. Nature (London) 269:521–522, 1977.
129. Hatcher VB, Lazarus GS, Levine N, Burk PG and Yost FJ. Biochim. Biophys. Acta. 483:160–171, 1977.
130. Bar–Shavit R, Kahn A, Wilner GD and Fenton JW. Science 220:728–731, 1983.
131. Ossowski L, Quigley JP and Reich E. In: Proteases and Biological Control (Eds. Reich E, Rifkin DB and Shaw E), Cold Spring Harbor Laboratory Press, Cold Spring Harbor, pp. 901–913, 1975.
132. Kalderon N. Proc. Natl. Acad. Sci. USA 76:5992–5998, 1979.
133. Moonen G, Brau–Wagemans MP and Selak I. Nature (London) 298:753–755, 1982.
134. Liotta LA, Foidart JM, Gehron–Robey P, Martin GR and Gullino PM. Lancet 2:146–147 1979.
135. Siegal GP, Barsky SH, Terranova VP and Liotta LA. Invasion Metastasis 1:54–70, 1981.
136. Barsky SH, Togo S, Garbisa S and Liotta LA. Lancet 2:296–297, 1983.
137. Albrechtsen R, Nielsen M, Wewer U, Engvall E and Ruoslahti E. Cancer Res. 41:5076–5081, 1981.
138. Nelles LP and Schnebli HP. Invasion Metastasis 82:113–123, 1982.

CHAPTER 22. HEMOSTATIC ALTERATIONS IN CANCER PATIENTS

RICHARD L. EDWARDS AND FREDERICK R. RICKLES

Previous chapters have documented the close relationship between activation of blood coagulation and the growth and metastasis of malignant tumors. A variety of tumor-related mechanisms have been shown to participate in the activation of the coagulation cascade and the initiation of platelet aggregation. In addition to playing a role in tumor homeostasis, these alterations can lead to the development of a "hypercoagulable state" with associated clinical and laboratory manifestations. This chapter will review the laboratory abnormalities and the associated clinical syndromes which accompany the hypercoagulable state in cancer patients.

I.   THROMBOEMBOLIC DISORDERS

The close relationship between neoplastic disease and clinically evident thromboembolic disorders (TED) has been well-established since Armand Trousseau (1) first reported the high incidence of thrombophlebitis in a series of patients with gastric cancer in 1865. Over the last 100 years, numerous additional reports have documented the occurrence in cancer patients of a wide variety of hemostatic or thromboembolic disorders including arterial and venous thrombosis, migratory thrombophlebitis, pulmonary embolism, nonbacterial thrombotic endocarditis and disseminated intravascular coagulation (DIC) (2).   In studies based on autopsy reports, the incidence of TED in cancer patients has been reported to range between 20 and 50%. Sproule (3) suggested that patients with pancreatic carcinoma were at particularly high risk for thromboembolic disease. In her study of 4,258 autopsies, evidence of widely disseminated TED was found in 31% of 16 patients with pancreatic carcinoma (body or tail) and 56% of those patients demonstrated evidence of at least one thrombosis at autopsy. In more recent studies, Thompson and Rogers (4) found a similar high incidence of TED in patients with pancreatic cancer. Ambrus and colleagues (5) have reported that thrombosis or bleeding constituted the second most common cause of death among hospitalized cancer patients.

Although autopsy studies have generally found a high incidence of TED in cancer patients, the incidence of clinically evident disorders is considerably less, ranging from 0 - 11%.   In 179 consecutive patients with pancreatic carcinoma, Anylan et al. (6) found none with evidence of TED while Hoerr and Harper (7) noted 2 patients with deep venous thrombosis (DVT) in a study of 100 patients with carcinoma of the pancreas, bile duct, duodenum or gall bladder. Other studies have demonstrated a higher incidence of TED, however. For example, Soong and Miller (8) reported 11 cases of clinically evident thrombosis in 100 unselected patients with disseminated malignancies. The apparent discrepancies among different studies may be caused by the known inaccuracies inherent in the clinical diagnosis of TED (9) or by the presence in cancer patients of other disorders which can mimic the clinical signs of TED. Such phenomena include embolization from nonbacterial endocarditis (10) or localized pain and swelling caused by direct tumor invasion.

Nevertheless, it is well known that TED can occur as a consequence of malignant disease. It has been estimated that 5 to 15% of all cases of DVT are associated with malignant disease. Moreover, TED is often the first indication of disease in an otherwise apparently healthy patient. In a study of 1,400 patients with DVT, Lieberman et al. (11) found 61 patients with cancer of whom half were treated for DVT before the diagnosis of cancer was made. Since hemostatic abnormalities may represent the first indication that malignant disease is present, early recognition of this potential association is important and may allow more timely diagnosis of the malignancy while it is in a relatively treatable stage. Several clinical characteristics are peculiar to TED associated with malignancy and have been reported by numerous authors. The "typical" DVT in a single extremity is less commonly reported in cancer patients than is migratory thrombophlebitis of numerous superficial veins. Moreover, when DVT occurs in cancer patients it more often involves unusual sites and tends to be resistant to standard therapy. Recurrent migratory superficial thrombophlebitis has been said to be virtually pathognomonic of cancer (12); however, others have found no prognostic or diagnostic difference between single versus multiple episodes of phlebitis (2).

It remains unresolved whether the specific tumor type plays an important role in determining the likelihood that TED will occur. Although patients with mucin-secreting tumors of the gastrointestinal tract have long been known to be prone to TED (3), other tumor types are also associated with an increased risk of TED. Table 1 lists the frequency in several large studies with which carcinomas of different organs have been reported to be associated with clinical evidence of TED. Although carcinoma of the pancreas has often been cited as having the greatest propensity for inducing TED (2,3,13), the series included in Table 1 reported a higher number of cases of TED in patients with carcinoma of the lung. The large number of lung cancer cases reported is undoubtedly due to the significantly increased prevalence of that tumor in comparison to other tumors such as pancreatic malignancy.

344

Table 1. Distribution of Tumor Types in Published Reports of Cancer
Associated with Clinically Evident Thromboembolic Disease.[a]

Tumor Type	Frequency of Tumor Type %
Lung	25.6
Pancreas	17.4
Stomach	16.8
Colon	15.2
Prostate	6.5
Ovary/Uterus	6.3
Gall Bladder	2.8
Breast	2.0
Kidney	0.4
Other	7.0

[a]Extracted from Sack et al. (2) and Ambrus et al. (5).

Other factors which may play a role in the apparent high
incidence of TED in some patients with cancer include the use of
chemotherapy and the availability of improved techniques for the
non-invasive diagnosis of TED. Chemotherapy may play an important
role in the initiation of TED in some patients. In one recent study
of 433 patients with breast cancer, there was a 5% incidence of
clinically detected TED during the period when the patients were
treated with chemotherapy. After chemotherapy was discontinued,
however, no further cases of TED were documented (14). Similarly,
patients with prostatic carcinoma have not been reported to have a
significantly increased risk of TED (13), but when treated with either
estrogens or chemotherapy, groups of patients appear to develop an
enhanced risk of thrombosis (11). Other conditions often associated
with neoplasia such as surgery, prolonged inactivity or impaired blood
flow due to local vascular obstruction can also increase the risk of
TED in cancer patients. Surgery has been shown to increase the risk
of TED more in cancer patients than in patients with non-malignant
disorders. In one study, Pineo and associates (15) noted a marked
increase in the incidence of TED following abdominal surgery in cancer
patients as compared to patients with non-malignant disorders (10 of
30 cancer patients developed TED versus 14 of 134 control patients
undergoing similar procedures).

II. HEMORRHAGIC DISORDERS

In addition to the ample evidence of localized TED, it is well known that patients with disseminated malignancies suffer an increased incidence of bleeding. Although local tumor growth can certainly result in bleeding by disrupting vascular integrity, it is apparent that most patients have varying degrees of DIC. In its most advanced form, DIC is associated with systemic thrombin activation and ensuing fibrin deposition throughout the vasculature. This sequence is then associated with ischemic organ damage, a microangiopathic hemolytic process and evidence of a bleeding disorder caused by consumption of clotting factors and platelets as well as activation of the fibrinolytic system. This fulminant type of DIC is not difficult to recognize, however, in more limited forms DIC may be associated with mild nonspecific abnormalities of coagulation tests and no clinical evidence of disordered hemostasis. Such mild abnormalities are common in cancer patients and have been said to be consistent with a form of "overcompensated" DIC (16). The laboratory manifestations of this limited form of DIC will be discussed below.

Although there is ample evidence for low grade DIC in cancer patients, the occurrence of overt DIC with consumption of platelets and clotting factors and a resultant bleeding diathesis is uncommon. In fact, bleeding from any cause has only been reported in 6 - 15% of patients with cancer (for review see 17). It has been said that whereas migratory thrombophlebitis is often an early sign of cancer, unexplained bleeding is generally a very late consequence which suggests the presence of widespread and usually untreatable disease (18).

Certain tumors appear to carry an increased risk for the development of overt DIC. Fulminant DIC frequently occurs during the treatment of promyelocytic leukemia (18,19). In this disorder, the DIC most commonly occurs soon after the initiation of cytotoxic chemotherapy and has been thought to result from tumor lysis with the resultant release of thromboplastin-like material from the cells (20,21). Overt DIC has also been reported to occur more commonly in patients with mucin-producing adenocarcinomas than in patients with other types of tumors (22,23). It must also be remembered that other conditions such as gram-negative sepsis or liver disease can contribute to the development of a bleeding disorder in chronically ill patients (24). Moreover, tumor involvement of the bone marrow or marrow suppression by chemotherapy can lead to decreased platelet production and a resultant hemostatic defect. Thus, there are many potential causes of bleeding in cancer patients, the most severe of which is DIC. The bleeding which occurs may be subtle and consist of mild bruising, petechiae or gingival bleeding or it may be fulminant with uncontrollable bleeding from venipuncture sites and fatal internal hemorrhage. Fortunately overt DIC has been reported to occur in only 9 - 15% of cancer patients including those in the high risk period after chemotherapy.

III. LABORATORY ABNORMALITIES

A. Routine Tests

The recognition that increased rates of TED and, conversely, bleeding are common in patients with cancer has led several authors to examine the coagulation system in those patients. Such studies have revealed a high incidence of abnormalities in routine blood coagulation tests performed on patients who demonstrate no clinical evidence of disordered hemostasis. In some studies, as many as 92% of cancer patients demonstrated at least one abnormal coagulation study (25,26). In a prospective study Sun and associates (25) reported finding at least 5 abnormal coagulation tests in 88 of 108 consecutive patients with a variety of tumor types. The most common coagulation abnormalities reported include elevated levels of fibrin/fibrinogen degradation products (FDP) (25,27), hyperfibrinogenemia (25,28) and prolongation of the prothrombin time or the thrombin time (25,26,29). Other abnormalities less commonly reported include hypofibrinogenemia, shortening of the partial thromboplastin time and positive tests for fibrin monomers (ethanol gelation or protamine sulfate tests).

In a variety of clinical studies the levels of specific coagulation factors have been reported to be normal, depressed or elevated in patients with cancer. Elevated levels of fibrinogen are observed in 30 - 50% of cancer patients and factor VIII levels are also often increased (29). Other studies have reported some patients to have increased levels of several factors while other patients have clearly depressed levels. Sun and colleagues (25) reported that 53% of their population of 108 cancer patients had depressed factor V levels while 33% had normal and 14% elevated levels. In the same patient group, there were none with depressed fibrinogen levels and 46% with clearly elevated fibrinogen levels. Conversely, in the Sack et al. (2) study of 182 patients with malignancy and chronic DIC, few had elevated fibrinogen levels at any time and there was a marked decrease in fibrinogen in those patients demonstrating thromboembolic episodes. These data support the hypothesis that there is a dynamic relationship between blood coagulation and neoplasia with most cancer patients demonstrating some evidence of DIC throughout the course of their disease. Cooper et al. (30) have proposed three levels of DIC: 1) a decompensated form in which FDP are elevated while fibrinogen, factors V and VIII and platelets are rapidly consumed and their levels are reduced, 2) a compensated state in which the rate of clotting factor and platelet consumption is moderate and their levels remain normal, and 3) an overcompensated state in which the rate of consumption is low while the rate of production is increased and therefore the platelet count or one or more of the factor levels becomes elevated. In any event, it is probable that the common event leading to most of the observed coagulation abnormalities in cancer patients is the activation of thrombin.

Quantitative and qualitative platelet abnormalities have also been observed frequently in patients with cancer. Thrombocytopenia has been reported to occur in as many as 27% of patients with advanced metastatic cancer (31). However, other studies of patients with less extensive disease who have not been exposed to marrow suppression by chemotherapy or radiation have found thrombocytopenia in only 4 - 11% of patients studied (25,26). While the exact mechanism of thrombocytopenia is not clear in all cases, several studies have documented either increased platelet destruction (32-34) or evidence for in vivo platelet activation and release with subsequent platelet consumption (35,36). The latter mechanism may therefore represent a manifestation of tumor-induced DIC.

Thrombocytosis has been reported much more frequently than thrombocytopenia in patients with cancer. Increased platelet counts have been found in 30 - 60% of untreated cancer patients (25,26,37,38) and may represent the end result of low grade DIC with "overcompensation." In this situation, it has been suggested that increased platelet consumption and the enhanced production of thrombopoietin has stimulated the marrow to produce platelets at an increased rate. In some cases the increase in platelet production more than offsets the accelerated destruction and results in the appearance of paradoxical thrombocytosis (26). The finding of increased thrombopoietic activity in the sera of cancer patients with thrombocytosis provides further support for this potential mechanism (39).

Although there is ample evidence to support the ability of tumor products to stimulate platelet aggregation in vitro and in vivo, few studies have examined platelet function in cancer patients. Davis and colleagues (38) have reported that some patients with advanced cancer demonstrate increased platelet aggregation following ADP stimulation in vitro and have correlated this abnormality with the presence of elevated levels of FDP. Other studies have supported the presence of hyperaggregable platelets in patients with carcinoma of the prostate receiving estrogen therapy (40) and in patients with gastrointestinal cancer (41). In the latter study, removal of the primary tumor was correlated with normalization of platelet aggregation studies. Nevertheless, since careful prospective studies of platelet function in cancer patients have not been done, it is difficult to assess the true incidence of primary platelet function abnormalities (excluding the potential effect of chemotherapy on platelet responses) in cancer or their clinical importance. Several recent reviews have provided more detailed consideration of the interactions between platelets and neoplastic cells (42,43).

B. Fibrinopeptide A Measurements

Since activation of blood coagulation is integral to the process of neoplastic growth and metastasis formation, sensitive methods for the detection of early stages of blood coagulation may be useful for detecting tumors and monitoring their progression. Although direct measurement of the levels of activated clotting factors in the plasma might allow identification of the "hypercoagulable state," such direct assays are not readily available at this time. Other approaches to the early detection of in vivo coagulation have included measurement of thrombin-antithrombin III complexes (44), direct measurement of plasma thrombin levels using a sensitive radioimmunoassay (45) and assay of plasma levels of fibrinogen-fibrin related antigen (46). Although potentially useful, little data is available regarding the results of these assays in cancer patients and the assays themselves are not readily available in most laboratories.

Measurement of the kinetics of fibrinogen turnover provides another method of assessing in vivo activation of the coagulation system. Many studies have shown that measurement of the half life of radiolabeled fibrinogen provides an effective approach to the detection of an increased fibrinogen turnover rate in vivo (47-49). Fibrinogen survival studies may be abnormal even in the presence of normal and elevated plasma fibrinogen levels, a situation most compatible with the "compensated" or "overcompensated" types of DIC. Several authors have studied fibrinogen survival in patients with a variety of malignant diseases and have reported increased fibrinogen turnover rates which were consistent with in vivo activation of blood coagulation (50-53). It must be remembered, however, that although increased turnover of labeled fibrinogen may parallel the intravascular deposition of fibrin, other possible causes include extravasation of fibrinogen into malignant effusions (54), fibrin deposition within the tumor (55) or fibrinogen degradation by other enzymes besides thrombin (56). This lack of specificity and the need to inject patients with a radioisotope and follow the decrease in labeled fibrinogen over time has limited the clinical usefulness of fibrinogen kinetic studies.

Another sensitive method for the detection of low grade activation of the coagulation system has become widely available since Nossel and others (57-58) developed a radioimmunoassay for fibrinopeptide A (fpA). Fibrinopeptide A is a 16 amino acid peptide which is cleaved from the A chain of fibrinogen by the enzyme thrombin. The plasma half life of this small peptide has been estimated to be less than 4 min, therefore fpA levels reflect the rate of ongoing blood coagulation and should provide an accurate estimate of the amount of thrombin present in the intravascular compartment. Plasma fpA levels, therefore, provide a dynamic measure of fibrinogen cleavage in vivo (52). Several studies have demonstrated an increase in fpA levels in virtually all patients with acute leukemia (52,59) and solid tumors (52,60,61). The increased levels of fpA were directly correlated with fibrinogen turnover rates in cancer patients (52), providing further support for enhanced fibrin deposition in those patients. These indicators of subclinical activation of blood coagulation may therefore reflect the interdependence of tumor growth and fibrin generation.

Several authors have now examined the relationship between the extent of tumor growth and the degree of activation of blood coagulation in a semi-quantitative fashion. Peuscher et al. (60) mesured fpA levels in 124 patients with various types of malignancy and found elevated levels in 93 of 98 (95%) of those with metastatic cancer while fpA was only elevated in 3 of 11 (27%) patients with limited primary disease and in 1 of 11 (9%) of those with disease in clinical remission. We have performed serial fpA determinations in 17 patients with acute leukemia. At the time of initial diagnosis, 15 of 17 (88%) had elevated plasma fpA levels (59). Following successful chemotherapy and reduction of tumor cell mass, fpA levels dropped, often into the normal range. Moreover, relapse of acute leukemia was associated with an abrupt increase in plasma fpA levels.

We have also studied the relationship between fpA level and tumor progression in a group of 50 patients with newly diagnosed solid tumors who were followed over a period of three years (61). The characteristics of the patient population are presented in Table 2. Fibrinopeptide A levels were elevated in 60% of patients at the time of entry into the study (Figure 1). Although a high initial fpA value had no prosnostic significance, failure of fpA levels to decrease during the initial 4 mo of treatment predicted a poor survival in those patients in whom serial fpA data was available for at least 4 mo (p 0.02). Disease progression was accompanied by an elevation of fpA levels which often preceded clinical evidence of progression by as much as two months. Serial studies also demonstrated a rise in fpA values during the month prior to death (Figure 2). It must be emphasized, however, that single determinations of fpA are of little clinical value in assessing tumor status since complicating factors such as infection, recent chemotherapy, poor venipuncture technique or acute TED can all cause elevation of fpA levels (61). Therefore, it is necessary to perform several sequential fpA determinations which show steadily increasing levels in order to predict disease progression or a poor prognosis in an individual patient.

Table 2. Patient Population.

Tumor Type	Extent of Disease[a]		Number of Patients
	Limited	Disseminated	
LUNG			
Squamous	9	2	11
Adenocarcinoma	4	8	12
Large Cell	7	1	8
Anaplastic	1	1	2
Small Cell	0	2	2
COLON	1	6	7
HEAD AND NECK	3	1	4
PROSTATE	0	4	4
ALL TUMOR TYPES	25	25	50

[a]For details of the stratification procedure see reference 61.

350

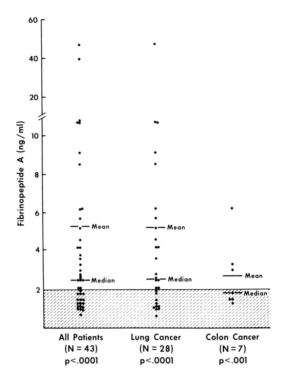

FIGURE 1. Initial Plasma Fibrinopeptide A Levels in Cancer Patients. Each dot represents the first fpA value determined in a patient after accrual to the study. The cross-hatched area represents the normal range.

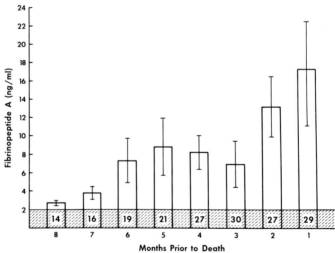

FIGURE 2. Fibrinopeptide A Levels Obtained in Cancer Patients during the Months Prior to Death. Each bar represents the mean ± 1 SEM of all fpA values determined during the indicated month prior to death. The numbers within the bars represent the number of patients who had fpA values measured.

The pathogenesis of the activation of coagulation in cancer patients has been under intense study for many years. Recent studies of fpA levels in patients with TED treated with heparin have provided some information regarding the origin of fpA in patients with cancer and inflammatory disorders. Yudelman and Greenberg (62) have reported that patients with TED occurring as a complication of cancer or inflammatory disease fail to normalize their plasma fpA levels following heparin therapy while patients with uncomplicated TED treated similarly do drop the fpA level to the normal range. Similar results have been reported by other investigators and support the clinical observation that the TED associated with cancer is particularly refractory to treatment with anticoagulant therapy (60-61).

The resistance of fpA levels to heparin treatment in cancer patients could be explained in several ways: 1) the fpA peptide may be cleaved from fibrinogen by a heparin-resistant proteinase produced in cancer patients (in place of thrombin), 2) thrombin generation in cancer patients is less susceptible to heparin (possibly because of some quantitative or qualitative abnormality in antithrombin III) or 3) thrombin-induced fibrinogen cleavage occurs predominantly in the extravascular compartment with subsequent leakage of fpA into the circulation. It is well established that alternative enzymes capable of fibrinogen cleavage exist and could be released by tumor cells (63) or activated leukocytes (56,64) in cancer patients. Tumor-associated plasminogen activators have been described and may result in the production of circulating plasmin in cancer patients. Since plasmin is capable of cleaving a peptide from fibrinogen which is similar to fpA but slightly larger, and since that peptide is capable of cross reacting in some fpA radioimmunoassays, concern has arisen regarding the specificity of fpA measurements in cancer patients. The fact that the extraction procedure used to process samples for most fpA assays eliminates the cross reacting peptide (58) along with the observation that Yudelman and Greenberg (62) were able to detect elevated fpA levels in cancer patients using an antibody which reacts poorly with peptides larger than fpA (62,64) supports the view that fpA is, in fact, the peptide measured in these studies. Thus, plasmin is an unlikely candidate for the enzyme responsible for the fpA elevation in cancer patients but another as yet unidentified heparin-resistant enzyme may exist (see also Chapter 12).

Intravascular generation of thrombin has been associated with a reduction of circulating antithrombin III levels in some patients with cancer (65). Since heparin works by complexing with and greatly augmenting the anticoagulant properties of antithrombin III, a marked decrease in antithrombin levels could account for the observation of relative heparin resistance in patients with cancer. However, most patients with cancer have been shown to have antithrombin III levels within the normal range (66) and Yudelman and Greenberg (62) were not able to demonstrate reduced antithrombin III levels in a group of cancer patients with heparin resistant fpA levels.

352

Wilner et al. (67) were able to demonstrate that fpA injected into extravascular sites is capable of leaking into the circulation and increasing the level of plasma fpA although less than 3% of the dose of fpA injected into the inflammatory site was recovered. Extravascular deposition of fibrin has commonly been observed in histologic examinations of tumor deposits. Since heparin is a large, charged polymer with little ability to diffuse from the circulatory system, extravascular fibrin deposition would readily explain the heparin resistance of plasma fpA levels. Moreover, we have reported that warfarin therapy is capable of reducing fpA levels to the normal range in most cancer patients studied (68). Since warfarin functions as an anticoagulant by causing the reduction of plasma levels of the functional forms of the vitamin K-dependent coagulation factors (II, VII, IX and X), this evidence would support the involvement of thrombin in the process leading to elevated plasma fpA levels.

IV. SUMMARY

The studies reviewed in this chapter support the view that thrombin activation is prominent in patients with malignant disease and results in fibrin deposition and elevation of plasma fpA levels. At least some of the fibrin deposition appears to occur extravascularly and therefore is resistant to the action of heparin. The degree of activation of coagulation in cancer patients is variable with many patients showing no clinical signs of TED or overt DIC. Nevertheless, most patients do exhibit laboratory evidence of subclinical activation of coagulation. While the most sensitive laboratory test is a radioimmunoassay for plasma fpA, other more routine tests often suggest the presence of compensated or overcompensated DIC in patients with cancer.

ACKNOWLEDGEMENT

These studies were supported in part by Research Grants CA-22202 and CA-30651 from the National Cancer Institute and the Medical Research Service of the Veterans Administration.

REFERENCES

1. Trousseau A. Clinique Medicale de l'Hotel-Dieu de Paris, The New Sydenham Society, London, England 3:94, 1865.
2. Sack GH Jr., Levin J and Bell W. Medicine 56:1-37, 1977.
3. Sproule EE. Am. J. Cancer 34:566-585, 1938.
4. Thompson CM and Roger RL. Am. J. Med. Sci. 223:469-475, 1952.
5. Ambrus JL, Ambrus CM, Mink IB and Pickren JW. J. Med. 6:61-64, 1975.
6. Anylan WG, Shingleton WW and Delaughter GD Jr. J. Am. Med. Assoc. 161:964-970, 1956.
7. Hoerr SO and Harper JR. J. Am. Med. Assoc. 164:2033-2044, 1957.
8. Soong BCF and Miller SO. Cancer (Philadelphia) 25:867-873, 1970.
9. Hull R, Hirsch J, Sackett DL, Powers P, Turpie AGG and Walker I. N. Engl. J. Med. 296:1497-1500, 1977.
10. Hefner RR Jr. Neurology 21:840-846, 1971.

11. Lieberman JS, Borrero J, Urdanetta E and Wright IS. J. Am. Med. Assoc. 177:542–545, 1961.
12. Durham RH. Arch. Intern. Med. 96:380–386, 1955.
13. Ambrus JL, Ambrus CM, Pickern J, Soldes S and Bross I. J. Med. 6:433–458, 1975.
14. Weese RB, Tormey DC, Holland JF and Weinberg VE. Cancer Treat. Rep. 65:677–679, 1981.
15. Pineo GF, Brain MC, Galkes AS, Hirsh J, Hatton MWC and Regoeczi E. Ann. N.Y. Acad. Sci. 230:262–270, 1974.
16. Owen CA Jr. and Bowie CJW. Mayo Clin. Proc. 49:673–679, 1974.
17. Peuscher FW. Neth. J. Med. 24:23–35, 1981.
18. Polliack A. Am. J. Clin. Pathol. 56:155–161, 1971.
19. Gralnick HR, Marchesi S and Givelber H. Blood 40:709–718, 1972.
20. Gralnick HR and Abrell E. Br. J. Haematol. 24:89–99, 1973.
21. Goualt-Heilman M, Chardon E, Sultan E and Josse F. Br. J. Haematol. 30:151–158, 1975.
22. Brain MC, Azzopardi JG and Baker LRI. Br. J. Haematol. 18:183–193, 1970.
23. Belt RJ, Leite C, Haas CD and Stephens RL. J. Am. Med. Assoc. 239:2571–2574, 1978.
24. Al-Mondhiry H. Thromb. Diath. Haemorrh. 34:181–193, 1975.
25. Sun NC, McAfee WM, Hum GJ and Weiner JM. Am. J. Clin. Pathol. 71:10–16, 1979.
26. Hagedorn AB, Bowie EJW, Elveback LR and Owen CA. Mayo Clin. Proc. 49:649–653, 1974.
27. Carlsson S. Acta Chir. Scand. 139:499–502, 1973.
28. Miller SP, Sanchez-Avalos J, Stefanski T and Zuckerman L. Cancer (Philadelphia) 20:1452–1465, 1967.
29. Rasche H and Dietrich M. Eur. J. Cancer 13:1053–1064, 1977.
30. Cooper HA, Bowie EJW and Owen CA Jr. Mayo Clin. Proc. 49:654–657, 1974.
31. Kies MS, Posch JJ, Giolma JP and Rubin RN Cancer (Philadelphia) 46:831–837, 1980.
32. Harker LA and Slichter SJ. N. Engl. J. Med. 287:999–1005, 1972.
33. Slichter SJ and Harker LA. Ann. N.Y. Acad. Sci. 230:252–261, 1974.
34. Johannson S, Kutti J and Olson LB. Acta Pathol. Microbiol. Scand. 86:505–511, 1978.
35. Bidet JN, Ferriere JP, Besse G, Collet PH, Gaillard G and Plagne R. Thromb. Res. 19:429–433, 1980.
36. Schernthaner G, Ludwig H and Silberbauer K. Acta Hematol. 62:219–222, 1970.
37. Levin L and Conley CL Arch. Intern. Med. 114:497–500, 1964.
38. Davis RB, Theologides A and Kennedy BJ. Ann. Intern. Med. 71:67–80, 1969.
39. Shaikh BS and Bullard V. Blood 50(Suppl. 1):252, 1977.
40. Jung SM, Isohisa I, Kinoshita K and Yamasaki H. Thromb. Haemostasis 46:30, 1981.
41. Yamamura T, Matsumoto H, Maruyama Y, Wada T and Yamanaka M. Thromb. Haemostasis 46:31, 1981.
42. Karpatkin S and Pearlstein E. Ann. Intern. Med. 95:636–641, 1981.
43. Zacharski LR, Rickles FR, Henderson WG, Martin JF, Forman WB, van Eeckhout JP, Cornell CJ and Forcier RJ. Am. J. Clin. Oncol. (in press), 1983.
44. Collen D and DeCock F. Thromb. Res. 5:777–779, 1974.
45. Shuman MA and Majerus PW. J. Clin. Invest. 58:1249–1258, 1976.
46. Merskey C, Johnson AJ, Harris JU, Wang MT and Swain S. Br. J. Haematol. 44:655–670, 1980.
47. Bettigole RE, Himelstein ES, Clifford GO and Mayer K. J. Nucl. Med. 10:322–323, 1969.

48. Collen D, Tytgat GN, Claeys H and Piessens R. Br. J. Haematol. 22:681–700, 1972.
49. Takeda Y. J. Clin. Invest. 45:103–111, 1966.
50. Mombelli G, Roux A, Haeberli A and Straub PW. Blood 60:381–388, 1982.
51. Lyman GH, Bettigole RE, Robson E, Ambrus JL and Urban H. Cancer (Philadelphia) 1:1113–1122, 1978.
52. Yoda Y and Abe T. Thomb. Haemostasis 46:706–709, 1981.
53. Robson E, Murawski GF and Bettigole RE. Thromb. Haemostasis 37:484–508, 1977.
54. Ruegg R and Straub PW. J. Lab. Clin. Med. 95:842–856, 1980.
55. Hiramoto R, Bernecky J, Jurandowski J and Pressman D. Cancer Res. 20:592–593, 1960.
56. Plow EF and Edgington TS. J. Clin. Invest. 56:30–38, 1975.
57. Nossel HL, Yudelman I, Canfield RE, Buttler VP Jr., Spanondis K, Wilner GD and Qureshi GD. J. Clin. Invest. 54:43–53, 1974.
58. Cronlund M, Hardin J, Burton J, Lee L, Haber E and Bloch KJ. J. Clin. Invest. 58:142–151, 1976.
59. Myers TJ, Rickles FR, Barb C and Cronlund M. Blood 57:518–525, 1981.
60. Peuscher FW, Cleton FJ, Armstrong L, Stoepman-van Dalen EA, van Mourik JA and van Aken WG. J. Lab. Clin. Med. 96:5–14, 1980.
61. Rickles FR, Edwards RL, Barb C and Cronlund M. Cancer (Philadelphia) 51:301–307, 1983.
62. Yudelman I and Greenberg J. Blood 59:787–792, 1982.
63. Strauli P, Barrett AJ and Baici A, Eds. Proteinases and Tumor Invasion, Raven Press, New York, 1980.
64. Bilzekian SB and Nossel HL. Blood 50:21–28, 1977.
65. Damus PS and Wallace GA. Thromb. Res. 6:27–38, 1976.
66. Rubin RN, Kies MS and Posch JJ. Thromb. Res. 18:353–360, 1980.
67. Wilner GD, Chatpar P and Horowitz J. J. Lab. Clin. Med. 91:205–213, 1978.
68. Rickles FR, Edwards RL and Zacharski LR. Proceedings of the 1981 International Istanbul Symposium, Istanbul, Turkey, in press, 1983.

CHAPTER 23. HISTORICAL OVERVIEW OF CLINICAL EXPERIENCE WITH ANTICOAGULANT THERAPY

BARNETT KRAMER

I. INTRODUCTION

Other chapters in this book delineate the considerable body of information untilizing in vitro and in vivo animal models which link the coagulation cascade to mechanisms of local growth and distant metastasis of cancer. The ultimate impact of such data, of course, depends upon its relevance to human malignancy and ultimately to therapy of human cancer. This chapter will, therefore, give an overview of the clinical observations and trials which have examined the effect of interruption of the coagulation mechanism upon the genesis and spread of human tumors. Despite a considerable number of studies, no definitive conclusions can be drawn and reasons for this will be discussed.

II. EARLY OBSERVATIONS AND HYPOTHESES

In 1878, Billroth (1) described microscopic intravascular tumor deposits associated with blood thrombi and postulated that these thrombi were involved in the pathogenesis of metastatic tumor growth. That such tumor deposits may be viable was suggested by Schmidt (2), Iwasaki (3) and Zacharski et al. (4) who described malignant cells in mitosis which were enmeshed in blood thrombi. A note of caution must be raised about this definition of "viability." Saphir (5) reported on the histologic examination of the lungs of 12 patients dying from various carcinomas. He did find microscopic tumor emboli in all cases, usually associated with organizing blood thrombi, and some containing mitotic cells. However, in the most mature appearing blood thrombi the emboli were necrotic leading Saphir to the conclusion that the organizing thrombi destroy tumor cells, thereby inhibiting metastases. O'Meara (6) suggested that even the local growth of a primary malignancy was intertwined with the coagulation cascade when he demonstrated fibrin at the advancing edge of cancer.

The above pathologic observations have generated several hypotheses. First, they suggested that fibrin deposition and the coagulation pathway are necessary both for local growth and distant spread of tumors in humans. Second, they suggested that interruption of the coagulation pathway may, therefore, be useful either prophylactically or therapeutically in cancer management. What follows is a discussion of the studies in humans designed to address these hypotheses.

III.   THE COAGULATION PATHWAY AND THE INCIDENCE OF CANCER

An obvious "experiment of nature" would be an investigation of the incidence of malignancy in patients with congenital clotting disorders. Forman (7) conducted such a study through a mail survey of physicians registered with the National Hemophilia Foundation.   He inquired about the incidence of malignancy in any patient with an inherited coagulation disorder. Of 325 questionnaires sent, 268 were returned. Responding physicians estimated that they had seen or had knowledge of a total of 10,500 patients, 61 of whom had a neoplastic disease. Although there was a slight preponderance of genitourinary tumors and soft tissue sarcomas among these 61 patients, the overall age adjusted incidence of malignancy was similar to an age and sex matched population. Moreover, there was not an unusually prolonged interval between diagnosis and appearance of clinically diagnosed metastases in the 61 patients; survival data were not reported. Hence, in this population of patients with coagulation disorders, the overall incidence and biologic behavior of malignancy was apparently not altered. However, because of the study design, most patients had classic hemophilia and virtually all patients had disorders of the intrinsic coagulation cascade. Disorders of the extrinsic coagulation cascade were excluded from this study because of their rarity.

Two other retrospective obsevational studies have explored a postulated protective effect of therapeutic anticoagulation against the onset of malignant disease. Michaels (8) reported on 540 patients, in a single private clinic in Manitoba, Canada, who received anticoagulation primarily for ischemic heart disease.   The mean duration of anticoagulation in this group was 35 mo with a range of 3 to 111 mo.   Comparing the incidence and mortality from malignant disease among these patients to incidence and mortality statistics in the general Manitoba population he found the same numbers of visceral cancers diagnosed as expected. Although there was a slight apparent increase in incidence of skin cancer over that expected, the apparent increase might be attributable to more frequent medical examinations in the study population than in controls. Only one death occurred in his study population compared to an expected mortality of 8 patients. In the author's opinion, this could not be explained by withholding anticoagulation in cancer patients once diagnosis of malignancy was made, nor could it be explained by a shortened clinical course due to death from underlying cardiovascular disease. Nevertheless, it was possible that malignancies were detected earlier in subjects under close observation for other medical reasons and, hence, the survival advantage was apparent rather than real. Indeed, in two patients the malignancy was diagnosed because of hemorrhage in an occult tumor while on anticoagulation. In addition, cancer mortality rates in a private patient population may be different from mortality rates experienced in the more heterogeneous general population. A second similar study was performed by Annegers and Zacharski (9) on a cohort of 378 patients anticoagulated for at least 6 wk after acute myocardial infarction. Forty malignancies were diagnosed vs the expected number of 39 over an observation period of 3,541 person-years. Moreover, the observed mortality from malignancy was not statistically different from that expected. Hence, neither of these two observational studies give strong support for therapeutic anticoagulation as prophylaxis against malignancy or metastasis of established malignant disease. Nevertheless, both studies involved relatively small numbers of patients, suggesting the possibility of sampling errors. The subclinical duration of malignant disease may extend over periods of years, i.e., far exceeding the duration of anticoagulation in these two groups. It would be surprising if anticoagulation for such a small fraction of this period would exert a major impact on the natural history of the malignancy.

IV. THERAPEUTIC TRIALS OF ANTICOAGULATION IN CANCER PATIENTS

A number of prospective therapeutic trials of anticoagulation in patients with established malignancy have been performed to determine any impact of anticoagulation on metastasis and survival. Unfortunately, most of the trials have been uncontrolled or have used historical controls. Moreover, various methods of antcoagulation were used in these trials and various criteria of response were reported thus making comparison of results difficult. In the following section (A), uncontrolled or historically controlled trials will be discussed. This will be followed by a section (B) on randomized and concurrently controlled trials. For the purposes of this discussion I have grouped uncontrolled and historically controlled trials. Although there is current controversy over the relative merits of trials with historical controls, I believe that constant changes in supportive and adjuvant care in medical oncology (of which anticoagulation is only one modality) make interpretation of such trials more difficult than that of concurrently controlled trials.

A. Uncontrolled or Historically Controled Trials (Table 1)

1. Warfarin trials. Hoover et al. (10) reported on a series of nine patients who underwent amputation with curative intent for osteogenic sarcoma. These patients were started on oral warfarin at least 7 da preoperatively and were kept on anticoagulant therapy for up to 6 mo following surgery. The target prothrombin time was twice baseline. The authors compared the survival of this group to 21 historical controls with osteogenic sarcoma, also operated upon for cure. Survival after 5-8 yr of follow-up in the anticoagulated patients was 56% vs a 14% survival at 5-11 yr in the controls (p = 0.04). However, since the control data were retrospective, it was impossible to compare the size of the primary tumors in the two series. Moreover, since the completion of this study it has become evident that certain histologic subtypes of osteogenic sarcoma have a more favorable prognosis than others, a factor not analyzed in this study.

Thornes (11) treated 96 patients with a variety of advanced malignancies with oral anticoagulants, 29 of whom responded for one to five years. In a subsequent study (12), he treated 20 patients with Hodgkin's disease and 10 patients with chronic myelogenous leukemia (CML) using a single alkylating agent. Warfarin was added as they became resistant to chemotherapy. He felt that 15 of the Hodgkin's

Table 1. Uncontrolled and Historically Controlled Trials of Anticoagulation in Human Neoplastic Disease.

Tumor Types	No. of Patients	Anticoagulant Regimen	Other Therapy	Result
Osteogenic Sarcoma (10)	9	Warfarin	Amputation	Increased survival (compared to historical controls)
Variety (11)	96	Warfarin	Varied	29 responses
Hodgkin's Disease (12)	20	Warfarin	Alkylator	15 responses
Chronic Myelogenous Leukemia (12)	10	Warfarin	Alkylator	6 responses
Pancreatic Adeno-carcinoma (13)	26	Warfarin	5-FU[a]	Lived "slightly longer" than expected
Variety (14)	4	Heparin		4 responses
Bronchogenic Carcinoma (15)	4	Heparin	CTX, 5-FU, 6-TG, MTX, VCR	4 responses
Bronchogenic Carcinoma (16)	14	Heparin	Same as above	7 responses
Breast Adeno-carcinoma (17)	1	Heparin	Tranexemic acid	Pleural effusion regressed
Variety (18)	19	Heparin ± Plasmin	CTX	0 responses
Bronchogenic Carcinoma (19)	27	Heparin	CTX	1 brief response
Non-small cell lung cancer (20)	16	Heparin	CTX, 5-FU, 6-TG, MTX VCR	0 responses

Table 1 Cont.: Uncontrolled and Historically Controlled Trials of Anti-coagulation in Human Neoplastic Disease.

Tumor Types	No. of Patients	Anticoagulant Regimen	Other Therapy	Result
Bronchogenic Carcinoma (21)	14	Heparin	CTX,5-FU, VCR,MTX	0 responses
Breast Adenocarcinoma (22)	10	Prolothan A	--	Tumors became softer, more mobile
Variety (23)	11	Plasmin (+ aspirin)	--	4 tumor regressions
Variety (24)	45	Fibrinolysins (variety)	Variety	No increase in survival
Variety (25)	6	Ancrod	--	4 responses
Xeroderma Pigmentosum (multiple skin cancers) (26)	9	Indomethacin	Prednisolone	8 responses
TOTAL	341 patients in 17 studies			

[a] CTX = cyclophosphamide; 5-FU = 5-fluorouracil; 6-TG = thioguanine; MTX = methotrexate; VCR = vincristine

patients and 6 of the CML patients "responded" as evidenced by decreased requirements for cytotoxic therapy to maintain disease stability.

Waddell (13) reported on 26 patients with pancreatic adenocarcinoma who were treated with weekly 5-fluorouracil and warfarin (designed to keep the serum prothrombin time about 30% of normal activity). The patients were considered to have lived "slightly longer" than a series previously reported by others. However, this series of patients were then used as historical controls for a subsequent set of 13 patients in his next clinical trial. These 13 patients received 5-fluorouracil with testolactone or spironolactone. This latter group had a survival rate far superior to the anticoagulated patients used as historical controls.

2. Heparin trials. A number of studies explored the use of heparin. Elias et al. (144) reported on four patients with refractory metastatic malignancies and elevated plasma fibrinogen levels. These patients were given heparin (20,000 - 30,000 units per da) by continuous intravenous infusion. Although they reported regression in all four patients, the regression was less than 50% in two of the three patients for whom measurements were given and no measurements were given for the fourth patient. Elias and Brugarolas (15) also reported on four patients with three cell types of metastatic bronchogenic carcinoma. All four patients received a week long chemotherapeutic regimen of cyclophosphamide, 5-fluorouracil, 6-thioguanine, methotrexate and vincristine. In addition, they were given continous intravenous heparin (30,000 - 40,000 units per da) for the week of chemotherapy. Although he did not give his criteria for tumor response, he noted a response in all four of his patients, two of whom had not responded to the same therapeutic regimen without heparin. Nevertheless, one patient died (of pneumonia) 11 da after the first course of chemotherapy. Elias et al (16) later reported on 14 patients with inoperable bronchogenic carcinoma who received the same set of cytotoxic agents as above and continuous heparinization during each course of chemotherapy. They reported a 50% response rate in this group compared to a 0% response rate in a prior series of 14 patients who had received the same chemotherapy without heparin. Again, their criteria for response are not delineated nor are the cell types in either of the two groups. The latter piece of information is critical since some cell types (e.g., small cell undifferentiated) are far more responsive to chemotherapy than others.

Astedt et al. (17) anecdotally reported a woman with breast cancer, pleural effusion and cerebral metastasis who was treated with heparin and tranexemic acid (a fibrinolytic inhibitor). Although the pleural effusion regressed and the brain metastasis resolved by brain scan, the patient had also been treated with whole brain irradiation before and after the anticoagulation therapy. The rationale in this study for using a fibrinolytic inhibitor was that the investigators had previously identified urokinase production by an ovarian tumor and, therefore, postulated that fibrinolysis was necessary for primary tumor growth.

In contrast to the above experiences with heparin are a series of negative studies with similar experimental design. Dahl (18) treated 19 incurable patients who had a variety of malignancies with cyclophosphamide and heparin, with or without plasmin. There were no responses in these patients. Edlis et al. (19) reported a Veterans Administration Lung Cancer Study Group (VALCSG) study in which 27 patients with a variety of bronchogenic lung cancer cell types were given continous intravenous heparin to achieve anticoagulation and then given cyclophosphamide. Heparin was begun 48 to 72 hr prior to chemotherapy and continued 24 hr after each course of chemotherapy. These courses were given every 3 wk. Because of significant bleeding problems in eight patients, only 19 of the 27 patients entered into study received at least one course of therapy. Of these 19, only one patient achieved a partial remission lasting four weeks. Rohwedder and Sagastume (20) reported another VALCSG study designed to reproduce Elias and coworkers' study of lung cancer described above (15,16).

Sixteen patients with non-small cell lung cancers were heparinized for eight days every four weeks while receiving Elias and coworkers' chemotherapy regimen (15,16). There were no partial remissions by today's standards (at least 50% tumor shrinking), but three patients had minimal objective improvement (less than one third shrinkage). None had improvement in performance status. Moreover, there was significant gastrointestinal blood loss which required transfusion in three patients. Jamieson and Angove (21) treated 14 patients with inoperable lung cancer (five of whom had small cell type) with a regimen of heparin as well as cyclophosphamide, 5-fluorouracil, vincristine and methotrexate in five day courses every five weeks. Patients were not anticoagulated between courses. There were no tumor regressions. However, four patients died before the end of the first course of chemotherapy, indicating the late stage of malignancy in many of these patients.

3. Miscellaneous anticoagulants. A variety of anticoagulant regimens besides warfarin derivatives or heparin have been tested. O'Meara and O'Halloran (22) described the use of Prolothan A (a protamine derivative) in 8 females and 2 males with advanced breast cancer. Clotting times and platelet counts in these patients were unchanged from baseline. All patients received Prolothan A twice per day for 14 da. It was felt that in each case the primary tumor became more mobile, better defined and firmer, usually with "decreased dimensions" (dimensions not supplied).

Larson et al. (23) performed a trial of plasmin in 11 patients with a wide variety of advanced malignancies. Several plasmin doses were employed. Each patient was treated with 1 g of aspirin as prophylaxis against the uniform onset of fever due to the use of porcine plasmin. A subjective improvement was reported in six patients and an objective tumor regression in four. However, criteria for regression were not defined and may have included major as well as minor regressions. Cliffton (24) described his personal experience using a variety of fibrinolysins in a study of 45 patients with a variety of malignancies. Although some tumor regression was observed, he felt there was no obvious increase in survival, concluding that fibrinolysins did not show great promise in this field. Williams and Maugham (25) treated six patients with widespread malignancy with ancrod, a defibrinating agent. Patients received no concomitant cytotoxic therapy. They noted temporary regression of a primary breast cancer and of a single lung metastasis from colon cancer, as well as a temporary neurologic improvement in a patient with spinal compression from metastatic colon cancer. A fourth patient with liver metastasis from rectal carcinoma experienced a decrease in liver size. However, the patient also had congestive heart failure and was simultaneously receiving digoxin and diuretics, raising the possibility of liver shrinkage from improved passive liver congestion. A precise definition of tumor regression was not reported.

Finally, Al-Saleem et al. (26) recently reported eight regressions of multiple skin cancers in nine xeroderma pigmentosum patients treated with the prostaglandin inhibitor indomethacin (25 - 100 mg per da). However, seven patients also received systemic prednisolone.

B. Concurrently Controlled Trials of Anticoagulation (Table 2)

In recent years, several concurrently controlled or randomized trials have appeared. Elias (27) randomized 25 patients with inoperable carcinoma of the lung to receive a regimen of cyclophosphamide, 5-fluorouracil, 6-thioguanine, methotrexate and vincristine in eight day courses every two weeks with or without continuous heparinization during the eight day courses. There were no responses in 13 controls vs 8 responses in 9 anticoagulated patients. The remaining three patients in the anticoagulated group are not discussed in this brief communication.

Thornes (28) randomized a series of 45 patients undergoing primary resection of adenocarcinoma of the rectum or colon to receive either streptokinase or saline, intraoperatively, immediately after tumor resection. A greater number of patients receiving streptokinase entered the study before control patients. Therefore, the study period was somewhat longer in the experimental group (58 mo compared to 34 mo). At the time of this report, there were 4 deaths due to recurrence in 23 control patients vs 3 deaths from recurrence in the 22 patients given streptokinase. Stanford (29) tested the utility of anticoagulation when added to a complex chemotherapeutic regimen of CCNU [1-(2-chloroethyl)-3-cyclohexyl-1-nitrosourea], cyclophosphamide, adriamycin, vincristine and methotrexate in 24 previously untreated patients with small cell carcinoma of the lung. Patients were randomized to chemotherapy alone or to chemotherapy combined with a complicated regimen of heparin, dextran and warfarin. Survival curves were not statistically different between the two groups. The median survival was 8.9 mo in the anticoagulated group vs 9.7 mo in controls.

A concurrently controlled but non-randomized study of warfarin in a variety of malignancies was reported by Thornes (12). One hundred twenty-eight patients with recurrent carcinomas received conventional therapy for their tumors. In addition, alternate patients with the same histologic diagnosis received warfarin. There was an apparent improvement in two year survival in the warfarin group (40.6% vs 17.8% in controls). There were, however, 15 significant bleeding episodes in the anticoagulated group: 3 ending in death, 12 requiring transfusion. The author states parenthetically that, although two year survival was improved in the warfarin group, when exacerbation of the underlying malignancy did occur patients died rapidly compared to patients not receiving anticoagulants.

D'Souza et al. (30) randomized 44 patients with Stage IV breast cancer to receive either monthly intravenous chemotherapy or oral chemotherapy (Endoxana, prednisone, 5-fluorouracil, methotrexate) plus warfarin (designed to double the prothrombin time) plus immunotherapy [levamisole, bacillus Calmette-Guerain (BCG)]. The warfarin/immunotherapy group demonstrated a significantly longer median survival (34 mo vs 17 mo). However, 15 of the 22 patients in the warfarin/immunotherapy group were switched to intravenous therapy because of inadequate response to the oral chemotherapy. Due to study design, it is difficult to know whether to attribute any positive results to the anticoagulation, the levamisole or the BCG.

Table 2: Concurrently Controlled Trials of Anticoagulation in Human Neoplastic Disease.

Tumor Types	No. of Patients	Anticoagulant Regimen	Other Therapy	Result
Bronchogenic Carcinoma (27)	25	Heparin	CTX, 5-FU, 6-TG, MTX, VCR[a]	0/13 responses vs 8/9 in study group
Colorectal Adenocarcinoma (28)	45	Streptokinase	Primary Surgery	Inconclusive
Small Cell Lung Cancer (29)	24	Heparin, Dextran, Warfarin	CCNU, CTX, A, VCR, MTX	No difference in survival
Variety (12)	128	Warfarin	"Conventional" for tumor type	Improved 2-year survival in study group (40.6% vs 17.8%)
Breast Adenocarcinoma (30)	44	Warfarin	Endoxana, prednisone, 5-FU, MTX, levamisole, BCG	Improved survival in warfarin/immunotherapy group
Small Cell Lung Cancer (31)	50	Warfarin	Radiation, CTX, VCR, MTX	Improved survival; response rates similar
Non Small Cell Lung Cancer; Colorectal Adenocarcinoma; Prostatic Adenocarcinoma; Head/Neck Cancer (32)	381	Warfarin	"Conventional" by cell type & stage	No improvement in response rate or survival
TOTAL	697 patients in 6 studies			

[a]CTX=cyclophosphamide;5-FU=5-fluorouracil;6-TG=thioguanine;MTX=methotrexate;VCR=vincristine;A=adriamycin;BCG=bacillus Calmette Guerain

The study on anticoagulation in malignancy which has probably received more attention than any others was conducted by the Veterans Administration Cooperative Study Group and reported by Zacharski et al. (31). The study design was a marked improvement over previous studies. Fifty patients with small cell carcinoma of the lung were randomized to receive or not to receive continuous warfarin anticoagulation along with their chemotherapy, which consisted of cyclophosphamide, vincristine and methotrexate. In addition, all patients received local chest irradiation to the primary tumor. The two study groups were well balanced for performance status as well as extent of disease (see also Chapters 24 and 26).

For undetermined reasons, a higher percentage of patients in the warfarin-treated group received prophylactic whole brain irradiation compared to controls. Of note, an additional 141 patients were screened at the participating institutions for study entry but were excluded for various reasons. The overall results showed similar response rates to chemotherapy between the 2 groups. However, the duration of remission was longer in the anticoagulated group and median survival was prolonged as well (50 vs 24 wk). Breaking down the survival by disease extent, a statistically significant difference was also present in the patients with extensive disease. However, the numbers of patients with extensive disease were quite small: 12 in the control group vs 13 in the warfarin-treated group. The number of complications due to bleeding was considerable in the anticoagulated group. There were 28 episodes of bleeding in 15 patients and there was one death from gastrointestinal bleeding, compared to one bleeding episode in each of four control patients (1 fatal). This study of small cell lung cancer was part of a larger study in the same cooperative group (32) in which 381 additional patients with a variety of malignancies (non-small cell lung cancer, colorectal carcinoma, prostatic cancer, head and neck cancer) were randomized to "standard" therapy for their malignancy ± long-term anticoagulation with warfarin (32). It is of interest that there was no significant improvement in response rate or survival for the anticoagulated group in any of the other malignant diseases.

C. Summary of Therapeutic Trials

All of the therapeutic trials of anticoagulation which are not controlled or historically controlled are summarized in Table 1. Concurrently controlled and randomized studies are summarized in Table 2. In all, 1,038 patients have been entered into 23 studies spanning a period from 1963 to the present. The response rates are widely variant, ranging from 0 to 100%. Therefore, after a period spanning two decades and the entry of well over 1,000 patients into a variety of experimental regimens of anticoagulation, we are still left with a confusing picture of the efficacy of anticoagulation for treatment of malignant disease.

1. Reported toxicities in therapeutic trials of anticoagulation for cancer. The studies of anticoagulation in neoplastic disease have, in some cases, engendered considerable toxicity. Sixty-one episodes of significant bleeding were discussed in the above studies and four

deaths were directly attributed to anticoagulation. The incidence of bleeding episodes within these studies varied from 0 to 60%. The above figures are probably a conservative estimate since a number of studies did not mention whether or not there were bleeding episodes.

Certainly, the argument can be made that chemotherapy itself entails considerable toxicity to the cancer patient, perhaps at least as great as the potential complications of anticoagulation. Nevertheless, in order to evaluate whether anticoagulation is worthwhile, that is in order to perform risk-benefit analysis, a better idea of benefits of anticoagulation is necessary. Possible reasons for lack of consensus on such benefits in the studies discussed here are outlined in the next section.

2. Comments on human trials to date. The myriad human trials of anticoagulation therapy described above demonstrate a confused state of affairs. For virtually every study design of any given tumor type which yields a positive result, there is a study of similar design which suggests little role for anticoagulation. The reasons for such inconclusive results can be grouped under two major categories: 1) true biologic ineffectiveness and 2) inadequate study design.

It may well be that the coagulation pathway plays little or no role in human malignancy. Nevertheless, as is detailed in other chapters of this book, evidence for an important role of coagulation in animal models is legion.

Hence, it is difficult to shrug off the inconclusive data in human clinical trials without seeking other possible explanations. It is conceivable that anticoagulation is an effective therapeutic maneuver in some tumors but not in others. Witness the disparate results among tumor types in the well-designed studies in the V.A. Cooperative Study performed by Zacharski and coworkers (Chapter 25). It is also possible that although tumor cell clumping (homotypic and heterotypic interactions) is an important mechanism of tumor metastasis and subsequent growth, anticoagulation is not sufficient to block these metastases. In other words, anticoagulation may have an antimetastatic potential but there are a variety of tumor "defense mechanisms" by which the neoplasm may bypass this therapeutic modality. There may be a spectrum of cell sensitivity within any given tumor (see Chapter 2). Finally, it is conceivable that adequate anticoagulation could, indeed, block metastasis of neoplastic disease, but that "adequate anticoagulation" would be fatal to the host. Along these lines, there are a number of tumor models in which cytotoxic chemotherapy is curative in a high percentage of cases but host toxicity limits these same therapeutic agents to a palliative or minimal role in humans.

Biological factors could be one reason for failure of anticoagulation therapy in humans. Equally important may be poor study design. It is clear that study designs have varied widely and the types of anticoagulants used have also been quite different. Most of the studies have used either no controls or historical controls. In addition, the bulk of reported studies include very few patients. Many of these patients are treated in a very late stage of their disease when it is well known that virtually any therapeutic maneuver is less effective. Moreover, many of the studies have grouped patients with a variety of cell types, thereby clouding the issue of whether certain cell types are more responsive to anticoagulation than others.

The level of anticoagulation necessary for antimetastatic therapy is not known in humans. Along these lines, virtually no study discusses what percentage of patients achieved clinically adequate levels of anticoagulation. Moreover, many of the studies, especially earlier ones, combine what would be considered inadequate chemotherapy by today's standards with the regimen of anticoagulation. Indeed, a number of studies did not employ chemotherapy at all, primarily because of the endstage status of their patient population.

Finally, many of these studies have different criteria of tumor response, thus making comparisons quite difficult. Perhaps even more importantly, most studies describe response rates rather than survival data. Although it is common to report response rates with cytotoxic chemotherapy trials, this is inadequate for a report of a modality whose primary mechanism of action is the prevention of metastasis. A more appropriate parameter to report would be ultimate survival or time from onset of therapy to recognition of metastasis, as in recent well-designed studies (32).

V. SUMMARY

In summary, there is a large data base of trials employing anticoagulation therapy for malignant disease in humans. Unfortunately, the data base is conflicting and inadequate. Although there is good in vitro and in vivo animal model evidence delineating a role for the coagulation cascade in neoplastic growth, human studies are inconclusive. Unfortunately, at this point after more than 1,000 patients have been studied over a two decade period, we are still not sure whether the reasons for the conflicting results are due to true ineffectiveness of anticoagulation therapy in humans or to deficiencies in study design. Hopefully, well-designed, randomized trials early in the course of disease can decide the issue.

REFERENCES

1. Billroth T. Lectures on Surgical Pathology and Therapeutics, translated from the 8th Edition, The New Sydenham Society, London, 1878.
2. Schmidt MD. Oie Verbreitungswege der Karzinome und die Beziehwag Generalisierter Sarkome zu den Leukaminschen Neubildungen. Gustav Fisher, Jena, 1903.
3. Iwasaki T. J. Pathol. Bacteriol. 20:85-104, 1915.
4. Zacharski LR, Henderson WG, Rickles FR, Forman WB, Cornell CJ Jr., Forcier RJ, Harrower HW and Johnson RO. Cancer (Philadelphia) 44:732-741, 1979.
5. Saphir O. Am. J. Pathol. 23:245-253, 1947.
6. O'Meara RAQ. Thromb. Diath. Haemorrh. (Suppl.) 28:137-142, 1968.
7. Forman WB. Cancer (Philadelphia) 44:1059-1061, 1979.
8. Michaels L. J. Med. 5:98-106, 1974.

9. Annegers JF and Zacharski LR. Thromb. Res. 18:399–403, 1980.
10. Hoover HC, Ketcham AS, Millar RC and Gralnick HR. Cancer (Philadelphia) 41:2475–2480, 1978.
11. Thornes RD. Br. Med. J. 1:110–111, 1972.
12. Thornes RD. J. Med. 5:83–91, 1974.
13. Waddell WR. Surgery 74:420–429, 1973.
14. Elias EG, Sepulveda F and Mink IB. J. Surg. Oncol. 5:189–193, 1973.
15. Elias EG and Brugarolas A. Cancer Chemother. Rep. 56:783–785, 1972.
16. Elias EG, Shukla SK and Mink IB. Cancer (Philadelphia) 36:129–136, 1975.
17. Astedt B, Mattsson W and Trope C. Acta Med. Scand. 201:491–493, 1977.
18. Dahl S. Onkologie (Basel) 20:35–38, 1966.
19. Edlis HE, Goudsmit A, Brindley C and Niemetz J. Cancer Treat. Rep. 60:575–578, 1976.
20. Rohwedder JJ and Sagastume E. Cancer Treatment Rep. 61:1399–1401, 1977.
21. Jamieson GG and Angove RC. Aust. N. Z. J. Med. 9:381–384, 1979.
22. O'Meara RAQ and O'Halloran MJ. Lancet 2:613–614, 1963.
23. Larsen V, Mogensen B, Amris CJ and Storm O. Dan. Med. Bull. 11:137–140, 1961.
24. Cliffton EE. J. L. State Med. Soc. 118:309–319, 1966.
25. Williams JRB and Maugham E. Br. Med. J. 3:174–175, 1972.
26. Al-Saleem T, Ali ZS and Qassab M. Lancet 2:264–265, 1980.
27. Elias EE. Proc. Am. Assoc. Cancer Res. 13:26, 1973.
28. Thornes RD. Cancer (Philadelphia) 35:91–97, 1975.
29. Stanford CF. Thorax 34:113–116, 1979.
30. D'Souza DP, Daly L and Thornes RD. J. Ir. Med. Assoc. 71:605–608, 1978.
31. Zacharski LR, Henderson WG, Rickles FR, Forman WB, Cornell CJ, Forcier J, Edwards R, Headley E, Kim S–H, O'Donnell JR, O'Dell R, Tornyos K and Kwaan HC. J. Am. Med. Assoc. 245:831–835, 1981.
32. Zacharski LR, Henderson WG, Rickles FR, Forman WB, Cornell CJ, Forcier J, Edwards R, Headley E, Kim S–H, O'Donnell JR, O'Dell R, Tornyos K and Kwaan HC. (submitted).

CHAPTER 24. RATIONALE FOR ANTICOAGULANT TREATMENT OF CANCER

LEO R. ZACHARSKI

I. INTRODUCTION

Strategies for therapeutic research in cancer are shaped by our current knowledge of tumor biology. This knowledge has led to understanding the importance of treating tumors early or when still localized, for example by surgical excision or radiotherapy, and of interrupting cell proliferation in more advanced tumors, for example by means of chemotherapeutic agents (1). By contrast, one property of neoplasia, namely the capacity for metastasis, has proven to be an elusive target of interventional therapy. Apparently the metastatic process depends upon the survival of specialized subpopulations of cells that possess specific properties that enable them to separate from the parent tumor, migrate through vascular channels to distant sites, attach to vessel walls, and then extravasate and proliferate (2). The resistance of the metastatic process to treatment suggests that properties other than proliferative potential are involved. These properties will require innovative therapeutic approaches.

A substantial volume of literature suggests that the ability of neoplastic cells to interact with the hemostatic mechanisms of the host is of importance in tumor metastasis. This evidence has been the subject of several recent reviews (3-7) and is presented in detail elsewhere in this volume. Neoplastic cells may be capable of inducing either clot formation or platelet clumping. Therapeutic measures that interfere with these reactions may result in limitation of metastasis.

The purpose of this paper is to present a concise overview of several kinds of coagulation-cancer interactions that have been recognized. This summary will provide a setting for assessing the significance of this interaction for therapeutic research using coagulation-inhibitory drugs in human malignancy. Because of the substantial literature on this subject, reference will be made when appropriate to recent reviews in which further detail will be found (3-7).

II. POSSIBLE TUMOR CELL INTERACTION WITH HEMOSTATIC MECHANISMS

A. Platelets

A number of different experimental tumor cell lines can induce platelet aggregation and the release reaction to varying degrees and by different mechanisms (4,6,7). This capacity appears to be related to the emergence on the tumor cell surface of aggregation-producing molecules that are associated with neoplastic transformation (see also Chapters 6, 7 and 12). Available evidence indicates that introduction of certain kinds of tumor cells into the vascular system may lead to clumping of platelets about the tumor cells and concomitant removal of platelets from the circulation.

Platelet-tumor cell interaction appears to be relevant to metastasis observed in certain experimental tumors (4,6,7). Pearlstein aand associates (8) found a correlation between the platelet-aggregating potential of a series of rat renal sarcoma cells lines and the metastatic potential of these lines upon in vivo injection (see also Chapter 11). Rendering experimental animals thrombocytopenic prior to tumor cell inoculation results in reduced metastasis (4,6,7) and platelet infusion reverses this effect. Similar reduction of metastasis in certain experimental tumor systems has been achieved with platelet-antagonistic agents such as various non-steroidal anti-inflammatory drugs, with drugs that inhibit phosphodiesterase and thereby produce elevated platelet cyclic AMP levels, with platelet-inhibitory prostaglandin derivatives and with nafazatrom which stimulates endogenous prostacyclin formation (7 and Chapter 14). In contrast, inhibition of endogenous prostacyclin or administration of platelet-stimulatory prostaglandin derrivatives enhances tumor metastasis (7). Certain platelet antagonists appear to reduce the adherence of circulating tumor cells to vascular endothelium, to increase tumor cell circulation time and to reduce the magnitude of the decrease in platelet count that follows inoculation of tumor cells (9).

The ability of platelets to enhance tumor metastasis may be explained by several mechanisms. Platelets attach to areas of endothelial damage and therefore might be present in areas where tumor growth has brough about such damage. When platelets surround embolic tumor cells within the circulation, they may serve as a bridge that allows the tumor cells to become attached to the vessel walls. Marcum and associates (10) have shown that platelet-aggregating Hut 20 tumor cells failed to attach to the walls of isolated, de-endothelialized rabbit aorta. By contrast, in the presence of platelets, large platelet-tumor cell thrombi formed that readily became arrested on the vessel wall. Induction of thrombocytopenia or administration of platelet antagonists may exert a beneficial effect by reducing one or more of the following: platelet clustering on tumor cells, the attachment of platelet-tumor cell emboli to vessel walls, the liberation of platelet growth factors that might enhance tumor cell proliferation or the participation of platelets in fibrin formation.

The limited data available on human malignancy indicate that certain cultured tumor cell lines are capable of inducing platelet aggregation and that platelets may cluster about tumor cells within vessels in vivo (4). Heightened platelet responsiveness to platelet aggregating agents, reduced platelet survival and evidence for in vivo platelet release has been observed in patients with cancer (4). An inverse correlation has recently been observed between the platelet aggregating potential of four small cell lung cancer cell lines maintained in continuous culture and longevity of the patients from whom the cells were derived (11).

Studies have only recently been initiated to determine the effects of platelet antagonistic drugs on cancer (4). It has been found that a conjugate of aspirin and acetaminophen has no effect on the course of breast cancer (12) and that aspirin alone has no effect on the course of resected carcinoma of the colon (13). By contrast, indomethacin has been implicated in regression of squamous cell carcinoma of the skin (14). In addition when compared with historical controls, treatment with the phosphodiesterase inhibitor RA-233 was associated with an apparent reduction in both recurrence and the appearance of distant metastases in a group of patients with a variety of localized sarcomas following resection (9).

B. Fibrin

While some tumor cell lines induce platelet aggregation, others have been studied for their clot-initiating properties (15). The cellular procoagulant may be either tissue factor or a different substance that activates factor X (see also Chapters 6, 7 and 12). Thrombi are commonly observed surrounding intravascular tumor cells in tissue sections (3) and fibrin appears to be present in association with deposits of viable tumor cells in a number of different experimental and human tumor types (3,16 and Chapter 8).

In general, maneuvers designed to enhance fibrin formation serve to augment tumor metastasis (3). These include injection of thromboplastin-containing cells along with the tumor cells, administration of anti-fibrinolytic agents and treatment with agents that activate plasma coagulation factors. By contrast, maneuvers designed to inhibit fibrin formation reduce tumor metastasis in certain experimental systems. Examples include treatment with warfarin, heparin or fibrinolytic enzymes. Talmadge and associates (17) found, in a series of chemically-transformed cell lines, that metastatic potential was directly correlated with procoagulant activity of cell lysates. Gilbert and Gordon (18) studied variants of the B16 melanoma. They observed a weak correlatiom between the metastatic potential of the cell lines and their procoagulant activity. Furthermore, when cells were harvested on successive days following plating and then injected into mice, a progressive decline in metastatic potential was observed. This decline was associated with a proportional decrease in procoagulant activity.

The ability of fibrin to enhance tumor growth and spread may be explained by several mechanisms. Fibrin forms when thrombin is generated in response to activation of the enzymatic coagulation cascade. Fibrin forms at sites of vessel damage, for example following trauma that results in egress of blood from the vascular compartment. Fibrin may also form at sites of inflammation in which increased permeability of vessels to plasma proteins results in accumulation of fibrinogen and enzymatic intermediates in the interstitial space. Should tumor cells within the circulation stimulate fibrin formation on their surfaces, adhesion to vessel walls may be facilitated. Fibrin surrounding intravascular or extravascular tumor deposits may also serve as a lattice upon which tumor cell proliferation may occur (3) or a protective barrier against host defense mechanisms (16).

Most observations on limitation of metastasis by anticoagulants have been made in experimental animal systems. However, a number of uncontrolled or poorly controlled studies have suggested that this approach may be of benefit in human malignancy as well (19). The improved survival with warfarin anti-coagulation that has recently been reported in patients with small cell lung cancer provides added reason for optimism (20).

III. DISCUSSION

The foregoing brief and obviously oversimplified discussion is presented in an attempt to summarize data that provide a scientific basis for testing anticoagulants for their ability to limit tumor metastasis. It is evident that considerable heterogeneity exists in the manner by which different neoplastic cell types interact with coagulation mechanisms and in the kinds of agents (anticoagulant versus anti-platelet) that will inhibit metastasis. Relationships are obviously complex. Furthermore, limited data are available for human malignancy. Therefore, the extent to which insights obtained from work in experimental animal tumors can be applied to human cancer is unknown. However, sufficient progress has been made to permit a preliminary analysis and interpretation of these data.

Although mechanisms are by no means completely worked out, the best information available suggests that the anticoagulant approach is unlike conventional approaches to cancer management. It is apparently neither a direct attack on tumor proliferation, as in chemotherapy, nor a means for enhancing host defenses that are presumed to be deficient, as in immunotherapy. Instead, the anticoagulant approach seeks to block certain host reactions that appear to be required for tumor cells to metastasize successfully.

The coagulation mechanism is easily seen to be beneficial to securing hemostasis when it is activated in response to tissue damage. By mounting a local coagulation response to tumor cells the host may be responding to a clot-promoting or platelet-aggregating stimulus (provided by the tumor cell) that is not usually present within the circulation much as it would to either tissue cells that are not ordinarily in contact with the blood or to a vascular prosthesis or microorganisms that are inserted into the blood stream. A comparison has been made between this response to an invading neoplasm and the response of the coagulation mechanism that occurs at a wound site (15). Viewed in this way, the coagulation response to cancer cells is "appropriate" but healing cannot ensue.

However, this may not be the entire story. Should blocking coagulation indeed prevent metastatic seeding, one might logically conclude that the response of the host through coagulation activation contributes positively to the "success" of the tumor. Stated otherwise, without this particular host response, the assault of the tumor might fail and the "wound" might cease to be a wound. It is unsettling to contemplate the possibility that tumor cells may usurp these special pathways of host response in order to provide for themselves a local environment that is conducive to their growth and spread. This view is unlike the usual concept that envisions the host as attempting (but with limited or no success) to counter tumor progression and that has prompted use of militaristic terms, such as "invasion", "resistance" and "host defenses" in describing the host-tumor interaction (21). By contrast, the coagulation hypothesis views the host-tumor interaction as a dynamic one in which cells that are not sufficiently different from normal to be recognized as "foreign" are allowed to flourish because the host provides suitable "culture conditions" for neoplastic cell growth.

It may be instructive to speculate on the significance of the coagulation or platelet-aggregating properties of neoplastic cells for malignant behavior. Neoplastic transformation obviously results in a dramatic reprogramming of the physiologic role these cells are to play. However, evidence indicates that individual cells within a tumor may be heterogenous with respect to their procoagulant (and other) properties. Apparently, phenotypic changes can take place in space and time within a tumor (22) that influence the degree and manner of its interaction with hemostatic reactions (8,17,18). Such adaptive variation could explain differences in aggressiveness of malignancies when comparison is made among tumor types or between different instances of the same tumor type occurring in different patients. It could also explain the evolution towards more aggressive and autonomous behavior that is all too often evident in cancer (22). It is possible that a mechanism related to interaction with blood coagulation reactions might explain the prolonged period of dormancy that sometimes exists between tumor resection and recurrence months or years later. For example, the appearance of a cell from within a larger population of slowly proliferating cells that has developed as its special phenotype the capacity to attract platelets to itself or to induce local fibrin formation could result in a survival advantage for the neoplasm with rapid expansion of that particular clone of cells. One mechanism by which this rapid expansion could take place involves a positive feedback loop in which a platelet-aggregating tumor cell attracts platelets to itself. The platelets, in turn, might deliver growth-promoting substances that allow rapid proliferation of tumor cells that are, like the parent cell, capable of aggregating platelets.

In conclusion, the anticoagulant approach to tumor management is based on evidence that activation of host coagulation reactions provides an altered local environment for tumor cells that accommodates their growth through metastatic dissemination. The tumor cell itself is viewed as orchestrating the host response through its platelet-aggregating or clot-inducing properties. Obviously much remains to be learned before the precise details as well as the practical consequences of this interaction are fully known for human malignancy. Evidence is currently fragmentary on the occurrence of platelets and fibrin at human tumor sites, on reaction pathways that may be involved and on the mechanisms of drug effects. However, a rationale now exists for carefully designed clinical trials of coagulation- or platelet-inhibitory drugs in human malignancy. It is noteworthy that several drugs are currently available for testing that are relatively inexpensive. Trials of this approach may be especially timely in tumor types for which current therapy is inadequate and future planning stalemated. It seems particularly reasonable to test the anticoagulant hypothesis in an attempt to delay or prevent metastatic seeding in patients whose disease appears to be localized, for example following surgical removal, but in whom the chances of subsequent recurrence are substantial.

REFERENCES

1. Zubrod CG. Cancer (Philadelphia) 30:1474-1479, 1972.
2. Poste G and Fidler IJ. Nature (London) 283:139-146, 1980.
3. Zacharski LR, Henderson, WG, Rickles FR, Forman WB, Cornell CJ, Forcier RJ, Harrower HW and Johnson RO. Cancer (Philadelphia) 44:732-741, 1979.
4. Zacharski LR, Henderson WG, Rickles FR, Forman WB, Van Eeckhout JP, Cornell CJ, Forcier RJ and Martin JF. Am. J. Clin. Oncol. 5:593-609, 1982.
5. Zacharski LR. In: Interaction of Platelets with Tumor Cells (Ed. Jamieson GA), Alan R. Liss, New York, pp. 113-129, 1982.
6. Karpatkin S and Pearlstein E. Ann. Intern. Med. 95:636-641, 1981.
7. Honn KV, Busse WD and Sloane BF. Biochem. Pharmacol. 32:1-11, 1983.
8. Pearlstein E, Salk PL, Yogeeswaran G and Karpatkin S. Proc. Natl. Acad. Sci. USA 77:4336-4339, 1980.
9. Gastpar H. Ann. Chir. Gynaecol. Fenn. 71:142-150, 1982.
10. Marcum JM, McGill M, Bastida E, Ordinas A and Jamieson GA. J. Lab. Clin. Med. 96:1046-1053, 1980.
11. Rosenstein R, Zacharski LR, Phillips PG, Pettengill OS, Del Prete SA and Sorenson GD. Fed. Proc. Fed. Am. Soc. Exp. Biol. 42:524, 1983.
12. Powles TJ, Dady PJ, Williams J, Easty GC and Coombes RC. Adv. Prostaglandin Thromboxane Res. 6:511-516, 1980.
13. Lipton A, Scialla S, Harvey H, Dixon R, Gordon R, Hamilton R, Ramsey H, Weltz M, Heckard R and White D. J. Med. in press, 1983.
14. Al-Saleem T, Ali ZS and Qassab M. Lancet 2:264-265, 1980.
15. Semeraro N and Donati MB. In: Malignancy and the Hemostatic System (Eds. Donati MB, Davidson JF and Garattini S), Raven Press, New York, pp. 65-81, 1981.
16. Dvorak HF, Orenstein NS and Dvorak AM. Lymphokines 2:203-233, 1981.
17. Talmadge JE, Starkey JR and Stanford DR. J. Supramol. Struct. Cell. Biochem. 15:139-151, 1981.
18. Gilbert LC and Gordon SG. Cancer Res. 43:536-540, 1983.
19. Zacharski LR. In: Malignancy and the Hemostatic System (Eds. Donati MB, Davidson JF and Garattini S), Raven Press, New York, pp. 113-127, 1981.

20. Zacharski LR, Henderson WG, Rickles FR, Forman WB, Cornell CJ, Forcier RJ, Edwards R, Headley E, Kim S-H, O'Donnell JF, O'Dell R, Tornyos K and Kwaan HC. J. Am. Med. Assoc. 245:831-835, 1981.
21. Strauli P. In: Proteinases and Tumor Invasion (Ed. Strauli P, Barrett AJ and Baici A), Raven Press, New York, pp. 1-13, 1980.
22. Dennis J, Donaghue T, Florian M and Kerbel RS. Nature (London) 292:242-245, 1981.

CHAPTER 25. THE DESIGN AND EXECUTION OF ANTICOAGULANT THERAPY TRIALS IN CANCER

LEO R. ZACHARSKI

I. INTRODUCTION

In order to overcome the limitations of traditional chemo-therapeutic, radiotherapeutic and surgical treatments for cancer, it might be possible to manipulate the host-tumor interaction to enhance the advantage of the host. With this approach, referred to as "biologic response modification," treatment is directed toward events at the host-tumor interface that are thought to be related to the success or failure of the tumor. For example, therapy may be designed to boost cellular or humoral immune responses to the tumor that are inadequate but potentially capable of forestalling malignant growth and spread.

An alternative set of reactions that occur due to host-tumor interaction are those caused by activation of blood coagulation (1,2). Neoplastic cells are capable of initiating the sequence of enzymatic reactions leading to fibrin formation or of inducing platelet clumping (see also Chapters 6-8,10-12). Also, coagulation reactions may occur at tumor sites in response to local tissue damage (3,4). Evidence obtained largely from studies of malignancy in experimental animals indicates that pharmacologic interference with fibrin formation or platelet reactions ameliorates the course of certain tumors (1,5). This has led to the hypothesis (discussed in greater detail elsewhere in this volume) that activation of coagulation by cancer modifies its local environment in a manner that is conducive to its perpetuation and dissemination (2). The host is viewed as responding to the invading neoplasm through its hemostatic mechanism much as it would to a wound (3). Unfortunately, by responding, the host may provide conditions necessary for adhesion of embolic tumor cells to vessel walls, growth factors for cell proliferation or a fibrin barrier that protects the tumor from host defenses. Other possibilities may also exist.

Little is known about the coagulation-cancer interaction in man and basic studies are needed to understand mechanisms. However, only therapeutic trials of anti-thrombotic drugs in cancer will provide insights into the significance, if any, of this interaction for patient well-being. Since testing the coagulation hypothesis may be attractive to investigators involved in systematic evaluation of cancer therapy, an examination of methods used to acquire information from clinical trials might be useful. No attempt will be made to present, as has been done by others (6-8), a comprehensive discussion of the many aspects of cancer protocol design. Rather, the purpose of this chapter is to focus on certain features of protocol design and execution that deserve individual consideration because of the special nature of the coagulation hypothesis and the drugs available for therapeutic trials.

II. EFFECTS OF REDUCED BLOOD COAGULABILITY ON CANCER

What happens to cancer when the clotting mechanism is blocked? There are at least three ways to answer this question. The first is to look for cancer in individuals in whom coagulation reactions are blocked because of an inherited defect. The second is to observe the occurrence of cancer in patients treated with anticoagulants for thrombotic disorders. The third is to examine the course of cancer patients purposely treated with anticoagulant drugs.

To test the effect that genetically defective hemostasis would have on malignancy, Forman (9) surveyed 10,500 individuals with hereditary hemorrhagic disorders and found 61 instances of malignancy. Not only was a reduced incidence and death rate from malignancy in this test population not found, but there appeared to be an excess of patients with soft tissue sarcomas. These data are subject to several interpretations. Differences may exist between the test and control populations which could influence the development and course of malignancy in bleeders that are independent of the faulty hemostasis. Such differences might include the geographic distribution of test subjects (they are more likely to be located in large metropolitan centers where interested investigators and adequate records exist), demographic features (such as differences in age or life style) and medical factors (for example, the effects of large amounts of blood products, commonly administered to patients with bleeding disorders, on tumor suppression or enhancement are unknown). A more serious limitation of studies of this kind is that the defect in the vast majority of patients with hereditary bleeding disorders is within the intrinsic, or Hageman factor-dependent, pathway of blood coagulation. Individuals with hemostatic defects in the extrinsic, or tissue factor-dependent, pathway of blood coagulation are much rarer yet this pathway may be activated by neoplastic cells (10). It is most unlikely that a sufficient sample size of test subjects with defects in the extrinsic pathway of coagulation is available to test adequately the effect of such defects on cancer. Studies of this kind are essential and the results would be of considerable interest, but negative findings should not lead to negative conclusions regarding the importance of coagulation-cancer interactions. In this context, reports of individuals with bleeding disorders who also have malignancy might contribute to our understanding of mechanisms by which tumors induce coagulation activation.

Michaels (11) sought for clues to the effects of drug-induced hypocoagulability on malignancy by examining 540 patients who had received oral anticoagulants for thromboembolic disease for at least three months. Analysis of 1,569 patient-years revealed the expected incidence of, but a reduced death rate from, malignancy. However, it could not be determined if patients who had an indication for anticoagulants had therapy withheld because of a coexisting malignancy or were withdrawn from treatment when a malignancy appeared.

In an attempt to pursue this question, 378 patients were identified who had been treated with oral anticoagulants for ischemic heart disease (12). These patients were followed for a total of 3,451 patient-years of which 1,510 were between the first and last dose of anticoagulant. The incidence of newly diagnosed, histologically confirmed malignancies in this population was the same as that expected from comparison with age and sex-specific tumor registry data. The mortality from malignancy in the experimental population was less than expected but not significantly so. Analysis of cancer mortality three years following initial anticoagulant treatment revealed that the deficit of cancer deaths occurred within the first three years. Thus, the apparent reduction in death rate was attributed to the fact that patients in the experimental group were cancer-free when placed on treatment. The interpretive problem was compounded when malignancies occurring in anticoagulant-treated patients were subdivided into histologic types. Thus, the subsets became very small and comparisons were virtually impossible.

The limitations of such surveys lie in the excessively optimistic expectation that observation of one clinical condition will provide information on another. Retrospective, epidemiologic approaches to the question of the effect of coagulation blockade on cancer do not seem to be the most effective ones. Fortunately, other approaches are available.

III. CLINICAL TRIALS OF ANTICOAGULANTS IN CANCER

Deliberate treatment of cancer patients with antithrombotic drugs should provide the strongest test of the coagulation hypothesis. Such undertakings must be guided by a written agreement describing prospectively the course of action to be taken and the manner in which data are to be collected, analyzed and reported (see Appendices I and II).

Protocols designed to evaluate anticoagulant effects on cancer should seek to satisfy three objectives (13). These include validity (are the results true?), applicability (are the results relevant beyond the confines of the study?) and efficiency (does the benefit outweigh the cost in terms of drug side effects and expense?). With regard to the last objective, it is reasonable to question the "superiority" of treatment that provides marginal improvement but is expensive, toxic and complicated to administer (14). The issue of cost becomes even more important when a choice must be made between two treatments of equal but incomplete efficacy. The true "cost" of anticoagulation in cancer, in terms of drug toxicity, remains to be determined. However, there is reason to suspect that such toxicity will be acceptable (based on current knowledge of agents available for testing) and that it will be unlike that of conventional cancer chemotherapeutic agents. Clinical trials are expensive but they usually are affordable. The only prohibitively expensive anticoagulant trial is one which produces questionable or invalid results.

How far the results of the few existing therapeutic trials of anticoagulants in cancer can be generalized is, at present, unknown. Caution is warranted in applying results obtained in one setting to patients in another for at least three reasons. One is because initial attempts at innovative treatment of any kind tend to be carried out in patients with advanced disease. Anticoagulant therapy is no exception (1,5). However, there is reason to suspect that the response of tumor cells that are primarily intravascular early in the disease (when embolic tumor cells have not yet given rise to metastases) may be different from the response when large extravascular tumor deposits exist (2). It is reasonable to postulate that a given drug might have value in limited disease even though it failed to affect advanced disease. A second reason relates to observations in experimental animal tumors that have revealed different patterns of responsiveness to antithrombotic drugs between tumor types (2). Thus, responses to a given drug may vary between different forms of human malignancy. Results obtained for one tumor type may not apply to another. The third is the possibility that patient populations in which anticoagulant trials are conducted may differ in undefined ways that would influence response.

A. The Case for Prospective, Randomized Anticoagulant Studies

Validity is the non-negotiable requirement for anticoagulant and all other cancer treatment studies (13). For a study to be valid, both false negative and false positive conclusions regarding control of the disease by treatment must be avoided. Investigators differ widely in their perception of the protocol complexity required to obtain valid results. The case for highly complex protocol design is that it stands the greatest chance of producing the highest quality data that is subject to fewest criticisms. However, such demands might require a protocol that is so cumbersome and restrictive that it is either prohibitively expensive or impractical to execute either because investigators cannot be persuaded to participate or because of poor patient or physician compliance during the conduct of the study. Few studies are so perfectly designed and executed that they are beyond criticism. Furthermore, some imaginative studies may produce findings that were not anticipated but raise questions of validity in retrospect. One element that certainly increases complexity and about which controversy exists is that of blinding. This issue will be considered later and will serve to illustrate the tension that exists between validity and feasibility.

At the other extreme, some would deny the necessity for more than the simplest protocol. Thus, a decision is made to treat a definite (or indefinite) number of patients in a certain way to see what happens. It is customary to adopt this approach for drugs that appear promising in animal tumors but which have never been given to patients (7). Typically, patients with various types of advanced malignancy are treated with increasing doses to ascertain the maximum tolerable dose (MTD) and possible antitumor effects. Promising leads are pursued by administering the MTD to larger number of patients with specific tumor types. Fortunately, considerable experience has already been gained for several anticoagulants available for trials in cancer (15) and the need for pilot studies to assess dose and toxicity for these well-known drugs is doubtful. Of course, adoption of newly developed agents, the dose and toxicity of which are uncertain, for use in human malignancy would require such cautious pilot studies. The concept of the MTD probably does not apply to anticoagulant trials since doses, such as for heparin and warfarin, required to achieve the desired pharmacologic effect are already known. Tumor cytotoxicity is not the goal of this treatment method. In fact, for certain platelet antagonists, such as aspirin (16) or nafazatrom (17), large doses may be less effective than lower doses. Thus, "more" is not necessarily "better" and may, in fact, be "worse."

Some investigators may be satisfied with data showing complete or partial remissions (CR or PR) or delay in disease progression in studies that do not include concurrent controls because the results can be compared with studies of similar patients treated in other ways (18,19). It is claimed that trials using concurrent controls are unnecessary because data available in the literature can be used for comparison, because clinically "interesting" (apparently meaning large) differences can be detected by this means and because progress can be made more expeditiously. Advocates go on to claim that many therapeutic advances have been made in uncontrolled trials and that it is the investigators' ethical responsibility to follow existing recommmendations (that is, data reported from other uncontrolled trials) if the best available therapy is to be given (18,19).

The hazards of accepting such a felicitous construct have been effectively documented (7,8,20-22). It cannot be assumed, much less proved, that a given population of patients is truly matched for prognostic factors with other reported populations. For unknown reasons the natural history of certain malignancies has appeared to change with time (23,24). The result of adherence to studies lacking concurrent controls has been the publication of misleading results. Either their value cannot be determined or they are proved subsequently to be erroneous in controlled trials (7,8,20-22).

Arguments for and against controlled trials are of key importance for studies of anticoagulants because it is unlikely that vast changes in the natural history of advanced cancer will be observed in the presence of antithrombotic drugs. However, small differences that some may regard as "uninteresting" (18,19) may be important because they would provide evidence for the existence of a coagulation-cancer interaction. This interaction might thus be exploited by selection of other coagulation-reactive drugs used individually or in combination, or by application of the same drugs with greater advantage in patients with early malignancy. Such small (but potentially important) differences would be difficult if not impossible to detect without concurrent controls.

Uncontrolled trials often rely upon end points other than survival, namely CR and PR (25), to judge efficacy. Aside from the fact that tumor measurements are crude, lack reproducibility and are relatively unreliable (26), it is not anticipated that the anticoagulant approach will cause tumor regression. Rather, this form of therapy appears to primarily affect metastatic seeding and tumor progression (2). Therefore, primary end points should be survival or disease-free interval in patients with limited disease who are treated in an adjuvant setting. The use of historical controls, especially for adjuvant studies, would be most unwise.

Another issue of theoretical importance is the diversity of conventional (cytotoxic and other) anti-cancer treatments that might be given in the course of an anticoagulant trial. The ever changing notion of what constitutes optimal therapy varies between institutions and even between investigators within an institution. Anticoagulants may interact with certain chemotherapeutic agents used for experimental tumors (1,16,27). It is not known whether such an interaction occurs in humans with malignancy. Since there is reason to suspect such an interaction, it would be hazardous to assume that standard treatment "known to be effective" would have no influence on the outcome of an anticoagulant trial. The safest way to avoid uninterpretable or erroneous results would be to adopt a prospective randomized study design in which investigators would agree to standard therapy.

Two prospective, controlled trials of coagulation-inhibitory drugs have been undertaken within the VA Hospital system. These are VA Cooperative Study #75 of warfarin (1) and VA Cooperative Study #188 of the platelet antagonist RA-233 (5). Because demographic differences from non-VA populations may exist that could influence the outcome, it would be unwise to use the data from these studies as a historical control for contemplated uncontrolled trials. Experience from VA Cooperative Study #75 (28,29) furnishes a concrete example of the dangers of using historical controls. While the survival values for certain tumors in this study were comparable to those reported previously, survival values for patients with advanced (Duke's D) colon cancer were not. Warfarin-treated patients with metastatic colon cancer had a median survival of 47 wk. This was considerably longer than the approximately 4 to 6 mo median survival observed in certain uncontrolled trials (for review see 30). Had a controlled trial not been done it might have been concluded that warfarin provided greater longevity than "expected" and that it would be unethical to withhold such treatment from patients with this disease (18). However, the median survival for concurrently randomized controls who were demonstrably similar to warfarin-treated patients was 41 wk (p = 0.79). In fact, the survival curves for control and warfarin-treated patients crossed eight times. Thus, data from controlled trials not only allow correct conclusions regarding the value of the treatment but also discourage the adoption of treatment (mistakenly considered effective) that may be associated with increased morbidity due to hemorrhagic complications.

The dilemma posed by the uncontrolled trial is further highlighted by a recent report of a trial of warfarin in advanced colon cancer in which a median survival of 19.2 mo (approximately 77 wk) was reported (30). Should this be taken as evidence that warfarin works in non-VA patients with colon cancer or as evidence for a change in the natural history of colon cancer favoring longer survival as has been observed for certain other malignancies (23,24)?

The experience from VA Cooperative Study #75 (28,29) serves to illustrate an equally dangerous problem of uncontrolled trials that is the opposite of that illustrated above for colon cancer: that of failing to observe a positive effect. For patients with small cell lung cancer (SCCL) entered into this study, median survivals of 49.5 and 23 wk, respectively, were observed for warfarin-treated and control patients (p = 0.018). This study was started in April of 1976 but was planned in earlier years. The combination chemotherapy regimen adopted as standard therapy was based upon the report of an uncontrolled trial in which cyclophosphamide, vincristine and methotrexate were associated with a median survival of 9.5 mo [approximately 38 wk (31)]. Had an uncontrolled trial of warfarin been undertaken it might have been concluded that the results were similar to or only modestly better than might be expected with chemotherapy alone. The lower survival time observed in the control group of the randomized trial of warfarin could have been construed as demonstrating the inferiority of the control group rather than the superiority of the warfarin-treated group. However, in a controlled trial of the same chemotherapy regimen reported subsequently (32), it was demonstrated that the earlier estimates of survival associated with this regimen were overly optimistic (31) and that the survival was, in fact, similar to that observed in the control group of the warfarin study. The conclusion that warfarin was associated with improved survival was strengthened by the observation that the survival observed in patients with SCCL who were encountered during the conduct of the warfarin trial (but not admitted to the study) was virtually identical to that of the control group (33).

In the foregoing section, the need for carefully planned, prospective, randomized trials using concurrent controls in evaluation of anticoagulant effects in cancer has been demonstrated. The temptation to perform further uncontrolled trials should be resisted.

B. Blinding of Anticoagulant Trials

Blinded studies, in which either the patient or the investigator or both are unaware whether the investigational drug is authentic or placebo, have advantages and disadvantages. A disadvantage is increased complexity and expense. More time is required to obtain informed consent because of the need to explain that blinding is required to reduce bias. Furthermore, placebo, as well as authentic drug, must be manufactured, stored and distributed. Additional study personnel apart from those who monitor therapy may be required to evaluate results.

Sometimes blinding may not be feasible. This issue was debated at length prior to the commencement of VA Cooperative Study #75. Initially a single-blind design was adopted with the study nurse or physician's assistant who recorded results blinded but the patient and the attending physician who monitored therapy unblinded. The decision to not have patient blinding was based upon the fact that important interactions occur between warfarin and certain other drugs that the patient might take, and that the experimental drug is known to be associated with a risk of bleeding which might be magnified with malignancy. These risks, plus the judgment that the primary end point (survival) would not likely be modified substantially by subjective factors, led to the conclusion that it would be best if patients knew the identity of the medication. In addition, certain practical limitations on patient blinding were imposed by the necessity for periodic prothrombin time determinations required for warfarin dose adjustment and the possible requirement for additional visits to the physician for this purpose. Blinding of nurses and physician's assistants employed by the study was intended to maintain objectivity in recording tumor measurements and toxic (bleeding) manifestations.

One year after the study began it was determined that unblinding of treatment to study personnel had occurred in 86% of patients due to inadvertent communication, observation of the stigmata or added venipunctures and the appearance of patients for otherwise unscheduled visits (among other reasons). The effort to maintain blinding was abandoned. It may not be feasible to blind cancer trials of warfarin because of these complexities.

The limitations related to warfarin may not apply to certain other drugs such as platelet antagonists (for example RA-233) that do not require blood tests for dose adjustment and that are associated with a much lower risk of bleeding. For such studies, the blinded approach should be seriously considered in order to avoid several problems. In an unblinded study, the investigator would know the regimen to which recently entered patients had been randomized and therefore could predict with reasonable accuracy the regimen to which the next patient might be randomized. This prediction might influence the decision to admit the patient to study. In unblinded studies confusion might arise over interpretation of side effects (for example nausea and vomiting) that could be due to the experimental drug, to other (for example cytotoxic) therapy or to the disease itself. Despite indoctrination, there might be a tendency of both patient and examiner to ignore or minimize bleeding complications occurring without anticoagulant treatment and to overemphasize bleeding episodes occurring in patients taking a drug that is "expected" to enhance bleeding. A blinded design would also be advisable should tumor measurements be primary end point parameters since judgment regarding the location of tumor margins may be somewhat subjective and arbitrary (26).

Another reason to blind anticoagulant studies in cancer when possible is that it allows evaluation of the relationship between patient compliance with treatment and outcome. Should anticoagulants inhibit metastatic seeding or otherwise delay tumor progression, as is suspected from work in experimental animals (2), close adherence to treatment over a maximum time would best achieve the goals of the study. In a drug trial reported recently (not in cancer), a significant association was, in fact, found between compliance with treatment and outcome (34). However, the study was performed in a double-blind manner and the same association between compliance and outcome was observed for placebo-treated patients. Obviously, some factor other than the drug contributed to the outcome in patients who were careful to take their medication. The implications for anticoagulant studies are obvious.

The blinded design may be criticized because complications can arise that require breaking of the code so that a decision can be made whether or not to discontinue the medication. This problem can be obviated by designing a protocol that permits either dose reduction or elimination of the study drug, that may be either active or placebo, recording of the reason for the dose alteration, and then reinstitution of the drug at a later time should the complication resolve. This plan is being followed in the double-blind trial of RA-233 that is currently underway (5).

Finally, it has never been demonstrated that a placebo effect is absent in cancer (35). Who is to say that hopes, beliefs and fears have no influence on outcome or that knowledge of treatment would have no influence on the intensity of care? Adoption of the blinded methodology is not, as some have claimed, a form of deception (36), but rather the opposite: a strategy to minimize the risk of deception of both patient and those conducting the study.

IV. DISCUSSION

Any attempt to prove superiority of one treatment over another must be regarded as a joint effort of both patient and investigator. Once established, this partnership requires continuous active participation by both parties until the test is concluded. This special relationship usually begins with a verbal and written introduction of the patient to the goals of the trial by both. This matter of informed consent is complex and evolving, and its goals imperfectly realized. Since the anticoagulant approach to cancer management is in its infancy, much thought should be given to the composition of informed consent documents. The content of these will depend on the particular agent and type of malignancy under investigation. Rather than considering this topic further here, informed consent documents used for the studies of warfarin and RA-233 are presented as Appendices I and II that follow.

Optimal conditions for executing a carefully planned prospective trial are provided by a multi-institutional cooperative group so that an adequate number of properly classified patients can be studied within a reasonable amount of time. There is probably no place for further uncontrolled trials of familiar anticoagulant drugs in cancer. Instead, prospective, randomized and (when feasible) blinded trials should be planned in which patients are properly classified according to histologic type of cancer and in which balance is achieved between treatment groups for factors of prognostic importance, such as stage of disease and performance status (6). The design of such studies must take into consideration the fact that the anticoagulant approach is unlike traditional (e.g., cytotoxic) approaches to tumor containment and also the mechanism by which the particular experimental drug interferes with hemostatic reactions. Therapeutic trials should, when possible, incorporate features that allow assessment of patient compliance with treatment and the effect of the drug on hemostasis. Innovative studies should seek to explore mechanisms of drug effects on the malignancy.

Protocols designed for simultaneous use of multiple anti-thrombotic drugs to achieve anticoagulation in initial trials should be deferred in favor of trials of single agents. The interpretive problems that arise from multi-drug trials are illustrated by two recent reports in SCCL. Stanford (37) reported no differences from control in a group of patients with SCCL randomized to receive heparin, dextran and warfarin. This contrasts with the beneficial effect observed for warfarin alone (33). While several explanations might be offered for these divergent findings, it is possible that either heparin or dextran (or both) might have negated a beneficial effect from treatment with warfarin alone. It has been shown in a particular experimental tumor model (38) that tumor growth and spread is reduced by the vitamin K antagonist phenprocoumon but paradoxically is increased by heparin and warfarin. The possibility that human SCCL may correspond to this experimental model is supported by findings of Jamieson and Angove (39) that heparin may accelerate the progression of SCCL. Once the results of treatment with individual anticoagulant agents are established, judicious studies of drug combinations may be considered.

Much information of potential value for the design of clinical trials of anticoagulants in cancer stands to be gained from further studies in experimental tumors. There has been a tendency in some experimental studies to focus on one aspect of the coagulation-tumor cell interaction (such as tumor cell-induced platelet aggregation) and to ignore other aspects (such as tumor cell-induced fibrin formation or fibrinolysis). It would be most helpful if such studies were expanded to explore the overall pattern of interaction as well as patterns of response to various coagulation-reactive treatments in order to define models that might prove useful for better understanding the coagulation-cancer interaction in man and for guiding the selection of individual (and possibly combinations of) agents for human trials.

It is most unlikely that the coagulation-cancer interaction is the only meaningful host-tumor interaction. However, existing evidence suggests that this interaction may be of importance for patient well being. The coagulation hypothesis seems to deserve testing under conditions that are least likely to provide misleading results. Because such studies are time consuming and expensive, it is desirable to maintain a registry of antithrombotic drug trials in malignancy (see Chapter 27). The purpose of such a registry would be to enhance communication between workers in this field in order to expedite planning and communication of results.

REFERENCES

1. Zacharski LR, Henderson WG, Rickles FR, Forman WB, Cornell CJ, Forcier RJ, Harrower HW and Johnson RO. Cancer (Philadelphia) 44:732-741, 1979.

2. Zacharski LR. In: Interaction of Platelets with Tumor Cells (Ed. Jamieson GA), Alan R. Liss, New York, pp. 113-129, 1982.

3. Dvorak HF, Orenstein NS and Dvorak AM. Lymphokines 2:203-233, 1981.

4. Farber E. Am. J. Pathol. 108:270-275, 1982.

5. Zacharski LR, Henderson WG, Rickles FR, Forman WB, Van Eeckhout JP, Cornell CJ Jr., Forcier RJ and Martin JF. Am. J. Clin. Oncol. 5:593-609, 1982.

6. Zelen M. Cancer Chemother. Rep. 4:31-42, 1973.

7. Livingston RB and Carter SK. In: Principles of Cancer Treatment (Eds. Carter SK, Glatstein E and Livingston RB), McGraw-Hill, New York, pp. 34-35, 1982.

8. Durant JR. In: Controversies in Oncology (Ed. Wiernik PH), John Wiley and Sons, New York, pp. 373-387, 1982.

9. Forman WB. Cancer (Philadelphia) 44:1059-1061, 1979.

10. Semeraro N and Donati MB. In: Malignancy and the Hemostatic System (Eds. Donati MB, Davidson JF and Garattini S), Raven Press, New York, pp. 65-81, 1981.

11. Michaels L. J. Med. 5:98-105, 1974.

12. Annegers JR. and Zacharski LR. Thromb. Res. 18:399-403, 1980.

13. Sackett DL. N. Engl. J. Med. 303:1059-1060, 1980.

14. Nelson RB. Forum on Medicine 594-600, September, 1979.

15. Zacharski LR. In: Malignancy and the Hemostatic System (Eds. Donati MB, Davidson JF and Garattini S), Raven Press, New York, pp. 113-127, 1981.

16. Verstraete M. Haemostasis 12:317-336, 1982.

17. Honn KV. Personal communication, 1983.

18. Gehan EA and Freireich EJ. N. Engl. J. Med. 290:198-203, 1974.

19. Gehan EA and Freireich EJ. Semin. Oncol. 8:430-436, 1981.

20. Byar DP, Simon RM, Friedewald WT, Schlesselman JJ, DeMets DL, Ellenberg JH, Gail MH and Ware JH. N. Engl. J. Med. 295:74-80, 1976.

21. Chalmers TC, Block JB and Lee S. N. Engl. J. Med. 287:75-78, 1972.

22. Gilbert, JP. N. Engl. J. Med. 291:1305-1306, 1974.

23. Hinds MW, Nomura AMY, Kolonel LN and Lee J. Cancer (Philadelphia) 51:175-178, 1983.

24. Dahlin DC. Mayo Clin. Proc. 54:621-622, 1979.

25. Green JA. Am. J. Med. 73:779-780, 1982.

26. Henderson WG, Zacharski LR, Spiegel PK, Rickles FR, Forman WB, Cornell CJ Jr., Forcier RJ, Edwards RL, Headley E, Kim S-H, O'Donnell JR, O'Dell R, Tornyos K and Kwaan HC. Cancer (Philadelphia) in press, 1983.

27. Carmel RJ and Brown JM. Cancer Res. 37:145-151, 1977.

28. Zacharski LR, Henderson WG, Rickles FR, Forman WB, Cornell CJ, Forcier RJ, Edards R, Headley E, Kim S-H, O'Donnell JF, O'Dell R, Tornyos K and Kwaan HC. Circulation 66:302, 1982.

29. Zacharski LR, Henderson WG, Rickles FR, Forman WB, Cornell CJ Jr., Forcier RJ, Edwards RL, Headley E, Kim S-H, O'Donnell JF, O'Dell R, Tornyos K and Kwaan HC. (submitted).

30. Chlebowski RT, Gota CH, Chan KK, Weiner JM, Block JB and Batemen JR. Cancer Res. 42:4827-4830, 1982.

31. Eagan RT, Maurer LH, Forcier RJ and Tulloh M. Cancer (Philadelphia) 33:527-532, 1974.

32. Maurer LH, Tulloh M, Weiss RB, Blom J, Leone L, Glidewell O and Pajak TF. Cancer (Philadelphia) 45:30-39, 1980.

33. Zacharski LR, Henderson WG, Rickles FR, Forman WB, Cornell CJ Jr., Forcier RJ, Edwards R, Headley E, Kim S-H, O'Donnell JF, O'Dell R, Tornyos K and Kwaan HC. J. Am. Med. Assoc. 245:831-835, 1981.

34. The Coronary Drug Project Research Group N. Engl. J. Med. 303:1038-1041, 1980.

386

35. Gilman AS, Goodman LS and Gilman A. The Pharmacologic Basis of Therapeutics, 6th ed. Macmillan, New York, pp. 46–47, 1980.
36. Editorial: Controlled trials: Planned deception? Lancet 1:534–535, 1979.
37. Stanford CF. Thorax 34:113–116, 1979.
38. Hagmar B. Acta. Pathol. Microbiol. Scand. 80:357–366, 1972.
39. Jamieson GA and Angove RC. Aust. N.Z. J. Med. 9:381–384, 1979

VA COOPERATIVE STUDY #75
Informed Consent Form
Explanation of Study

While much progress has been made in cancer treatment, therapy in many patients is far from perfect. The best surgical, radiation therapy and drug management available does not always prevent growth or recurrence of the tumor.

For this reason the Federal Government sponsors research into new and better forms of cancer therapy. You are being asked to participate in such a project. Studies in experimental animals during the past 10 or 15 years have shown that the growth and spread of tumor is linked to the ability of the blood to clot. It seems that the mechanism which is so helpful when we are cut or scratched may be harmful when the clot forms around the growing tumor. It may be that the clot helps the tumor to grow or that the clot prevents the body from destroying the tumor. Medications which reduce blood coagulation are known as anticoagulants. Studies have shown that when anticoagulants are given to animals with malignancy, growth of the malignancy is retarded or prevented.

It is interesting that anticoagulants have been safely given to patients to control excessive clotting (thrombosis) for over 20 years. It may be that these same medications will be of benefit to cancer patients but this has not been demonstrated. The study which you are invited to participate in is designed to investigate this question.

All patients will be give the very best treatment modern medicine has to offer. This treatment varies with different types of tumors. In some cases this may be surgery, in others radiation therapy, and in others various medications or combinations of these. No treatment which you need for any reason will be withheld although you are requested to obtain all or as much of your medical care as possible here. This includes care for problems related or unrelated to your malignancy. If you must see a doctor nearer your home, please ask him to contact us for details of your medical history and treatment.

As has been said, anticoagulant medications reduce the ability of the blood to clot. Too much medication can therefore lead to excessive bleeding, such as bleeding into urine or bowels, coughing up blood, nosebleeds, vaginal bleeding, etc. Under very unusual circumstances such bleeding may be fatal but the chances of this are extremely small. However, bleeding complications can be prevented by adjusting the dose so that no bleeding is likely with every-day activities. Very rarely allergic reactions to this medication occur. It is our opinion that the risks of anticoagulation are very small in comparison to the possible benefits we are looking for. Further instructions on the use of anticoagulants will be given in the event that you are placed on this medication.

If you wish to participate in this study you will be assigned randomly to one of two different treatments. One of these alternatives will be the very best treatment currently available. The other alternative will be treatment with the best treatment currently available plus anticoagulant medication. In either case you will be examined as frequently as necessary to assure that treatment is optimal. You are to understand that once assigned to a given group you cannot choose to change to another group.

388

As in all chronic disease, treatment for tumors must continue on a long-term basis. However, you should understand that if you decide not to participate in this study or to withdraw from the study at any time the best treatment currently available will continue to be given to you. You should understand that this study may be of benefit to cancer patients but may not necessarily be of benefit to you. You will be followed in this study for a minimum of 3 years. We ask that if you move during this time that you notify us of your new address.

If you are to receive the anticoagulant drug you should be aware of the information on the following pages.

INFORMATION FOR PATIENTS WHO RECEIVE ANTICOAGULANT THERAPY

These are the instructions you will receive should you be placed on anticoagulant therapy. The mechanics are simple, and it is very important that you understand the reasons for therapy, dosage, and the effects of overdose. Under continuous supervision, you should have no side effects from your medication; however, it is important to follow instructions carefully.

"Anticoagulant" may be a new word to you. An "anticoagulant" is a substance that reduces the ability of the blood to clot. The medicine you are taking is called warfarin (Coumadin®).

HOW THE DRUG WORKS

Your blood contains a number of different protein clotting factors which are all necessary if you are to stop bleeding normally following injury. Four of these clotting factors are made by the liver only when you body contains an adequate amount of vitamin K. The anticoagulant drug you are taking is a vitamin K antagonist, which means that it temporarily makes some of the vitamin unavailable to your body. Your blood level of these four clotting factors is thereby reduced to about 10-20% of the normal level. This amount is adequate to prevent bleeding with everyday life and still provide protection against the formation of abnormal clots (thrombi or emboli) in your body.

DETERMINING DRUG DOSAGE

The drug you are taking is called warfarin. The brand name of the variety of warfarin you have received is Coumadin. Pink Coumadin tablets contain 5 milligrams of warfarin. Purple Coumadin tablets contain 2 milligrams of warfarin. Both tablet sizes are creased down the middle (scored). Scored tablets may be divided in two equal parts by placing a knife edge in the crease and pressing down, while holding the table firmly by its edges against a flat surface. Thus, half of a purple tablet is 1 milligram and half of the pink tablet is 2½ milligrams. A dose of 6 milligrams could be accomplished by taking one pink and one-half of a purple tablet.

REGULATING YOUR ANTICOAGULANT DOSAGE

This is accomplished by having a prothrombin time test performed about every two weeks. Your doctor will contact you after he receives the test result, and will give you the dosage of Coumadin for the next two weeks. If you cannot come to the laboratory on the day you are to have your prothrombin time, it is <u>very important</u> that you call your doctor, explain the delay, and arrange for a new appointment time. Drawing the blood sample for the prothrombin time test takes only a few minutes, and you are then free to resume your usual daily schedule. A regular time should be arranged to receive your doctor's telephone call with your dosage instructions.

TAKING YOUR DAILY MEDICATION (WARFARIN)

Take the required number of tablets at the same time each afternoon, for example, four o'clock, and mark on a calendar that you have taken your medication. On the day of the prothrombin time determination, do not take the day's dose until you have heard from your doctor. If you have not heard from him by three o'clock, call your doctor for instructions.

DIET

Please avoid the following foods entirely: Cabbage, brussel sprouts, cauliflower, spinach, broccoli and liver. Please take a constant amount daily of milk and green salads. Eat what you want, but eat the <u>same amount</u> each day.

ALCOHOL

You are permitted to have one or two drinks per day <u>but no more</u>. The ingestion of greater amounts of alcohol may irritate the lining of your stomach and expose you to the danger of bleeding.

DRUGS

Many drugs are recognized to make patients more sensitive or more resistant to Coumadin®. It is <u>essential</u> that the doctor who is regulating your Coumadin dosage know <u>in advance</u> of any new drugs you are given by other physicians. If you <u>stop</u> taking a drug you must also inform your doctor. Finally, many patent medications that can be purchased without a prescription will affect your anticoagulant therapy. Examples are aspirin, Bufferin®, Excedrin®, Anacin®, and regular Alka-Seltzer®. In summary, don't take <u>any drug</u> unless your doctor has given his approval.

ABNORMAL BLEEDING

Although the risk of significant bleeding is small, it is always a possibility for patients receiving anticoagulants. By following a few simple rules, the chance of having this uncommon complication is minimized.

Inform your doctor promptly if any of the following happens:

1. Excessive bleeding after cuts, as during shaving. For that matter any bleeding that does not stop itself with reasonable promptness.

2. Excessive menstrual bleeding.

3. The sudden appearance of "black and blue spots" on the skin.

4. Bleeding from the nose or mouth.

5. The appearance of red or dark-brown urine.

6. The appearance of red or black bowel movements.

Should any such symptoms appear, don't become alarmed. Call your doctor. He knows how to treat such things effectively.

GENERAL INSTRUCTIONS

If you should be in an accident and feel you have been injured, call your doctor.

Carry a card, that will be given, in your purse or wallet. It states that you are receiving Coumadin anticoagulant medication and gives your doctor's name, address and telephone number.

If you should develop an infection, nausea, vomiting, diarrhea or any other illness, let your doctor know.

PROTHROMBIN TIME VISITS

1. Arrive at the laboratory in the morning without breakfast.

2. Bring your bottle of Coumadin tablets.

3. If you are not going to be home the remainder of the day, tell the doctor where he may reach you.

4. Tell the doctor if any unusual bleeding has occurred.

This project has been approved by the Research and Education Committee of this VA hospital and our Human Studies Committee.

APPENDIX II

VA COOPERATIVE STUDY #75
Information Sheet About the Study of
ANTICOAGULANTS IN THE RX OF CA (RA-233)

While much progress has been made in cancer treatment, therapy in many patients is far from perfect. The best surgical, radiation therapy and drug management available does not always prevent growth or recurrence of the tumor.

For this reason the Federal Government sponsors research into new and better forms of cancer therapy. You are being asked to participate in such a project. Studies in experimental animals during the past 10 to 15 years have shown that the growth and spread of tumors is linked to the ability of the blood to clot. It seems that the mechanism which is so helpful when we are cut or scratched may be harmful when the clot forms around the growing tumor. It may be that the clot helps the tumor to grow or that the clot prevents the body from destroying the tumor. Studies have shown that when anticoagulants are given to animals with cancer, growth of the tumors is slowed or stopped at least for a while.

Anticoagulants have been safely given to patients to control excessive clotting (thrombosis) for over 20 years. It may be that these same medications will be of benefit to cancer patients, but this has not been demonstrated. The study which you are invited to participate in is designed to investigate this question.

The usual treatment for cancer varies with different types of tumors. In some cases this may be surgery, in others radiation therapy, and in others various single medications or combinations of medications. No treatment which you need for any reason will be withheld although you are requested to obtain all or as much of your medical care as possible here. This includes care for problems related or unrelated to your cancer. If you must see a doctor nearer your home, please ask him to contact us for details of your medical history and treatment.

Should you participate in this study, you will be receiving the treatment known at this time to be best for your particular type of tumor. In addition, you will be assigned to a group of patients that will receive one of the following treatments: an anticoagulant drug called RA-233; or a placebo (a harmless, inactive substance in drug form). This assignment will be done randomly (i.e., like a toss of a coin).

It is not yet known whether the anticoagulant treatments will have a positive effect on your disease. The study results will be closely watched. If a clear advantage to one treatment is found, each patient in the study will be given the option to receive this treatment.

RA-233 has been used in Europe to treat cancer but has not been tested in this country. While results so far are promising, there is no definite proof that it is effective in treating cancer. It is such proof that we are trying to obtain in this study. You will be asked to take 2 pills 3 times each day. This medication is not known to produce any unpleasant side effects except for occasional headache and lowering blood pressure. The drug works on tiny cells in the blood called platelets which are required for blood coagulation. It is believed these platelets may also contribute to the growth and spread of cancer. In order to study the effects that the medication is having, you will be asked to give a blood sample at monthly intervals for special tests.

As in all chronic (continuing, persistent) disease, treatment for cancer must continue on a long-term basis. You will be examined at regular intervals to be sure that your treatment is the best suited to your needs. You will have all of the benefits of any other VA patient. In fact, if you decide not to continue in this study, you may withdraw at any time and continue to receive all other treatment that you may need. If you stay in this study, we anticipate that you will be on your new treatment for the duration of the study (5 years), or until the course of your illness requires that your physician withdraw you from the study, temporarily or permanently.

Should you move from this area, we will ask that you inform us of your new address.

While you are in this study group, we ask that you report any unusual changes in your condition to your doctor at the VA. He should be called in the event that you are in an accident or are injured.

While all other medications are available for use, we ask that you avoid medications that contain aspirin if possible. These include Bufferin®, Excedrin®, Anacin® and regular Alka-Seltzer®, among many. You may freely use Tylenol® on occasions that you might otherwise have used aspirin.

This project has been approved by the Research and Development Committee and the Human Studies Committee of this VA Hospital.

You should understand that this study may benefit future cancer patients but may or may not benefit you.

CHAPTER 26. EXPERIMENTAL AND CLINICAL EXPERIENCE WITH PYRIMIDO-PYRIMIDINE DERIVATIVES IN THE INHIBITION OF MALIGNANT METASTASIS FORMATION

HELMUTH GASTPAR, JULIAN L. AMBRUS, WILHELM van EIMEREN

I. INTRODUCTION

The fate of disseminated tumor cells in the circulation is largely determined by their physiochemical surface properties which are foreign to the blood and conditioned by the thromboplastic activities intrinsic to the tumor cell (1). The term "cancer cell stickiness" (2) describes a tumor-specific, population-variable property of the circulating tumor cells in terms of an increased tendency to adhere to foreign surfaces (3). Cell populations with a high degree of stickiness have a correspondingly high thromboplastic activity and transplantation rate (4,5).

In former investigations we were able to demonstrate that malignant tumors with a high frequency of metastasis formation correlate with a low incidence of circulating tumor cells in the peripheral blood. In contrast, in neoplastic diseases which metastasize only infrequently the percentage of free-floating tumor cells in venous blood was significantly higher. Possibly the disseminated tumor cells of metastasizing cancers are more sticky than the cells of non-metastasizing ones, resulting in a greater tendency to adhere to vascular endothelium (6). Using intravital capillary microscopy and microcinematography, it has been demonstrated in animals that sticky tumor cells and tumor cell-platelet complexes are able to adhere to normal vascular endothelium. Within minutes parietal microthrombi occur, immediately stabilized by a fibrin network upon which further platelets and leukocytes gather (7-9).

Experimental data suggest that development of metastases from blood-borne cancer cells in some instances is closely related to disseminated intravascular coagulation (3). The immediate decrease in the number of circulating platelets following intravenous injection of Walker 256 carcinosarcoma cells in rats (6) represents the hematological counterpart to the morphological findings of tumor cells associated with platelet clusters arrested in the pulmonary arterioles and capillaries (10,11). The demonstration of fibrin monomers in the blood of the animals indicates that intravascular fibrin formation is accompanied by the consumption of platelets (12).

We have demonstrated that platelet aggregation may also occur in response to human cancer cells during their circulation in the blood (7). Patients with metastatic cancer have a permanent reduction in platelet survival and increased platelet consumption (13). Moreover, it was demonstrated recently that human and animal platelets contain a growth-promoting factor for certain malignant cell lines which is released during thrombin- or collagen-induced aggregation (14-16). On the other hand, purified plasma membrane vesicles shed by several tumor cell lines induce immediate platelet aggregation in vitro (17, see also Chapter 10).

II. THE EFFECT OF PYRIMIDO-PYRIMIDINE DERIVATIVES ON CELL GROWTH AND METASTASIS FORMATION IN ANIMALS

Gasic and Gasic (18) observed in 1962 that pretreatment of mice with neuraminidase resulted in a significant reduction in the frequency of pulmonary metastases after intravenous injection of tumor cells. Further studies showed that neuraminidase induced marked thrombocytopenia in the animals and that the antimetastatic effect of neuraminidase could be abolished by platelet transfusion (19).

We were able to demonstrate (7) that pretreatment with the platelet aggregation inhibitors dipyridamole and several other pyrimido-pyrimidine derivatives, such as mopidamole (RA 233) and VK 744 [2-(2-aminoethyl)amino-4-morpholinothieno(3,2-d)pyrimidine-dihydrochloride] significantly reduced the number of lethal tumor cell emboli in rats after intravenous injection of 1,000,000 Walker 256 carcinosarcoma cells (Figure 1).

At the same time, these substances, in a dose dependent manner, reduced the tendency of the circulating tumor cells to adhere to the endothelium of the mesenteric vessels [observed by intravital capillary microscopy (Figure 2)] and to reduce the platelet count (Figure 3) (6). Similar findings were obtained with the aggregation inhibitors bencyclane, pentoxifylline, sulfinpyrazone, the methyl-pyrazoline derivative nafazatrom and the pyrimido-pyrimidine derivative RX-RA 69 [8-benzylthio-4-morpholino-2-piperizino-pyrimido (5,4-d)pyrimidine] (21-24). Also we were able to show that the pyrimido-pyrimidine derivative mopidamole (Figure 4), as well as bencyclane, pentoxifylline and nafazatrom in therapeutic doses significantly increased the circulation time of intravenously injected ^{32}P-labeled Ehrlich ascites tumor cells in mice (25-28).

A very important role in the regulation of energy metabolism of platelets is played by cyclic AMP (29). The pool of cAMP is controlled by two enzymes, adenylate cyclase (AC) and cAMP-phosphodiesterase (PDE). The fact that inhibitors of AC and/or activators of PDE activate platelet aggregation and conversely activators of AC and/or inhibitors of PDE inhibit platelet aggregation suggests an important role for cAMP in the mechanisms of platelet aggregation (30). Pyrimido-pyrimidine derivatives, dipyridamole, mopidamole and RX-RA 69, as well as the methylxanthine derivative pentoxifylline are well known inhibitors of PDE and thereby cause an increase in the cAMP level of platelets (31,32), especially of the membrane-related cAMP (32). However, at therapeutic doses the above drugs have only a moderate and short-lasting in vitro effect on cAMP levels of human platelets and on platelet aggregation.

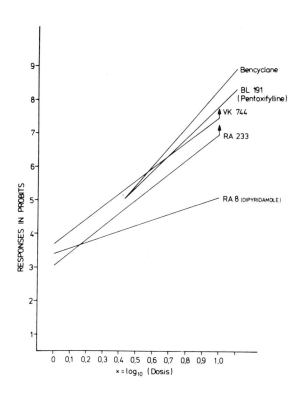

FIGURE 1. Probit Regression Lines for the Effect of Bencyclane, Pentoxifylline and Three Pyrimido-Pyrimidine Derivatives, Dipyridamole (RA 8), Mopidamole (RA 233) and VK 744, on Prevention of Mortality due to Cancer Cell Embolism after Intravenous Injection of 1,000,000 Walker 256 Carcinosarcoma Cells in Rats. The arrows at the top of the RA 233 and VK 744 lines indicate 100% response rates. [From Gastpar (20) with permission.]

396

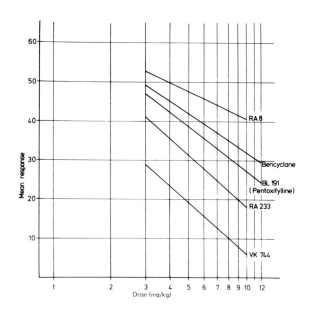

FIGURE 2. Dose-Response Relationship for the Effect of Bencyclane, Pentoxifylline and the Three Pyrimido-Pyrimidine Derivatives, Dipyridamole (RA 8), Mopidamole (RA 233) and VK 744, on Cancer Cell Stickiness to Vascular Endothelium in the Mesentery of Surviving Rats (cells/cm^2) after Intravenous Injection of 1,000,000 Walker 256 Carcinosarcoma Cells. [From Gastpar (20) with permission.]

This discrepancy between low in vitro and comparatively high in vivo activity of these substances may be explained by the observations that dipyridamole (34,35), pentoxifylline (36) and nafazatrom (37) at therapeutic doses stimulate the biosynthesis and/or release of prostacyclin (PGI$_2$) from the vessel wall, which in turn stimulates platelet AC resulting in further elevation of cAMP levels in platelets (see Chapters 13 and 14). It may be speculated, therefore, that an endothelial cell-platelet interaction is required for the full activity of these derivatives, and probably mopidamole, in vivo (36). Dipyridamole, pentoxifylline and nafazatrom increase $\overline{PGI}_2$ synthesis and/or release which in turn elevates cAMP synthesis in the platelets.

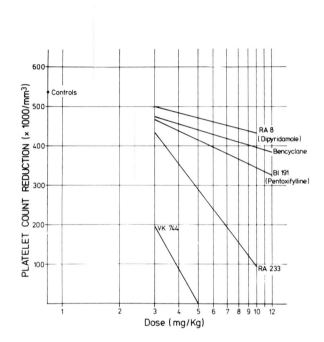

FIGURE 3. Dose-Response Relationship for the Effect of Bencyclane, Pentoxifylline and the Three Pyrimido-Pyrimidine Derivatives, Dipyridamole (RA 8), Mopidamole (RA 233) and VK 744 on Platelet Count Reduction in the Venous Blood of Surviving Rats after Intravenous Injection of 1,000,000 Walker 256 Carcinosarcoma Cells. [From Gastpar (20) with permission.]

The cAMP level, stimulated in this manner, may be further increased by the inhibitory effect on platelet PDE evoked by dipyridamole, mopidamole, RX-RA 69 or pentoxifylline (Figure 5).

398

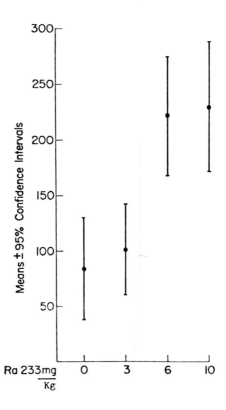

FIGURE 4. Effect of Various Doses of Mopidamole (RA 233) on the Circulation Time (min) of 25,000,000 Intravenously Injected, ^{32}P-Labeled, Polyploid Ehrlich Ascites Tumor Cells in Mice. [From Ambrus et al. (25) with permission.]

Cyclic AMP, however, has not only a major influence on the integrity of the platelets, but also controls the arrest of mitosis by chalones (38). Transformed cells show a lower concentration of cAMP than corresponding normal cells (39) and the addition of exogenous cAMP derivatives to culture media inhibits cell division (40-42). In various cultured tumor cells it was found that cAMP derivatives induced an inhibition of proliferation (43-45), sometimes causing a revertance of transformed tumor cells to more normal appearances (46,47). The PDE activity of leukemic lymphocytes has been shown to be 5 to 10 times greater than that of normal lymphocytes (48), and in human tumor biopsies certain types of PDE activities have been shown to be higher than in corresponding normal tissue from the same patient (49).

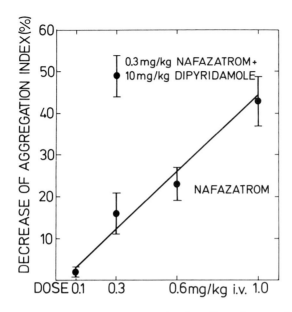

FIGURE 5. Inhibition of ADP-Induced Platelet Aggregation In Vivo by Nafazatrom in Stumptailed Monkeys (Macaca arctoides). Potentiating effect by simultaneous application of dipyridamole. Decrease of aggregation index by 10 mg/kg/i.v. dipyridamole alone in the same animals: 5.0 ± 1.3% (26).

There is some evidence to suggest that aggregation inhibitors have a stimulating effect on cAMP synthesis in vivo and an inhibiting action on PDE. Dipyridamole, mopidamole, RX-RA 69 and pentoxifylline may also act directly on tumor cells by inhibiting their cAMP turnover. The results of recent investigations by our group point in this direction, showing that ^{3}H-thymidine incorporation into human leukemic and other neoplastic cells (50) and the growth of these cells in culture media (51) were inhibited by the pyrimido-pyrimidine derivative mopidamole (Figures 6 and 7).

The addition of mopidamole to a culture of a human promyelocytic leukemic cell line (HL-60) resulted in differentiation to normal appearing cells (50). Not only morphologic maturation was noted but evidence of enzymologic differentiation (lysozyme activity) was also induced by mopidamole exposure (Table 1). This maturation appeared to be a permanent phenotypic change since inoculation of treated cells into nude mice did not result in neoplastic growth (52).

400

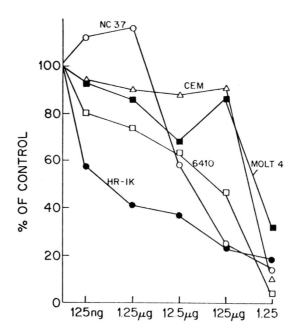

FIGURE 6. Effects of Mopidamole (RA 233) on In Vitro Cell Growth. ³H-thymidine incorporation results expressed as percentage of untreated control cell incorporation. Molt-4F: Acute lymphoid leukemia (T-cell); CCRF-CEM: Acute lymphatic leukemia (T-cell); 6410: Acute myeloid leukemia (B-cell); Hr-IK Burkitt's lymphoma (B-cell, carries EB virus); NC-37: Normal lymphocyte (B-cell, carries EB virus). [From Biddle et al. (51) with permission.]

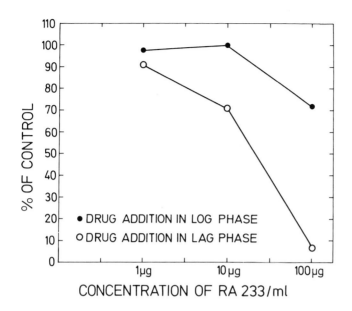

FIGURE 7. Effect of Mopidamole (RA 233) on In Vitro Cell Growth of Daudi (Burkitt's lymphoma, B-cell, carries EB virus). Results expressed as a percentage of control cell population increase. [From Biddle et al. (51) with permission.]

Table 1. Myeloid Differentiation in Human Promyelocytic Leukemia (HL-60) Cells after 6 Days Treatment with RA 233[a].

RA 233 mg/kg	Cell x 10^7/100 mm Petri dish	% Morpho- logically mature cells	Lysozyme Activity[b]
0.000	3.4	10	3
0.025	3.5	13	3
0.250	0.5	73	17

[a][From Ambrus et al. (50) with permission.]

[b] μg equiv./10 ml/10^7 cells

Furthermore, we demonstrated (Figure 8) that mopidamole, administered orally, is able to significantly diminish spontaneous lung metastases in syngenic Wilms' tumor (nephroblastoma) of the rat, the C1300-neuroblastoma of the mouse and the HM-Kim mammary carcinoma of the

402

rat. Mopidamole has no effect on the NIH-renal adenocarcinoma of the mouse (50). Similar effects were obtained with pentoxifylline (53) and the PGI$_2$-releasing agent nafazatrom (26, see also Chapter 14). Interestingly, none of these substances were able to inhibit metastasis formation by the NIH-renal adenocarcinoma of the mouse.

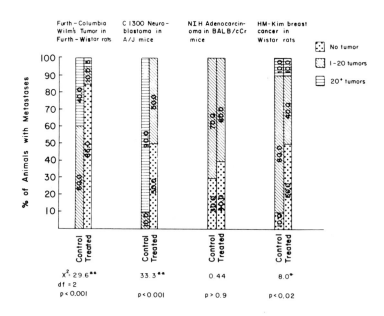

FIGURE 8. Effect of Daily Oral Doses of 100 mg/kg Mopidamole (RA 233) on the Frequency of Spontaneous Lung Metastases in Four Syngeneic Animal Tumors, 3-4 Weeks after Transplantation. [From Ambrus et al. (26) with permission.]

Recent experiments demonstrate (Table 2) that in a number of human neoplastic cells lines growth will be inhibited by mopidamole and also by human fibroblast interferon (HFIF). If the substances are combined a marked potentiation of the inhibitory effect occurs (50). This may be related to the finding that HFIF stimulates AC and therefore can increase cAMP production, while mopidamole in turn prevents cAMP decomposition by inhibition of PDE. From current experiments it appears that mopidamole also potentiates the ability of interferon to increase natural killer cell activity in mice (52). If low level interferon production is part of the normal antitumor defense mechanism of the host, potentiation of this effect by pyrimido-pyrimidine derivatives may be an additional mechanism by which mopidamole exerts an antitumor – antimetastasis effect.

Table 2. Effect of Human Fibroblast Interferon (HFIF) and RA 233 on In Vitro Cell Growth.

Cells	Drug Concentration	% of Untreated Controls ± S.D.	% Control Expected if Additive
DAUDI	0.001 mg/ml RA 233	91 ± 3	48
	50 ref. U/ml HFIF	53 ± 4	
	RA 233 + HFIF	36 ± 2	
ES-1	0.01 mg/ml RA 233	66 ± 4	32
	50 ref. U/ml HFIF	48 ± 3	
	RA 233 + HFIF	13 ± 5	
LMCaP	0.1 mg/ml RA 233	80 ± 2	61
	100 ref. U/ml HFIF	76 ± 2	
	RA 233 + HFIF	32 ± 3	
RT-4	0.1 mg/ml RA 233	86 ± 2	50
	100 ref. U/ml HFIF	58 ± 4	
	RA 233 + HFIF	37 ± 5	
HT-29	0.1 mg/ml RA 233	16 ± 2	12
	100 ref. U/ml HFIF	75 ± 4	
	RA 233 + HFIF	2 ± 1	
BG-27	0.1 mg/ml RA 233	65 ± 3	56
	100 ref. U/ml HFIF	86 ± 3	
	RA 233 + HFIF	33 ± 5	

Drugs administered during the lag phase of cell growth. Results expressed as a percentage of control cell population increase. ES-1: Malignant melanoma; LMCaP: Prostatic carcinoma; RT-4: Transitional bladder cell carcinoma; HT-29: Colon adenocarcinoma; BG-27: Diploid foreskin fibroblastic sarcoma. [From Ambrus et al. (50) with permission.]

Preliminary experiments also suggest that in certain neoplastic conditions red cell membrane deformability is impaired. This may contribute to capillary plugs resulting in disturbances of the microcirculation of tumors. Impaired penetration of chemotherapeutic agents and decreased oxygenation with a consecutive decrease in radiation sensitivity could result. Because mopidamole and related compounds have been shown to decrease impaired red cell deformability this effect may also contribute to an enhanced chemotherapeutic and radiation sensitivity of certain malignant tumors after mopidamole treatment (52).

404

III. CLINICAL RESULTS OF METASTASIS PROPHYLAXIS IN MALIGNANT HUMAN
      TUMORS USING THE PYRIMIDO-PYRIMIDINE DERIVATIVE MOPIDAMOLE
      (RA 233)

On the basis of our in vivo findings in animal tumors using
several aggregation inhibitors and on the basis of the good clinical
tolerance of the pyrimido-pyrimidine derivative mopidamole we
initiated a long-term clinical study. For the past ten years we have
been studying metastasis prophylaxis using mopidamole in a total of 38
patients with primary soft tissue sarcomas and malignant lymphomas of
the head and neck region (Table 3). We are referring to a very
carefully selected group of patients, tumor stage classification
$T_1N_1M_0$, in whom no indications of distant metastasis existed, as
determined clinically by X-rays, lymphograms, scintigraphs or in
selected case by surgical exploration. The primary tumors were
treated by surgical excision when possible followed by radiation
therapy.

Table 3. Histological Tumor Diagnoses of 38 Matched Pairs Treated
with Pyrimido-Pyrimidine Derivative, Mopidamole (RA 233).

Number of 38 Patient Pairs	Diagnosis	Diagnostic Equivalent[a]
19	Retothelial sarcoma	Large cell "histiocytic" lymphoma
6	Lymphosarcoma	Lymphocytic lymphoma
5	Hodgkin's sarcoma	Hodgkin's disease
2	Melanosarcoma	Melanoma
2	Anaplastic sarcoma	Undifferentiated sarcoma
2	Spinocellular sarcoma	Spindle cell sarcoma
1	Angioplastic sarcoma	Angiosarcoma
1	Rhabdomyosarcoma	Rhabdomyosarcoma

[a]Editors opinion

The patients received mopidamole in a daily oral dose of 3 x 500
mg (or 3 x 250 mg when under 16 years of age). The derivative was
administered until side effects occurred, recurrent tumor growth at
the original site was observed or metastases were identified.
Otherwise, the above mentioned dose schedule was continued for a

period of five years. Mopidamole was well tolerated in spite of the extensive duration of treatment. Possible drug related side effects were observed in only three cases.

For the past five years we have followed a comparable patient control group. This group of 38 matched pairs was comparable for the following factors: (1) age (± 5 years); (2) sex; (3) site of tumor; (4) histologic tumor type; (5) surgical procedures; (6) radiation therapy techniques and doses used; (7) time of surgery (± 6 month). From a statistical point of view, the use of these criteria made our matching technique obviously free of bias.

The study is now completed. Sixteen patients were under prophylactic treatment with mopidamole over the full five year time period, with a follow-up at 82 - 126 mo. These patients are without metastases or tumor relapse. Another group of nine patients terminated the prophylactic treatment for various reasons after 20 - 46 mo but remained under clinical surveillance. Of these, only one patient developed metastases 22 mo after termination of treatment. In the other eight patients, neither recurrent tumor growth nor development of metastases has occurred over a period of 79 - 126 mo. In 24 patients of the mopidamole group (63.2%) neither relapse nor metastases occurred over a five year period. Within a period of 3 - 59 mo, the tumor relapsed or metastases developed in the remaining 14 patients (36.8%), six have subsequently died (16.8%). Six of the 38 patients in the control group (15.8%) exhibited no recurrence of tumor growth or development of metastases. In the remaining 32 patients, relapse of tumor growth or metastases were observed within a period of 7 - 39 mo (84.2%). Seventeen of these 32 patients (44.7%) have subsequently died.

Using the life table technique (54), analysis showed a highly significant difference between the two groups (p ≤ 0.001): metastases in the mopidamole group occurred significantly later and to a lesser extent than in the untreated group (Figure 9), and the survival time of the patients in the mopidamole group was significantly prolonged (Figure 10). The general significance of the antitumor and antimetastatic effect of mopidamole, however, has to be substantiated in other human malignant tumors as well. Randomized prospective studies involving multiple institutions in several countries have been initiated utilizing mopidamole in patients with breast, lung, ovarian and prostatic carcinomas and malignant melanoma.

IV. CONCLUSIONS

The pilot clinical study to evaluate relapse and metastases in soft tissue sarcoma and malignant lymphoma of the head and neck region has been completed. Long-term treatment with mopidamole was initiated because this pyrimido-pyrimidine derivative has been shown to inhibit platelet aggregation. The aggregation of platelets by circulating tumor cells appears to be part of the early stages of the metastatic process. It seems, however, that other related mechanisms are also involved in the clinical results obtained:

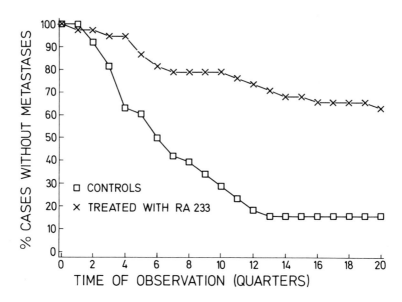

FIGURE 9. Cumulative Relation between Observation Period (quarters) after Surgery and Manifestation of Metastases or Relapse on the Basis of 38 Matched Pairs with Sarcoma or Malignant Lymphoma of the Head and Neck Region (life table technique, 54; z_{38} = 6.1, p $\leq$ 0.001).

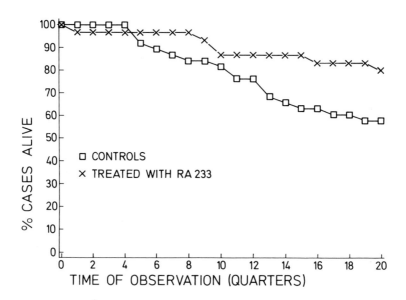

FIGURE 10. Cumulative Relation between Observation Period (quarters) and Survival-Time on the Basis of 38 Matched Pairs with Sarcoma or Malignant Lymphoma of the Head and Neck Region (life table technique, 54); z_{38} = 2.9; p = 0.006).

(a) Mopidamole, and other related derivatives, probably inhibit platelet aggregation by inhibition of PDE-induced decomposition of cAMP and may stimulate the synthesis and/or release of PGI_2 from the vessel wall which in turn increases cAMP synthesis. The latter mechanism was definitely shown only for the related pyrimido-pyrimidine derivative dipyridamole and the methylaxanthine derivative pentoxifylline. Increased cAMP levels inhibit platelet aggregation probably by causing phosphorylation of contractile proteins associated with the cell membrane.

(b) Increase in cAMP levels by mopidamole also results in direct inhibition of mitotic rate.

(c) Mopidamole-increased cAMP levels promote a reverse transformation in human promyelocytic leukemia cells which appears to be a permanent phenotypic change.

(d) Mopidamole potentiates the antimitotic effect of interferons and their natural killer cell activating activity.

(e) Mopidamole and related compounds have been shown to decrease impaired red cell deformability. This effect may contribute to increased chemotherapeutic and radiation sensitivity of certain malignant tumors.

REFERENCES

1. Gastpar H. Med. Welt 27: 1737–1741, 1976.
2. Coman DR. Cancer Res. 21: 1336–1338, 1961.
3. Strauli P. Thromb. Diathes. Haemorrh. Suppl. 20: 147–160, 1966.
4. Koike A. Cancer (Philadelphia) 17: 450–460, 1964.
5. Kojima K and Sakai I. Cancer Res. 24: 1887–1891, 1964.
6. Gastpar H. Hematol. Rev. 3: 1–51, 1972.
7. Gastpar H. Thrombos. Diath. Haemorrh. Suppl. 42: 291–303, 1970.
8. Gastpar H, Graeber F, Herrmann A and Loebell E. Arch. Ohren Nasen Kehlkopfheilkd. 178: 534, 1961.
9. Wood S Jr., Holyoke ED and Yardley JH. Proc. Can. Cancer Res. Conf. 4:167–223, 1961.
10. Jones DS, Wallace AC and Frazer EE. J. Natl. Cancer Inst. 46: 493, 1971.
11. Warren BA and Vales O. Br. J. Exp. Pathol. 53: 301–313, 1972.
12. Hilgard P. Br. J. Cancer 28: 429–453, 1973.
13. Abrahamsen AF. Z. Krebsforsch 86:109–111, 1976.
14. Cowan DH and Graham J. Prog. Clin. Biol. Res. 89:249–266, 1982.
15. Hara Y, Steiner M and Baldini MG. Cancer Res. 40:1212–1216, 1980.
16. Lipton A, Kepner N, Rogers C, Witkoski E and Leitzel K. Prog. Clin. Biol. Res. 89:233–246, 1982.
17. Gasic GJ, Catalfamo JL, Gasic TB and Avdalovic N. In: Malignancy and the Hemostatic System (Eds. Donati MB, Davidson JF and Garattini S), Raven Press, New York, pp. 27–36, 1981.
18. Gasic G and Gasic T. Proc. Natl. Acad. Sci. USA 48:1172–1177, 1962.
19. Gasic G, Gasic T and Stewart C. Proc. Natl. Acad. Sci. USA 61:46–52, 1968.
20. Gastpar H. In: Neue Aspekte der Krebsbekampfung (Ed. Krokowski E), Thieme, Stuttgart, pp. 111–130, 1979.

21. Gastpar H. Fortschr. Med. 91:1322-1328, 1973.
22. Gastpar H. Thromb. Res. 5:277-290, 1974.
23. Gastpar H. Fortschr. Med. 96:1823-1827, 1978.
24. Gastpar H. Ann. Chir. Gynaecol. Fenn. 71:142-150, 1982.
25. Ambrus JL, Ambrus CM and Gastpar H. J. Med. 9:183-186, 1978.
26. Ambrus JL, Ambrus CM, Gastpar H and Williams P. J. Med. 13:35-47, 1982.
27. Gastpar H, Ambrus JL and Ambrus CM. J. Med. 9:265-268, 1978.
28. Gastpar H, Ambrus JL and Thurber LE. J. Med. 8:53-56, 1977.
29. Schneider W. In: Platelets: Production, Function, Transfusion and Storage (Eds. Baldini MG and Ebbe S), Grune & Stratton, New York, pp. 177-185, 1974.
30. Reuter H and Gross R. In: Collagen Platelet Interaction (Ed. Gastpar H), Schattauer, Stuttgart, pp. 87-94, 1978.
31. Salzmann EW and Weisenberger H. Adv. Cyclic Nucleotide Res. 1:231, 1972.
32. Stefanovich V. Res. Commun. Chem. Pathol. Pharmacol. 5:655, 1973.
33. Amer MS and Mayol RF. Biochim. Biophys. Acta 309:149-156, 1973.
34. Blass KE, Block HU, Forster W and Ponicke K. Br. J. Pharmacol. 68:71-73, 1980.
35. Massoti G, Poggesi G, Galanti G and Neri Serneri G. In: Collagen Platelet Interaction (Ed. Gastpar H), Schattauer, Stuttgart, pp. 87-94, 1978.
36. Weithmann KU. IRCS Med. Sci.-Biochem. 8:293-294, 1980.
37. Carreras LO, Chamone DAF, Klerckx P and Vermylen J. Thromb. Res. 19:663-670, 1980.
38. Iversen OH. In: Homeostatic Regulator (Eds. Wolstenhome GEW and Knight J), Churchill, London, pp. 29, 1969.
39. Sheppard JR. Nature (London) 236:14-18, 1972.
40. Heidrick ML and Ryan WL. Cancer Res. 30:376-378, 1970.
41. Smets LA. Nature (London) New Biol. 239:123, 1972.
42. Wijk R van, Wicks WD and Clay K. Cancer Res. 32:1905-1911, 1972.
43. Gericke D and Chandra P. Hoppe-Seylers Z. Physiol. Chem. 350:1469-1471, 1969.
44. Keller R. Life Sci. 11:485-500, 1972.
45. Ryan WL and Heidrick ML. Science 162:1484-1492, 1968.
46. Johnson GS, Friedman RM and Paston I. Proc. Natl. Acad. Sci. USA 68:425-429, 1971.
47. Sheppard JR. Proc. Natl. Acad. Sci. USA 68:1316-1320, 1971.
48. Hait WN and Weiss B. Biochim. Biophys. Acta. 497:86-100, 1977.
49. Stefanovich V, Ambrus JL, Ambrus CM, Karakousis C and Takita H. J. Med., (in press).
50. Ambrus JL, Ambrus CM, Gastpar H, Huberman E, Montagna R, Biddle W, Leong S and Horoszewicz J. Prog. Clin. Biol. Res. 89:97-111, 1982.
51. Biddle W, Montagna RA, Leong SS, Horoszewicz J, Gastpar H and Ambrus JL. Pathol. Biol., (in press).
52. Ambrus JL, et al. unpublished experimental data.
53. Gordon S, Witul M, Cohen C, Williams P, Gastpar H, Murphy GP and Ambrus JL. J. Med. 10:435-443, 1979.
54. Cutler SJ and Ederer F. J. Chronic Dis. 8:699, 1961.

CHAPTER 27. CURRENT CLINICAL TRIALS WITH ANTICOAGULANT THERAPY IN THE MANAGEMENT OF CANCER PATIENTS

WALLEY J. TEMPLE AND ALFRED S. KETCHAM

I. INTRODUCTION

During the last 100 years clinicians and investigators have nurtured a growing suspicion that tumors profoundly alter coagulation function in humans. Accumulation of encouraging clinical and experimental data mandates that properly designed clinical trials be performed to determine the value of anticoagulants in the management of the cancer patient. One must appreciate the historical development in this field to evaluate the current prospective randomized clinical trials with an appropriate perspective.

II. HISTORICAL OVERVIEW

As early as 1862 Armand Trousseau made the poignant observation, "Should you, when in doubt as to the nature of an affection of the stomach, should you when hesitating between chronic gastritis, simple ulcer, and cancer, observe a vein become inflamed in the arm or leg, you may dispel your doubt and pronounce that there is a cancer" (1). Many clnicians have since confirmed these observations and to this day, Trousseau's sign is an eponym for the syndrome migratory thrombophlebitis. In fact the appearance of an episode of idiopathic thrombophlebitis warrants a search for an occult cancer.

A. Clinical Background

A number of clinical syndromes have been associated with active cancers, principally migratory thrombophlebitis, thromboembolism, thrombotic non-bacterial endocarditis and acute or chronic disseminated intravascular coagulation (DIC) (2). These complications may be more common than we realize. One retrospective study of 506 deaths in cancer patients attributed hemorrhage or thrombosis as the key precipitating factor in 18% and a contributing factor in another 43% (3). However, clinically recognized coagulopathies are generally noted in less than 10% of cancer patients.

Far more significant than these dramatic, but relatively infrequently recognized clinical syndromes, are the subclinical abnormalities in patients with active cancers. These changes are not usually detected by the routine coagulation profile of prothrombin time (PT), partial thromboplastin time (PTT) and platelet count (4).

In-depth examination of these patients' coagulation function with fibrinogen consumption tests (5), platelet survival times (2), fibrin breakdown products (4) or fibrinopeptide A (6), often reveals a continuing process of both excess coagulation and fibrinolysis (2-4,7,8). In promyelocytic leukemia, virtually all patients have ongoing clinical or subclinical DIC (2). The frequencies of these subclinical coagulopathies vary according to the parameters measured and the population of cancer patients studied. Most in-depth analyses, however, report at least 50% of all patients with active cancers are associated with easily detectable coagulation abnormalities (2,4-7,9).

O'Meara was the first investigator to explore this phenomena in the laboratory (10). He compared the reaction of citrated plasma to addition of normal tissues or cancer tissues and found that only with the latter did clotting regularly occur. He also prepared a saline extract from these cancers which had similar thromboplastic properties to the cancer tissues and called it the "cancer coagulative factor" (11). Lawrence et al. (12) expanded on these experiments by injecting crude human tumor preparations intravenously into rabbits. In 75% of the animals this resulted in lethal thrombosis of the right heart and pulmonary outflow tracts. However, death could be prevented by prior treatment with the anticoagulants heparin, dicoumarol or soybean trypsin inhibitor. Current investigators have now identified a number of coagulation reactive tumor properties, which include platelet activating surfaces, release of procoagulant A acting on factor X, plasminogen activators and release of tissue factors acting on factor VII (7,13).

The significance of these observations with respect to the growth and spread of a tumor was first suggested by Bilroth in 1878 (14). Using the then relatively embryonic tool of microscopy, he noted live tumor cells within an embolic thrombus and questioned whether it could be associated with the development of a metastasis. In a more extensive study, Iwasaki (15) in 1915 noted the frequent association of tumor cells with emboli in cancer patients. Willis (16) in 1934 actually noted a metastatic invasive focus of tumor cells on a vessel wall surrounded by a thrombus. Further studies in the late 1940's and early 50's by Saphir (17), Durham et al. (18), Morgan (19) and Winterbauer et al. (20) documented such findings in more detail. However, they continued to question whether a thrombus was a host defense mechanism designed to contain the growth of tumor cells or whether it was a significant factor in the pathogenesis of metastasis. The answers to these provocative clinical and pathologic observations are now being unraveled in the laboratory.

B. Research Background

In 1958 Wood (21) published a landmark paper on the pathogenesis of a metastasis and the involvement of the coagulation system. Using cinemicroscopy of a rabbit ear chamber, he recorded the sequence of metastasis formation after i.v. injection of V2 carcinoma cells. By painstaking examination of over 100,000 filmed sequences, he documented four stages in the development of an i.v. induced metastasis. The tumor cells initially adhered to the capillary endothelium and were very quickly covered by a thrombus. Thereafter, the cells extruded through the capillary endothelium and the break was repaired by regenerating endothelium. The extraluminal metastasis was often established within 12-24 hr of the initial adhesion. These elegant studies were completed by examining the effect of the anticoagulants heparin, warfarin and arvin (an inhibitor of factor XIII) on the development of a metastasis (22). The tumor cells adhered to the endothelium even in the presence of therapeutic levels of anticoagulants. However, as might be expected, no thrombus entrapped these cells and they soon detached and were swept back into the circulation. This latter event correlated with a decrease in systemic metastasis.

Approximately ten studies have reported that warfarin anticoagulation was effective in reducing both spontaneous and artifically induced metastasis in various animal models (23). Ketcham and associates (24-28) conducted extensive studies of spontaneous metastasis. Warfarin treatment during the course of tumor growth consistently reduced spontaneous metastasis between 30-75%, depending on tumor model and study design. Hilgard (29 and Chapter 17) has reported that a significant reduction of spontaneous metastasis was produced either by warfarin treatment or by hypoprothrombinemia induced by a vitamin K deficient diet. Brown (30) also showed that warfarin decreased spontaneous metastasis. Warfarin's anticoagulation effects are due to decreased synthesis of vitamin K dependent coagulation proteins. Therefore, Brown (30) examined concomitant warfarin and vitamin K therapy. This resulted in a normal prothrombin time and did not decrease the incidence of metastasis. Therefore, in his model, anticoagulation was the main axis in reducing i.v. induced metastasis and an additional cytotoxic effect of warfarin was not detectable. However, all these authors did note an inhibition of primary tumor growth rate with warfarin treatment. By specifically controlling for this effect, Brown (30) concluded that warfarin's antimetastatic effect was not due to inhibition of tumor growth.

As originally suggested by Wood (21), the major locus of action of warfarin in decreasing metastasis appears to reside in its effects on the coagulation system. However, other mechanisms of action have been reported which may contribute to the overall effect. In vitro, the drug has been shown to uncouple oxidative phosphorylation (31), to slow or synchronize tumor cells in culture (32) and to decrease the synthesis of ribosomal RNA (33). In subsequent reports, Wood and his co-workers (34) also noted that warfarin selectively inhibited the locomotion of tumor cells. After reviewing his earlier studies, he felt that this may have been as critical as the antithrombotic effect in preventing tumor cell invasion of the capillary endothelium.

The work of Gullino (35) and Franks et al. (36) identifies the importance of normal tissue stroma in the physiology and growth of a tumor. Theoretically one can hypothesize that anticoagulants interfere with the fibrin platelet stroma commonly seen in tumors (37). This effect may account for the decreased growth of the primary tumor with anticoagulation as observed in animal (9,25,26,29,30) and clinical (38,39) studies.

Researchers have similarly been intrigued with the effect of platelet active agents on metastasis. The work of Jones et al. (40) and Sindelar et al. (41) implicated platelet aggregation in the pathogenesis of experimental metastasis. In their electron microscopic studies of lung tissue following intravenously injected tumor cells, large aggregates of platelets with very little fibrin were found surrounding the tumor cell emboli. Hilgard's (42) experiments subsequently showed that circulating platelets rapidly disappeared after intravenous tumor cell injection, thus emphasizing the magnitude of this interaction. Gastpar (43) expanded these observations with a study of the effects of pyrimido pyrimidine compounds on the thromboplastic effect of tumors. These compounds interfere with the primary wave of platelet aggregation. In his rat models these substances were shown to markedly diminish mortality if given prior to intravenous injection of tumor cells. Subsequently Gasic et al. (44) found that various manipulations of platelets altered the incidence of metastasis. Neuraminidase- or platelet antibody-induced thrombocytopenia or aspirin treatment reduced the incidence of lung colony formation from tail vein injected tumor cells. Especially interesting were his observations that tumors, even of the same line and histology, had variable platelet aggregating activities. This property correlated inversely with the degree of thrombocytopenia in reducing metastasis. His work also included the corollary observation that fibroblast-induced platelet aggregation would result in an increase in metastasis when injected intravenously with tumor cells.

Of particular relevance in the story of platelets and metastasis has been the recent work of Honn et al. (45). Using the syngeneic B16 murine melanoma model, he found that prostacyclin decreased lung colony formation by 70%. The effect of this powerful inhibitor of platelet aggregation was augmented by 23% when combined with the phosphodiesterase inhibitor theophylline. On the other hand, 15-hydroperoxyarachidonic acid, a chemical that decreases prostacyclin production, increased intravenously induced metastasis by 250%. In other studies Sloane et al. (46,47) correlated the activity of a cathepsin B-like enzyme in two B16 melanoma variants with their lung colonization potential. Cathepsin B's close homologue papain is a powerful platelet aggregating agent, an effect which is inhibited by prostacyclin (48). Since a cathepsin B-like cysteine proteinase is also released by human tumors, pharmacologic manipulation of the prostacyclin system has obvious clinical potential in suppressing metastasis or tumor induced coagulopathies. This work is supplemented by that of Fitzpatrick and Stringfellow (49) who noted prostaglandin D_2, another prostaglandin inhibitor of platelet aggregation, to be in higher concentration in the B16F1 melanoma with its lower lung colonizing capability as compared to the B16F10 line of higher capability. Therefore, the variable colonization potential demonstrated by the B16 melanoma tumor lines may act through more than one biochemical pathway in activating or inhibiting platelet aggregation. These correlations confirm one's suspicion of a complex nature through which tumors may interact with the coagulation system.

The potential of other coagulation reactive drugs in reducing metastasis is less well documented. The value of heparin as a prophylactic agent for metastases remains somewhat controversial. Kircuita et al. (50) and Agostino and Cliffton (51) documented beneficial effects using heparin in animal models. However, Hagmar (52), Boeryd (53) and Boeryd and Rodenstam (54) could not repeat these observations in their murine rhabdomyosarcoma model. It may well be that the latter tumor implants by other mechanisms, however, many of their experiments have major technical deficiencies such as the use of a large intravenous tumor challenge and small numbers of animals with a high experimental mortality rate. Also when studying the effects of heparin on spontaneous metastasis, they discontinued heparin prior to amuputation of the tumor in order to reduce mortality.

The effect of fibrinolytic agents on metastasis also needs to be confirmed. Cliffton (55) consistently found that administration of streptokinase, prior to challenge in either spontaneous or artificial model systems, reduced metastasis 30-50%. He also established the corollary that agents inhibiting fibrinolysis, such as diet induced hyperlipidemia, administration of epsilon amino caproic acid or trasylol, increased the incidence of experimental metastasis. In view of the evidence supporting the beneficial effect of coumadin and platelet active agents on metastasis, it would not be surprising if the value of either of these two classes of agents will ultimately be confirmed in selective situations.

III.   COMPLETED CLINICAL TRIALS

The experimental data have provided a basis for investigating the relevance of anticoagulants in the treatment of human cancer. In fact a number of studies have been reported. However, until recently they were so poorly designed that enthusiasm in this area was significantly dampened. This factor, coupled with the current research emphasis on adjuvant chemotherapy, delayed significant development in this field until the last few years. The study that sparked interest for the serious clinical consideration of this modality was reported by Michaels in 1964 (56). In 540 patients anticoagulated for myocardial infarcts for a total of 1,569 patient years, the expected number of cancers were diagnosed. However, of the ten potentially lethal tumors that developed, only one metastasized. Annegers and Zacharski (57) have recently concluded a similar retrospective study of 378 patients treated for 3,541 patient years. Although their findings were not statistically significant, only fourteen patients died of metastatic cancer in the anticoagulated group as compared to twenty in a matched control population. Of the many non-randomized and uncontrolled studies that followed, Thorne's (39) reports were notable. In 128 cancer patients who had failed on conventional therapy, the addition of anticoagulants increased the two year survival from 18% in the untreated patients to 40% in the treated group. He subsequently described promising preliminary results using a short infusion of streptokinase perioperatively in curable colon cancer patients. However, there was no confirmation with a follow-up report. Dramatic results, which also have to be confirmed by others, were reported by Gastpar (43). He described the use of RA 233 as a surgical adjuvant in a variety of head and neck sarcomas or lymphomas. The 38 treated patients had an 80% projected three year survival as compared to 6% of patients in the matched pair controls.

In the past four years, five well designed studies using warfarin or platelet active agents have been completed. The most encouraging and provocative reports detailed the use of warfarin both as a surgical adjuvant and as an adjunct to standard therapy. Hoover et al. (58) reported on nine consecutive osteosarcoma patients who were amputated for cure in a Phase II trial. Therapeutic warfarin was started preoperatively and continued for six to twelve months postoperatively as the only adjuvant agent. Five of the nine patients were free of disease at five years, one having had a resection of a solitary metastasis. The historical control patients had a 15% five year survival. Zacharski et al. (13,59) reported the first prospective randomized trial examining 50 oat cell cancer patients. They were randomized to receive standard chemotherapy and radiation with or without the addition of warfarin. Survival was increased from a mean of 26 wk to 50 wk with the adjunctive use of warfarin. These two studies on anticoagulants are pivotal as they have ushered in the new era of well designed prospective Phase I, II and III trials. A second randomized prospective trial, performed by Conroy et al. (60), compared cyclophosphamide with or without adjunctive warfarin in lung cancer patients. Although results were not of note overall, warfarin significantly increased progression free survival in the small subset of patients with limited disease.

The results of two prospective trials using platelet active agents were not as encouraging. Lipton et al. (61) randomized 84 colon cancer patients to routine follow-up or to receive aspirin 600 mg twice daily, and found no benefit. Unfortunately treatment was delayed for up to eight weeks after surgery. This factor and an inadequate sample size does not convincingly rule out the use of this or other platelet active agents as a potential adjuvant in this disease. Powles et al. (62) randomized 180 Stage II or anaplastic breast cancer patients to receive placebo or benoral (an aspirin paracetemol compound) for a period of eighteen months post-surgery. Although thromboxane levels were significantly decreased by this therapy, no difference was detected between the two groups after three years of follow-up. Although this is a reasonable sample size, it would have been more instructive if therapy had been started prior to surgery. A long-term follow-up is mandatory to confirm these preliminary results.

IV. SUMMARY OF CURRENT CONCEPTS FOR CLINICAL STUDIES

From this brief critique one can understand the impetus to continue with clinical trials using anticoagulants as an adjunct in cancer treatment. In order to judge the validity of design of ongoing and planned future trials, it is appropriate to reflect a moment on the basic tenets and insights that may be extracted from this research.

Warfarin appears to be the agent of choice, but platelet active agents are emerging as alternatives for study in these trials.

Significant alterations in patient survival may result from one or a combination of activities of these coagulation reactive drugs. The growth of a primary tumor or its metastasis may be slowed by direct cytostatic or cytotoxic action of these agents, or they may interfere with development of normal tumor stroma. Survival may also be prolonged by reversing the coagulopathy that develops in many of these patients with active tumors. Finally, they may act by reducing or preventing metastasis from the primary when used as a surgical adjuvant or prevent a metastasis from a metastasis when used as an adjunct to chemotherapy. In the former instance treatment started prior to surgery and continued uninterruptedly to some point after surgery would be the ideal design.

The patient populations most suitable for this type of manipulation are those with tumors having frequent clinical and subclinical association with distrubed coagulation function such as lung, stomach, prostate, pancreas, colon and ovarian tumors or leukemias (1-3). All these tumors would provide excellent material using anticoagulants as an adjunct to effective chemotherapy. However, colon and ovarian cancer are perhaps the best tumors in which to study their potential as a surgical adjuvant. Besides having documented thromboplastic properties, they are of intermediate aggressiveness in terms of metastasis. Because of these tumors' marginal ability to spread, either as a result of inherent cellular properties or as a result of fairly effective host defenses in man, one would predict that metastasis could be significantly altered by anticoagulation. It is likely that in more aggressive tumors such as lung, stomach or pancreas, significant amounts of subclinical metastatic deposits are already present and their marked affinity to develop metastasis would overwhelm any effect provided by anticoagulants. Therefore, marked improvement of survival in these tumors would have to rely on additional modes of therapy (59).

As animal studies indicate there is a marked variability of each tumor type to react with the coagulation system. Therefore, future clinical trials will be benefited by identifying the potentially susceptible tumors to this treatment. Similarly, tests to determine the locus or loci of entry of each tumor into the coagulation cascade would eliminate the current empirical approach to treatment design. A preliminary report published by Malone et al. (63) promises development in this area. He assayed the activation and inhibition (AI) of fibrinolysis and expressed the two activities as a ratio. Tumors that were associated with metastasis had a significantly higher AI ratio.

A. Current Clinical Trials

The six clinical trials in progress incorporate the above principles in their design to the degree that the state of the art allows. Three Phase I studies are examining the platelet active agent nafazatrom. The remaining studies are Phase III trials. Two of these focus on the use of warfarin or RA 233 as an adjunct to the treatment of incurable lung or colon cancer. The remaining two are testing the value of warfarin used as a surgical adjuvant in curable colon cancer patients.

Nafazatrom (Bay g 6575) is one of the most potent platelet active antithrombogenic agents known, acting via the generation of prostacyclin (see Chapter 14). The Phase I trials will document toxicity of nafazatrom but each has a unique emphasis on the biology of this agent. The study directed by Haas et al. concentrates on the pharmacokinetics of this drug at various doses (Figure 1). Both serum and urine levels are frequently monitored. The dosage range will begin at $0.25 \text{ g/m}^2/\text{day}$ and escalate in increments to $16 \text{ g/m}^2/\text{day}$ until significant toxicity intervenes. Although the study conducted by Warrell et al. is examining a similar population of cancer patients, they are only scrutinizing patients who have documented subclinical coagulopathies (Figure 2). Patients with gross evidence of DIC, or who have normal platelet survival, are not eligible. The facility of nafazatrom to reverse the thromboplastic effects of cancers will be documented in doses starting at $225 \text{ mg/m}^2/\text{day}$ and terminating at $4725 \text{ mg/m}^2/\text{day}$. If beta thromboglobulin or fibrinopeptide A serum levels return to normal during treatment, platelet survival will again be measured. Phase I studies are not designed primarily to determine response but these studies will also monitor this parameter.

The VA cooperative study group headed by L. Zacharski is conducting the first prospective trial using the platelet active agent RA 233 (Figure 3). Three tumors will be examined: small cell carcinoma of the lung, non-small cell carcinoma of the lung and metastatic colon cancer. After being stratified for the amount of disease, they will be randomized to receive four drug polychemotherapy with or without the addition of RA 233. Approximately 300 patients have already been entered on study. Aside from testing this promising agent, this study is particularly valuable because of its extensive documentation of hematologic function in these patients with active tumors on a monthly basis. One would expect that this in-depth dynamic study of hemostasis during tumor regression and progression will lead to a better understanding of the pathophysiology of tumor induced coagulopathies. Hopefully this knowledge will lead to the tailoring of anticoagulation according to the tumor/host responses. The second study in lung cancer patients is examining the use of adjunctive warfarin in oat cell cancer patients with measurable disease beyond the lungs and supraclavicular area. This study randomized patients to three treatment arms: MACC polychemotherapy with or without warfarin and MACC polychemotherapy alternating with MEPH polychemotherapy (Figure 4). The coagulation profile in this study will be limited to monitoring of the prothrombin time. Although this study uses a different chemotherapy combination than that reported by Zacharski et al. (59), it will be particularly important if it confirms the synergistic action of warfarin with chemotherapy in oat cell cancer patients.

The two remaining Phase III studies are looking at the adjuvant potential of warfarin in surgically resected colon cancer patients having lesions that are high risk for recurrence. As no effective adjuvant chemotherapy is available, this is a particularly attractive patient population to study. The multi-center European trial directed by White is based at the Royal Marsden Hospital, London, England. Colon cancer patients are randomized in a two tiered fashion

PHASE I
PHARMACOLOGIC EVALUATION OF NAFAZATROM
HAAS, CD, BAKER, LH, SAMSOM, MD, YOUNG, JD,
VAITKEVICIUS, V· WAYNE STATE UNIVERSITY, DETROIT, MI.

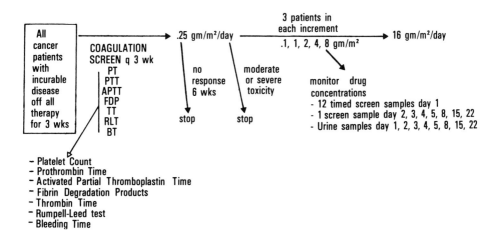

- Platelet Count
- Prothrombin Time
- Activated Partial Thromboplastin Time
- Fibrin Degradation Products
- Thrombin Time
- Rumpell-Leed test
- Bleeding Time

FIGURE 1. A Phase I Trial Concentrating on the Toxicity and Pharmacokinetics of the Platelet Active Agent, Nafazatrom. This investigation is being piloted by Haas and his co-workers at Wayne State University School of Medicine in Detroit, Michigan. Patients who have incurable or cancer uncontrollable by conventional therapy will be included. All therapy must have been stopped 3 wk prior to inclusion in the trial and expected life span must exceed 4 wk. Multiple sequential serum drug levels and urinary excretion rates will be measured at each of the doses ranging from 1 $g/m^2/da$ to 16 $g/m^2/da$, should no major toxicity intervene. The first two groups will be started at 0.25 $g/m^2/da$ or 0.5 $g/m^2/da$ and escalated to 1 $g/m^2/da$. The drug will be given as a single oral dose. Tumor responses will be followed throughout the study and if there is no response after 6 wk patients will be removed from the study.

418

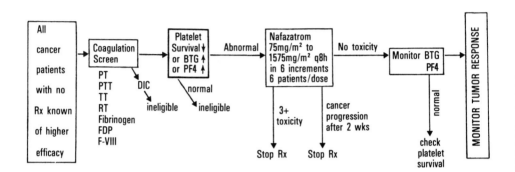

CLINICAL EVALUATION OF
THE ANTI-METASTATIC COMPOUND NAFAZATROM (BAY g 6575)
IN PATIENTS WITH ADVANCED CANCER
Warrell, RS, Bockman,RS
Memorial Sloan Kettering - New York,NY

PT = Prothrombin time
PTT = Partial Thromboplastin time
TT = Thrombin time
RT = Reptilase time
FDP = Fibrin breakdown products
PF4 = Platelet Factor 4
BTG = Beta thromboglubin

DIC defined as:
FDP>40 mg mcg/ml
Fibrinogen <100 mg/dl
FACTOR VIII: <40 mcg/ml

FIGURE 2. A Phase I Trial Studying the Platelet Active Agent
Nafazatrom. This investigation is being performed by Warrell and
Bockman at the Memorial Sloan-Kettering Hospital in New York. This
study will concentrate on the toxicity and the effect on coagulation
parameters of this drug. All patients with advanced cancer who are
not candidates for protocols of higher efficacy will be considered.
These patients will then be further selected by coagulation tests.
Only those without disseminated intravascular coagulation but with a
decrease in platelet survival (less than 80% of normal) or an increase
in beta thromboglobulin will be treated. Toxicity of doses ranging
from 75 mg/m² given orally every 8 hr up to 1575 mg/m² given every 8
hr will be studied. If fibrinopeptide A or beta thromboglobulin
levels, measured at two weekly intervals, return to normal, platelet
survival will then be restudied. Tumor responses will be measured and
if the tumor progresses after 2 wk of therapy the patient will be
removed from the study.

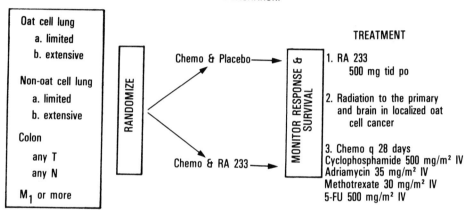

PROSPECTIVE RANDOMIZED
RA 233 - TRIAL IN ADVANCED LUNG &
COLON CANCER
VA COOPERATIVE STUDY 188
CHAIRMAN L. ZACHARSKI

FIGURE 3. The VA Sponsored Phase III Trial Examining the Adjunctive Role of the Pyrimido Pyrimidine Derivative RA-233 to Polychemotherapy. All lung cancer patients with small cell or non-small cell tumors and metastatic colon cancer patients will be randomized to treatment with polychemotherapy with placebo or with RA-233. Stratification of patients to extent of disease will result in four subgroups in the lung cancer patients. Every 4 wk, extensive testing of coagulation parameters will be performed. Over one hundred patients will be required in each group to provide meaningful results. Investigators from 12 VA hospitals are participating. The Executive Planning Committee includes: Zacharski L, Rickles F, Forman WB, Henderson WG, Cornell CJ and Forcier RJ.

420

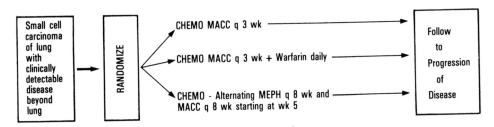

PROTOCOL 8084
SMALL CELL CARCINOMA OF THE LUNG
EXTENSIVE DISEASE,
CANCER & LEUKEMIA GROUP B
CHAIRMAN CHAHINIAN P., NORTH WG
CANCER AND LEUKEMIA GROUP B

Small cell carcinoma of lung with clinically detectable disease beyond lung → RANDOMIZE →

CHEMO MACC q 3 wk ⟶

CHEMO MACC q 3 wk + Warfarin daily ⟶

CHEMO - Alternating MEPH q 8 wk and MACC q 8 wk starting at wk 5 ⟶

Follow to Progression of Disease

STRATIFICATION:
    Male, female
    Performance 0-1
    Status 2-3

MACC= Methotrexate 30 mg/m² IV
       Adriamycin 40 mg/m² IV (max 450 mg/m²)
       CCNU 30 mg/m² IV
       Cyclophosphamide 400 mg/m² IV

MEPH= Mitomycin-C 7 mg/m² IV
       Etoposide 40 mg/m² IV x 3 days
       Cisplatin 50 mg/m² IV
       Hexamethylmelamine 100 mg/m² po x 14 days

WARFARIN = Maintain P.T. 2-2½ x control

FIGURE 4. A CALGB Directed Phase III Trial in Lung Cancer Patients Including Warfarin Anticoagulation in One of the Three Study Arms. The study chairmen are: Chahinian P and North WG. Only patients with small cell cancer of the lung which has extended beyond the lungs and supraclavicular nodes will be included. Patients must not have had previous chemotherapy. Survival using a single four drug regimen, MACC with or without warfarin will be compared to an alternating regimen of MACC and MEPH. The neurophysin levels of vasopressin and oxytocin will also be followed every 9 wk to document their value in monitoring tumor response. Treatment will be continued for at least two cycles and until disease progresses outside the CNS. In the polychemotherapy MACC and warfarin treated patients, only MACC will be discontinued in the face of progressive disease. Survival will be followed in all patients.

421

(Figure 5). Prior to surgery all patients are randomized to surgery alone or in combination with a 5 hr infusion of 250,000 IU of urokinase given immediately postoperatively. After pathologic staging, Duke's B and C patients are then eligible for a second randomization to receive no further treatment or warfarin

FIRST INTERNATIONAL UROKINASE/WARFARIN
TRIAL IN COLORECTAL CANCER
CHAIRMAN H. WHITE - ROYAL MARSDEN HOSPITAL
LONDON, ENGLAND

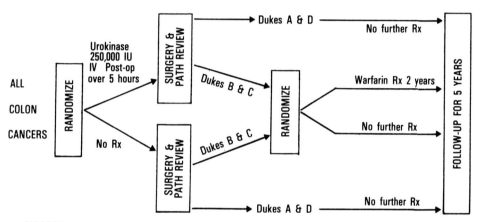

STRATIFY:

1. Prophylactic
   low dose heparin

2. No prophylactic
   heparin

FIGURE 5. The International European Phase III Study of Adjuvant Urokinase and Warfarin Anticoagulation in Duke's B and C Colon Cancer Patients. Randomization will be done in a two tiered fashion which will result in four treatment groups. The first tier will randomize to no treatment or a urokinase infusion postop. After staging, all Duke's B and C patients will be subsequently randomized to no treatment or to warfarin anticoagulation for two years. Separate consideration of patients treated with prophylactic low dose heparin or therapeutic heparin in the event of thromboembolism will be done. However, these patients will remain on study. A five year follow-up documenting relapse rates and survival will complete this study. The study coordinators and the respective countries are: Cattan A - France; Clery AP - Ireland; Merkle P - Germany; Mutzner F - Switzerland; Rickett J, Thomson H, Wellwood J and White H, Chairman - England and Van Overbeeke A - Netherlands.

anticoagulation for two years. Therefore, four treatment permutations will be generated requiring at least 450 Duke's B and C patients to provide statistically meaningful results. At this point well over 200 patients have been accrued to this protocol.

The Southeastern Cooperative Group Study chaired by Temple et al. (Figure 6) is examining a similar population of high risk colon cancer patients. This protocol, however, is somewhat different. Prior to resection all colon cancer patients are randomized to surgery only or to receive parental warfarin which will be started one day prior to surgery and continued until pathologic staging is completed. Only in those patients with Stage II and III tumors (TNM Classification) will oral warfarin be continued uninterruptedly for one year. Although warfarin treatment is started in this trial one day prior to surgery, full anticoagulation will not be achieved until two to three days postoperatively. The ideal schedule in both of these surgical adjuvant studies would be to have therapeutic anticoagulation present prior to surgery in order to duplicate the optimal design outlined in animal models. Nevertheless, the possibility of intraoperative bleeding would surely lead to an unacceptable incidence of postoperative intra-abdominal hematoma with subsequent abscess or alternatively, anastomotic suture line bleeding or hematoma with breakdown. Therefore, a relatively short hiatus of normal coagulation perioperatively is included in both these studies as a safety factor. This does theoretically leave an increased chance for metastasis to develop as a result of tumor cell seeding during operative manipulation (64). The development underway of potent platelet active agents, which may not result in clinical bleeding problems, should improve the design of these studies in the future. Despite this quandry, the design of these two studies represents a synthesis of the literature supporting an adjuvant role for warfarin in these patients.

V. SUMMARY

Laboratory studies, clinical research and clinical reports examining the effects of anticoagulants in the treatment of cancer have provided a framework for the conduct of well designed prospective trials. The accumulated data leave no doubt that anticoagulation with biologic response modifiers will prove a significant factor in the management of cancer patients. As the science of the pathophysiology of coagulation unfolds, the infrastructure for the use of anticoagulants in a more sophisticated fashion, i.e., blocking specific pathways, at specific times, and in specific doses, is beginning to be elaborated. In addition, new and powerful agents are being developed that will provide innovative ways of manipulating coagulation parameters in patients with active cancer. In the meantime it is hoped that the current trials, using relatively empiric treatment regimens, will verify the value of this therapy in cancer patients.

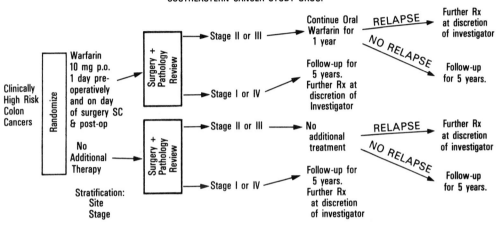

**PHASE III SURGICAL WARFARIN ANTICOAGULATION
STUDY FOR STAGE II & III ADENOCARCINOMA OF THE COLON
CHAIRMEN: W.J. TEMPLE, A.S. KETCHAM, G.H. HILL, Y.S. AHN
SOUTHEASTERN CANCER STUDY GROUP**

DEF. Stage II T_3-T_5,N_0-M_0
     Stage III Any T, N_1-M_0

FIGURE 6.   A Phase III Trial of Adjuvant Warfarin in Stage II and III
Colon Cancer Patients.   This multicenter trial (GI 82 351) will be
conducted by members of the Southeastern Cancer Study Group.   The
study chairmen are Temple WJ, Ketcham AS, Ahn YS – University of Miami
and Hill GH – New Jersey Medical School, Newark, NJ.   All potentially
curable and resectable colon cancer patients will be randomized to
surgery only or to receive warfarin starting one day prior to surgery
and continued intraoperatively and postoperatively.   The empiric dose
of 10 mg of warfarin will be given subcutaneously one day
preoperatively and on the day of surgery.   The dose will then be
adjusted in the postoperative period to maintain a prothrombin time of
two to two and one-half times normal.   Only patients who have
pathologic stagge II or III tumors, as outlined by the American Joint
Committee for Cancer Staging and End Results Reporting, will be
continued in the study.   However, all patients initially randomized in
the study will be followed five years for relapse and survival.

The philosopher, Goethe, in 1793 stated that "The most beautiful discoveries are not made so much by man as by the period ... They mature in the course of time just as the fruits fall from the tree at the same time in different gardens." So it is with these trials which are evaluating anticoagulants for the treatment of human cancers.

REFERENCES

1. Sack Jr., GH, Levin J and Bell WR. Medicine 56:1-37, 1977.
2. Rasche H and Dietrich J. Eur. J. Cancer 13:1053-1064, 1977.
3. Brodsky I, Fuscaldo AA and Fuscaldo KE. In: Oncologic Med. Clinical Topics and Practical Management. (Ed. Sutnick AI and Engstrom PF), Baltimore Union Park Press, pp. 247-259, 1967.
4. Miller SO, Sanchez-Avalos J, Stefanski T and Zucherman L. Cancer (Philadelphia) 20:1452-1465, 1967,
5. Lyman GH, Bettigole RE, Robson E, Ambrus JL and Urban H. Cancer (Philadelphia) 41:1113-1122, 1978.
6. Rickles RR, Edwards RL, Barb C and Cronlund M. Cancer (Philadelphia) 51:301-307, 1983.
7. Caprini JA and Sener SF. Ca Cancer J. Clin. 32:162-172, 1982.
8. Peck SD and Reiquam CW. Cancer (Philadelphia) 31:1114-1119, 1973.
9. Kies MS, Posch Jr., JJ, Giolma JP and Rubin RN. Cancer (Philadelphia) 46:831-837, 1980.
10. O'Meara RAQ and Thornes RD. Ir. J. Med. Sci. 423:106-112, 1961.
11. Thornes RD and O'Meara RAQ. Ir. J. Med. Sci. 428:361-365, 1961.
12. Lawrence EA, Bowman DE, Moore DB and Bernstein GI. Surg. Forum 3:694-698, 1953.
13. Zacharski LR, Henderson WG, Rickles FR, Forman WB, Cornell, Jr. CJ, Forcier RJ, Harrower HW and Johnson RO. Cancer (Philadelphia) 44:732-741, 1979.
14. Billroth T. Translated from the 8th ed. London, New Sydenham Society, 1978.
15. Iwasaki T. J. Pathol. Bacteriol. 20:85-105, 1915.
16. Willis RA. The Spread of Tumours in the Human Body. J. and A. Churchill, London, 1934.
17. Saphir O. Am. J. Pathol. 23:245-253, 1947.
18. Durham JR, Ashley PF and Dorencamp D. J. Am. Med. Assoc. 175:757-760, 1961.
19. Morgan AD. J. Pathol. Bacteriol. 61:75-84, 1949.
20. Winterbauer RH, Elfenbein BI and Ball WC, Jr. Am. J. Med. 45:271-290, 1968.
21. Wood, Jr., S. Arch. Pathol. 66:550-568, 1958.
22. Wood, Jr., S. J. Med. 5:7-22, 1974.
23. Maat B and Hilgard P. Cancer Res. Clin. Oncol. 101:275-283, 1981.
24. Ketcham AS, Wexler H and Minton JP. J. Am. Med. Assoc. 198:157-164, 1966.
25. Ryan JJ, Ketcham AS and Wexler H. Ann. Surg. 168:163-168, 1968.
26. Ryan JJ, Ketcham AS and Wexler H. Science 162:1493-1494, 1968.
27. Ryan JJ, Ketcham AS and Wexler H. Cancer Res. 29:2191-2194, 1969.
28. Millar RC and Ketcham AS. J. Med. 4:23-31, 1974.
29. Hilgard P. Br. J. Cancer 35:891-892, 1977.
30. Brown JM. Cancer Res. 33:1217-1224, 1973.
31. Martius C and Nitz-Litzow D. Biochim. Biophys. Act. 13:289-290, 1954.
32. Lisnell A and Mellgren J. Acta Pathol. 57:145-153, 1962.
33. Kirsch WM, Schulz D, Van Buskirk JJ and Young EE. J. Med. 5:69-82, 1974.
34. Thornes RD, Edlow DW and Wood, S, Jr. Johns Hopkins Med. J. 123:305-316, 1968.

35. Gullino PM. Prog. Exp. Tumor Res. 8:1-25, 1966.
36. Franks LM, Riddle PN, Carbonell AW and Gey GO. J. Pathol. 100:113-119, 1969.
37. Hiramoto R, Bernecky J, Jurandowski J and Pressman D. Cancer Res. 20:592-593, 1960.
38. Hilgard P and Thornes RD. Eur. J. Cancer 12:755-762, 1976.
39. Thornes RD. J. Med. 5:83-91, 1974.
40. Jones DS, Wallace AC and Fraser EE. J. Natl. Cancer Inst. 46:493-504, 1971.
41. Sindelar WF, Tralka TS and Ketcham AS. J. Surg. Res. 18:137-161, 1975.
42. Hilgard P. Br. J. Cancer 28:429-435, 1973.
43. Gastpar H. J. Med. 8:103-114, 1977.
44. Gasic GJ, Gasic TB, Galanti N, Johnson T and Murphy J. Int. J. Cancer. 11:704-718, 1973.
45. Honn KV, Cicone B and Skoff A. Science 212:1270-1272, 1981.
46. Sloane BF, Honn KV, Sadler JG, Turner WA, Kimpson JJ and Taylor JD. Cancer Res. 42:980-985, 1982.
47. Sloane BF, Dunn JR and Honn KV. Science 212:1151-1153, 1981.
48. Honn KV, Cavanaugh P, Evens C, Taylor JD and Sloane BF. Science 217:540-542, 1982.
49. Fitzpatrick FA and Stringfellow DA. Proc. Natl. Acad. Sci. USA 76:1765-1769, 1979.
50. Kiricuta I, Todorutiu C, Muresian T and Risca R. Cancer (Philadelphia) 31:1392-1396, 1973.
51. Agostino D and Cliffton EE. Arch. Surg. 84:449-453, 1962.
52. Hagmar B. Acta Pathol. Microbiol. Scand. (Section A) 80:357-366, 1972.
53. Boeryd B. Acta Pathol. Microbiol. Scand. 65:395-404, 1965.
54. Boeryd B and Rudenstam C. Acta Pathol. Microbiol. Scand. 69:28-34, 1967.
55. Cliffton EE. Fed. Proc. Fed. Am. Soc. Exp. Biol. 25:89-93, 1966.
56. Michaels L. Lancet 2:832-835, 1964.
57. Annegers JF and Zacharski LR. Thromb. Res. 18:399-403, 1980.
58. Hoover, Jr., HC, Ketcham AS, Millar RC and Gralnick HR. Cancer (Philadelphia) 41:2475-2480, 1978.
59. Zacharski LR, Henderson WG, Rickles FR, Forman WB, Cornell, Jr., CJ, Forcier RJ, Edwards R, Headley E, Kim S, O'Donnell JR, Dell R, Tornyos K and Kwaan HC. J. Am. Med. Assoc. 245:831-835, 1981.
60. Conroy JF, MacIntyre JM, Brodsky I, Elias EG and Skanloff RB. Cancer (Philadelphia) (in press).
61. Lipton A, Scialla S, Harvey H, Dixon R, Gordon R, Hamilton R, Ramsey H, Weltz M, Heckard R and White D. J. Med. 13:419-429, 1982.
62. Powles TJ, Dady PJ, Williams J, Easty GC and Coombes RC. Adv. Prostaglandin Thromboxane Res. 6:511-516, 1980.
63. Malone JM, Wangensteen SL, Moore WS and Keown K. Ann. Surg. 190:342-349, 1979.
64. Griffiths JD. Ann. R. Coll. Surg. Engl. 27:14-44, 1960.

430